By No Extraordinary Means

Medical Ethics series

David H. Smith and Robert M. Veatch, series eds.

By No Extraordinary Means

The Choice to Forgo
Life-Sustaining Food and Water

Expanded edition

EDITED BY JOANNE LYNN, M.D.

INDIANA UNIVERSITY PRESS

Bloomington & Indianapolis

Manufactured in the United States of America

Library of Congress Cataloging-in-Publication Data

By no extraordinary means : the choice to forgo life-sustaining food and water / edited by Joanne Lynn.—Expanded ed.
    p. cm.—(Medical ethics series)
    Bibliography: p.
    Includes index.
    ISBN 0-253-20517-4 (pbk.) ISBN 0-253-33659-7
    1. Terminal care—Moral and ethical aspects. 2. Artificial feeding—Moral and ethical aspects. 3. Dehydration (Physiology) —Prevention—Moral and ethical aspects. I. Lynn, Joanne.
II. Series.
R726.B9   1989
174'.24—dc19   89-30769
                                     CIP

1 2 3 4 5 93 92 91 90 89

CONTENTS

Part III   Perspectives on the Law

Part IV   Special Considerations
for Particular Populations

Part V *In re* Claire C. Conroy: A Case Study

Foreword

by Julia and Joseph Quinlan, with Paul Armstrong, J.D.

In the near decade since the landmark case involving Karen Ann Quinlan we have come to know firsthand the importance of clear articulation of the sacred notions implicit in the right of terminally ill individuals and their families to make fundamental treatment decisions.

So, too, we have been blessed with the knowledge and friendship of those who, through their special wisdom, courage, and experience, have contributed significantly to the perception and understanding of the ongoing scientific, medical, and moral dilemmas which continue to capture the interest and empathy of the world.

In this spirit, we are privileged to commend to the attention of readers of this book the signal contributions of the various authors and their articles. Each, while keenly aware of the sacredness of human life, seeks to recognize the role and limits of individual autonomy and integrity and at the same time honor the precepts and responsibilities of civilized society. This uniquely human and unifying thread pervades the differing positions of the authors and thus renders the collective work invaluable to all of us who continue to meet and labor to resolve the contemporary conundrums of the medical enterprise.

Contributors

Edward J. Bayer, S.T.D., is Director of Continuing Education, The Pope John XXIII Medical-Moral Research and Education Center, coeditor of *Handbook on Critical Life Issues* (1982) and *Handbook on Critical Sexual Issues* (1983) and author of the forthcoming book *Rape within Marriage: A Moral Analysis Delayed* (University Press of America, 1985).

Dan W. Brock, Ph.D., is Professor and Chairman of the Department of Philosophy, Brown University. He was Staff Philosopher for the President's Commission for the Study of Ethical Problems in Medicine and Biomedical and Behavioral Research and has written numerous articles on political philosophy and biomedical ethics.

Daniel Callahan, Ph.D., is a cofounder and Director of The Hasting Center.

Alexander M. Capron, LL.B., is Topping Professor of Law, Medicine, and Public Policy at the University of Southern California. He served as Executive Director of the President's Commission for the Study of Ethical Problems in Medicine and Biomedical and Behavioral Research.

Ronald A. Carson, Ph. D. is Kempner Professor and Director of the Institute for the Medical Humanities, University of Texas Medical Branch at Galveston. Dr. Carson is a Fellow of the Hastings Center and author of numerous essays and articles on subjects in the medical humanities.

Robert C. Cassidy, Ph.D., is the Director of the Clinical Values Program and an Assistant Professor in the Department of Family Medicine, University of Medicine and Dentistry of New Jersey—Rutgers Medical School. His doctorate in the philosophy of religion is from Princeton University.

James F. Childress, B.D., M.A., Ph.D., is Commonwealth Professor of Religious Studies and Professor of Medical Education at the University of Virginia. He is the author of several books in biomedical ethics, including *Principles of Biomedical Ethics* (with Tom L. Beauchamp) and *Who Should Decide? Paternalism in Health Care,* and of numerous articles.

Ronald Cranford, M.D., is Associate Physician in Neurology at Hennepin County Medical Center and Associate Professor of Neurology at the University of Minnesota. He serves as Chairman of the Ethics and Humanities Committee of the American Academy of Neurology and was coeditor of *Institutional Ethics Committees and Health Care Decision-Making.*

John J. DeLaney, Jr., J.D., is an attorney with the law firm of Young, Rose & Millspaugh, Roseland, New Jersey, and served as guardian *ad litem* for Claire Conroy.

Joel Frader, M.D., is Assistant Professor of Pediatrics at Children's Hospital and the University of Pittsburgh School of Medicine.

Ron Landsman, J. D., is a partner in the law firm of Landsman and Laster in Washington, D.C.

Joanne Lynn, M.D., is an Associate Professor in the Division of Geriatric Medicine at George Washington University Medical Center and Medical Director of The Washington Home and Hospice. She served as Assistant Director of the President's Commission for the Study of Ethical Problems in Medicine and Biomedical and Behavioral Research and directed its work on the report *Deciding to Forego Life-Sustaining Treatment.*

David A. Major, M.D., has been the Associate Chairman for Education and Director of the Division of General Internal Medicine at Hahnemann University in Philadelphia, where he was Professor of Medicine. He is an active member of the Society for Health and Human Values and has established a teaching program in medical ethics at Hahnemann. He is currently at Pennsylvania Hospital holding a faculty appointment at the University of Pennsylvania.

Russell L. McIntyre, Th.D., is Associate Professor of Medical Ethics in the Department of Environmental and Community Medicine of the University of Medicine and Dentistry of New Jersey—Rutgers Medical School.

Gilbert Meilaender, Ph.D., is Associate Professor and Chairman of Religion at Oberlin College.

Kenneth C. Micetich, M.D., is Assistant Professor of Medicine in the Section of Hematology-Oncology at Loyola University Stritch School of Medicine.

Michael A. Nevins, M.D., F.A.C.P., is a physician specializing in internal medicine, cardiology, and geriatrics in Woodcliff Lake, New Jersey. He is the Governor for New Jersey of the American College of Physicians.

Merry O'Brien, R.N., B.S.N., has been a staff nurse at The Washington Home Hospice for the past four years.

Joseph Rodriguez, J.D., is the Public Advocate for the State of New Jersey and was active in arguing and briefing the *Conroy* case before the Appellate Division and the New Jersey Supreme Court.

Phyllis Schmitz, R.N., B.S.N., has been a staff nurse at The Washington Home Hospice for the past four years.

Bernard L. Siegel, J.D., is Deputy District Attorney for Investigations for the city of Philadelphia. He was formerly First Assistant District Attorney, Erie County, Pa., and Deputy Attorney General, Pennsylvania Department of Justice.

Mark Siegler, M.D., F.A.C.P., is Professor of Medicine and Director of the Center for Clinical Medical Ethics at the University of Chicago-Pritzker School of Medicine. He is a Fellow of The Hastings Center and serves as a consultant on ethical issues to the American College of Physicians. He serves on the editorial board of the *American Journal of Medicine,* the *Archives of Internal Medicine,* the *Journal of Medicine and Philosophy,* and is the Associate Editor of the second edition of the *Bibliography of Bioethics.*

Patricia H. Steinecker, M.D., is Associate Professor of Medicine in the Section of Hematology-Oncology at Loyola University Stritch School of Medicine.

William I. Strasser, J.D., is a partner in the law firm Donohue, Donohue, Costenbader, & Strasser, in Nutley, New Jersey, and represented Claire Conroy's nephew Thomas Whittemore. He is also a member of the New Jersey Commission on Legal and Ethical Problems in the Delivery of Health Care.

Jeff Stryker served as Research Analyst in the Biological Applications Program of the Congressional Office of Technology Assessment and on the staff of The President's Commission for the Study of Ethical Problems in Medicine and Biomedical and Behavioral Research.

David Thomasma, Ph.D., holds the Father Michael I. English, S.J., Chair of Medical Ethics and is the Director of the Medical Humanities Program at Loyola University Stritch School of Medicine.

Alan J. Weisbard, J.D., is Assistant Professor of Law at the Benjamin N. Cardozo School of Law, Yeshiva University, in New York City. He also serves as Visiting Assistant Professor at the Albert Einstein College of Medicine of Yeshiva University and as Senior Adjunct Associate of The Hastings Center. He previously served as Assistant Director of The President's Commission for the Study of Ethical Problems in Medicine and Biomedical and Behavioral Research.

Jacqueline J. Glover, Ph.D., is Assistant Professor of Clinical Ethics in the Department of Health Care Sciences at George Washington University. She is also Philosopher in Residence at the Children's Hospital National Medical Center.

By No Extraordinary Means

Joanne Lynn, M.D.

Introduction and Overview

Some years ago as I was about to leave Nairobi to work in a remote part of Kenya, an experienced Peace Corps volunteer told me, "Everyone is worried about the dramatic dangers of life in Africa—the elephants, lions, and such. You would do well to ignore those. It is the little things—the mosquitoes, schistosomes, and ants—that really pose a danger." Those who analyze decision-making issues in health care would do well to follow similar advice.

As recently as a few years ago, the center stage of concerns about how to make health care decisions was occupied by the allocation of renal dialysis and the elimination of haughtily paternalist practices by physicians. These big and dramatic issues were certainly important and the experience gathered in those areas is valuable. But the issues with more overall impact upon the scope and content of health care are the uncounted thousands of "little choices." These are the things that, when added up, have a profound impact upon care, levels of health, and costs, but which are often decided without much reflection. This book is dedicated to such an issue. Techniques to supply nutrition and hydration to patients who cannot or will not eat or drink have been developed over the past century and are now in use for a wide array of patients. Probably the means used to secure adequate nutrition and hydration are appropriate for most of these patients and the benefits have been substantial. However, some patients probably should not receive these treatments, even though forgoing them may well lead to an earlier death. Which patients should forgo medical procedures that provide food and water, and how should the decision be made?

I first confronted this issue in caring for a profoundly demented lady nearly one hundred years of age who had retained, from among her lifelong skills, largely only those necessary for ambulation and cantankerousness. She had outlived all family and friends but was a much loved character in a nursing home, despite her needs for extensive care and her loud objections to any disruption in her routine. She did well there for many years. Finally, as these things go, her illness progressed or something changed so that she suddenly stopped eating. My long indoctrination into modern medicine suggested a neat resolution—she was fed by nasogastric tube and an evaluation was undertaken to find any reversible cause for her problem. She was miserable. She fought the insertion of the tube and the restraints, and she quickly lost trust in her old friends among the caregivers. No reversible cause was found and her agony was unremitting. Finally, her caregivers decided as a group to stop the torture and to care for her in whatever humane ways presented themselves. She died rather suddenly three weeks later, with no evidence of antecedent distress, having eaten virtually nothing in those weeks. However, she walked freely among her friends and seemed to enjoy herself.

At about the same time, I found myself working in a hospice, where very few of the patients received artificial nutrition or hydration despite very little intake. Gradually, the staff and I noticed that the suctioning apparatus that our hospital experience indicated would be needed frequently to help ease respiratory troubles near death was rarely used.[1] Also, we noticed that patients who remained quite alert until death often reduced their intake dramatically in the final few days before death and were sometimes puzzled by their own lack of hunger or thirst.[2] In fact, if their lips and mouths were kept moist with ice chips or lubricant, patients who were quite dehydrated remained comfortable. It occurred to us that the medical circumvention of this pattern by supplying artificial nutrition and especially artificial hydration could be harmful in causing more respiratory distress as well as in imposing the annoyances of tubes and needles. Other hospice personnel have since confirmed our observations.

However, to stop nutrition and hydration is disquieting. Patients are likely to die more quickly and certainly. And the procedures to provide nutrition and hydration are, for the staff, usually so simple. The burdens of feeding interventions are more substantial for the patient—Ron Landsman notes that artificial feedings are "no picnic"—but the patients' discomfort is frequently disregarded because caregivers react unreflectively to physiological abnormalities without considering whether doing so actually helps the patient.

My colleagues and I were faced with troubling questions. What if our assessments were wrong? What if patients actually suffered without artificial nutrition and hydration? How could we be sure that decisions would always be made with great care? How would society view a failure to provide these basic essentials for life, especially in a nursing home setting where it is so easy to believe allegations of abuse?

Once the issue of providing or forgoing artificial nutrition and hydration had been identified, it turned up frequently. The issue had always been present, but the responses had been so automatic that it had seemed to be rare. However, the literature in ethics, medicine, nursing, and law said almost nothing about this issue.[3] Even textbooks describing the procedures for normalizing nutrition and hydration gave no guidance as to the appropriate recipients.

In 1982, an infant with Down syndrome and esophageal atresia with tracheoesophageal fistula (abnormalities of the esophagus and the trachea that preclude normal eating and predispose to pneumonia) died during court proceedings without having received nutrition and hydration. Although death was principally caused by aspiration pneumonia, the ensuing public reaction made clear that not feeding the infant was unacceptable, though it left much unclear about what else should count as defensible practice.[4]

In 1983, two well-known cases involving the possibly justifiable discontinuing of medical means for supplying nutrition and hydration came to court. One was a criminal prosecution of two physicians in Los Angeles for stopping intravenous fluids sustaining a patient with profound anoxic brain injury caused by a cessation of heartbeat after a routine surgery.[5] The other arose when the nephew of a severely demented, elderly, nursing home resident applied to the chancery court for authorization to have a nasogastric tube withdrawn, although the patient could not eat enough to sustain life.[6] In each of these cases, the initial judge to hear the case allowed the discontinuation of artificial feeding; the first appellate ruling reversed with blistering language, suggesting that such a course could well be murder; and the next level of appeal reversed again, allowing at least some forgoing of food and water. In both cases, the final ruling made clear that withdrawing nutrition and hydration in some cases would be correct and endeavored to set forth substantive and, in the latter case, procedural guidance for practitioners faced with this problem. The discussion that these cases touched off in the affected professional and academic communities has led to a number of publications and a growing consensus that some circumstances warrant withholding nutrition and hydration[7] and that such a decision requires great caution.[8]

As part of the learning process essential to forming, defining, and guiding the growth of consensus, the Society for Health and Human Values sponsored a conference on March 23 and 24, 1984, in Philadelphia. The papers collected for this book have grown out of that conference, which brought together an unusually broad array of interested parties to consider the wisdom of alternate approaches.

Why has this issue surfaced at this time? Some of the techniques have been available for decades.[9] One might expect to find evidence of distress over whether or not to use gastrostomies or to give fluids by subcutaneous infusion for fifty years or more, but there is no such discussion in the literature. Perhaps the recent focus upon supportive care for dying persons has illuminated issues that previously would have been ignored as part of a more general denial of the problems of dying. Perhaps there are so many more elderly and so many are resident in institutions where these techniques are more readily available and where choosing whether or not to apply them is also more public. Perhaps there is a growing humility, a recognition of limits that allows professionals more readily to acknowledge that interventions are not always helpful.

These are "laudable" reasons for the unquestioned application of artificial nutrition and hydration to have become an issue at this time. There are also some troubling possibilities. Perhaps we now focus upon this issue because it offers a way to eliminate those who Callahan calls the "biologically tenacious."[10] Those who are so severely disabled as to be candidates for long-term artificial feeding are most often unappealing and easily discriminated against by the "temporarily able-bodied" who dominate society. Perhaps even more important, recent recognition that costs of health care must not continue to grow at present rates may well have led to pressures to reduce expenditures that are widely seen as being of limited benefit to society. It is very expensive to provide long-term support to patients who, because of physical and mental disabilities associated with old age or with congenital abnormalities, cannot eat in the normal way. Although the artificial feeding itself is often fairly inexpensive, the costs of the lives that it allows to continue are large and are often borne by the public generally, so that these costs are quite apparent. Society might welcome a reduction of this costly burden, especially if it can seem to be justified by appeal to factors other than the crass and demeaning one of finances. Callahan raises the specter that not providing nutrition and hydration could become the "non-treatment of choice" if it is allowed at all.[11]

What problems have surfaced as a result of having raised these issues publicly? Foremost for health care professionals has been concern over whether forgoing nutrition and especially hydration might constitute murder or assisting suicide and thus be subject to possible criminal sanctions. While courts have thus far failed to construe this choice as criminal, they probably could. This illuminates a hazy borderline that has long existed but has been almost studiously ignored: when any forgoing of a life-sustaining treatment predictably eventuates in an earlier death, the strict definition of murder or suicide will have been met. It has been a convention that medical decisions will not be construed in this way,[12] but it is an unspoken convention. When the option chosen is only dubiously "medical," since it can readily be understood by anyone and is so akin to ordinary means of eating and drinking, the convention may not protect the professionals involved from the scrutiny of those concerned with enforcing the criminal law.

Another problem is that there is very little empirical data about the effects on patients of using or of not using artificial feeding techniques. The observations of the current era give this little attention, since virtually all patients receive the treatment as a matter of course. And the observations of past eras likewise gave patients' experience of dehydration and fatal malnutrition little attention, perhaps because they could not be prevented. There is, for example, no empirical study reported that aims to define ideal hydration for patients near death. There is not even an empirical study of the current patterns of use and nonuse of the feeding and hydration techniques. This dearth of information elsewhere makes the anecdotal reports of O'Brien and Schmitz and the initial survey of Micetich, Steinecker, and Thomasma in this volume especially significant.

A third concern is that even the most carefully drawn guidelines and well-developed understandings are no better than is their application in the hands of the average decision-maker. Although good arguments exist as to who should not receive medical nutrition and hydration procedures, these guidelines could be applied so thoughtlessly as to cause the premature death of many severely dependent and defenseless persons. Daniel Callahan calls this the "klutz factor."[13] A prudent society would do well to weigh the likelihood and magnitude of such errors before allowing actions justified by rational arguments.

A final concern is that allowing or requiring that some patients should not be fed will cause decay in our moral life. This concern ranges from the risk that life itself will be held less dear if it can be lost in this way, to the fear that health care practitioners will lose a very important aspect of their social and self identity if they are party to this sort of death. These concerns arise because the giving of food and water and the food and water themselves have very powerful symbolic meanings that must be accommodated in any public policy concerning this practice.

The symbolism of having given food and water is sometimes quite separate from having achieved physiologically adequate nutrition and hydration. Caring concern and steadfastness may well best be conveyed through hand feeding, even if it is certain to be physiologically inadequate.[14] And using artificial means to ensure adequate nutrition and hydration may serve to increase isolation and suffering for a patient. Ordinarily, both normal physiology and compassion are important, but sometimes one or the other is not very significant. In assessing the arguments proffered by the authors herein, one should bear this distinction in mind, for a risk or a benefit that is said to accrue from "forgoing food and water" sometimes applies only to forgoing medically adequate nutrition and hydration and other times only to forgoing normal oral feeding.

This book represents an endeavor to collect the best of current thought on these subjects, to engender some reflections on aspects that have not previously been published, to provide authoritative source material to assist those who are concerned about the outcome of this discussion, and to give some guidance to those who are faced with a decision regarding a person for whom they care.

With deepest gratitude, the editor and the Society for Health and Human Values acknowledge the valuable and unpaid contributions of those who spoke at the conference and who so graciously agreed to collaborate on this book. Our thanks go also to the organizations who joined to sponsor the conference: the American Academy of Pediatrics, the American College of Osteopathic Pediatricians, the American Health Care Association, the American Society of Law and Medicine, the Center for the Study of Aging, Concern for Dying, Hahnemann University, the Hastings Center, the National Congress of Hospitals Governing Boards of the American Hospital Association, the Office on Aging and Long Term Care of the Hospital Research and Educational Trust of the American Hospital Association, the Presbyterian Church U.S.A., the Society for the Right to Die, the Society of Teachers of Family Medicine, and the University of Medicine and Dentistry of New Jersey. We appreciate the excellent secretarial services provided by Cheryl Betts of George Washington University. Editing and footnoting of the manuscripts depended heavily upon the skills and dedication of Jeff Stryker.

It is the hope of the Society for Health and Human Values that this collection will prove useful in developing the best standards to guide responses to this difficult subject. It is the hope of the editor that others who are troubled by the choices which present themselves when patients cannot eat or drink will find some assistance herein.

NOTES

1. Reporting the same observation is Marion B. Dolan, "Another Hospice Nurse" *Nursing83*, 51 (January 1983).

2. Joyce V. Zerwekh, "The Dehydration Question," *Nursing83* 47–51 (January 1983).

3. The only article addressing this topic before 1983 seems to be Carson Strong's "Can Fluids and Electrolytes be 'Extraordinary' Treatment?" *J. Med. Ethics* 7:83–85 (1981).

4. *In re* Infant Doe, No. GU 8204–004A (Cir. Ct. Monroe County, Ind., April 12, 1982) *writ of mandamus dismissed sub nom.* Infant Doe v. Baker, No. 482–5–140 (Sup. Ct. Ind., May 27, 1982); John E. Pless, "The Story of Baby Doe" (letter), *N. Engl. J. Med.* 309:664 (1983); see also chapter 17.

5. Barber v. Los Angeles County Superior Court, 195 Cal. Rptr. 484, 147 Cal. App. 3d 1006 (1983); Jonathan Kirsch, "A Death at Kaiser Hospital," *Calif. Mag.* 79–175 (November 1982).

6. *In re* Conroy, 98 N.J. 321, 486 A.2d 1209 (1985). ᵛ

7. See, e.g., Joanne Lynn and James F. Childress, "Must Patients Always be Given Food and Water?" *Hastings Cent. Rep.* 13:17–21 (October 1983); *In re* Hier, 18 Mass. App. 200 (1984).

8. See, e.g., Gilbert Meilaender, "Against the Stream," *Hastings Cent. Rep.* 14:11–13 (December 1984); Mark Siegler and Alan J. Weisbard, "Against the Emerging Stream: Should Fluids and Nutritional Support be Discontinued?" *Arch. Intern. Med.* 145:129–131 (1985).

9. Intravenous infusions saved victims of cholera in 1831. Richard J. Duma, "Thomas Latta, What Have We Done? The Hazards of Intravenous Therapy," *N. Engl. J. Med.* 294:1178–1180 (1976).

10. See chapter 6.

11. Daniel Callahan, "On Feeding the Dying," *Hastings Cent. Rep.* 13:22 (October 1983).

12. President's Commission for the Study of Ethical Problems in Medicine and Biomedical and Behavioral Research, *Deciding to Forego Life-Sustaining Treatment*, Washington, D.C.: U.S. Government Printing Office (1983), 35–39, 80.

13. See chapters 6 and 11.

14. Encouraging oral intake can be quite time-consuming. See chapter 3.

Part I The Issues

Alexander Morgan Capron, LL.B.

1 Historical Overview:
Law and Public Perceptions

DYING, PUBLIC POLICY, AND PRIVACY RIGHTS

Once, really not all that long ago, death was familiar. In this sense it was a public matter. Although most deaths occurred at home, they were still something that other people observed and participated in; they were not secret, hidden, or taboo. Rather, they were part of life for the living—part of the future that was understood and anticipated for all.

In recent years, death has become more public in the physical sense of occurring increasingly in hospitals and other health care facilities, which today are the site of about eighty percent of all deaths. Yet while this factual shift to public deaths was occurring, death as a concept became private, almost shameful in the world as we construct it verbally. Perhaps because death remained the ultimate reminder of the failure of medicine, it came to be regarded as not a fit subject for the biomedical sciences. As for nonscientists, death was obscured by a fascination with death-denying trappings, such as the ceremony and pomp of funerals that employ elaborate crypts, the manicured graveyards with names like Forest Lawn, and, even more notably, cryonics, which places the body into allegedly "suspended animation," the ultimate denial of death's sting.

This intriguing and ironic mixture of public and private issues was underscored by the intervention of the courts in a series of significant cases. Even as the courts asserted their authority over decisions about death—and thereby moved the issues more and more clearly onto a public stage—they insisted that the decisions were encompassed within patients' "right of privacy." The result is almost Newspeak: a matter is made *public* in order to protect it as a matter of *privacy*, first labeled thus by the New Jersey Supreme Court in *Quinlan*.[1]

Broadly construed, *Quinlan* recognizes that patients have a right to choose whether or not to avail themselves of particular medical intervention, and that in order to preserve this right for incompetent patients, guardians may make such decisions on behalf of patients who are unable to decide directly for themselves. *Quinlan* is subject, however, to a narrower reading that may have originated in the factual setting of the cases on reproductive freedom in which the United States Supreme Court first articulated this right of privacy.

Through laws prohibiting or restricting abortion, states had sought to protect the lives of fetuses against the threat posed were their mothers to terminate the pregnancies. In the landmark case of *Roe v. Wade*[2] the United States Supreme Court announced a balance between women's interests in their own lives and the State's interest in protecting the potentiality of human life, as well as in protecting the health of pregnant women. The Court held that the State's interest in preventing abortion grows as the woman approaches term and eventually becomes compelling enough in Fourteenth Amendment terms to justify restricting a woman's right to privacy regarding abortion.

In adopting the right of privacy from the abortion cases, the *Quinlan* opinion also borrowed the balancing test which the Supreme Court had used for abortion cases. Whatever the validity of this approach to right of privacy in the context of abortion, this waxing-and-waning approach to the right of privacy may seriously distort the protections for patients that the *Quinlan* opinion and the reports of the President's Commission[3] intended to achieve. This can be seen, indeed, from the Appellate Division's opinion in the *Conroy* case.[4] On the one hand, that opinion suggests that the deeper a person's coma or the closer he or she is to death, the less worthy his or her life is of respect, which is simply not true. The law plainly regards it as wrong to kill, even when a person's remaining life would probably be very brief or otherwise impaired. Thus, the balancing approach would underprotect some patients because it would diminish their "right to privacy" because of severe disability. It would treat them, in other words, like an unborn fetus.

On the other hand, the Appellate Division would also overprotect the lives of some patients at the expense of their other interests. Claire Conroy could not be allowed to die, in this court's view, because her diagnostic category was not the same as Karen Quinlan's (that is, a persistent vegetative state). Whatever the proper result in Miss Conroy's case, there surely are patients suffering from cancer and other life-threatening illnesses who may not wish, and may not be well-served by, prolongation of the dying process. It would be ironic, indeed, if patients who are aware of the world, and hence of pain, were under a stronger requirement to continue treatment that may be painful, while at the same time deeply comatose patients who are unaware of pain could be spared such treatment. A competent patient with cancer who decided to discontinue the chemotherapy believed by his physicians to offer his only hope of overcoming an otherwise fatal disease would be exercising his "right to privacy"—that is, his authority to decide whether to accept or reject medical interventions. There should be no suggestion in the law that a patient's right to make this choice only arises when he or she becomes permanently unconscious or is near death despite medicine's best efforts to prolong life.

A patient's right to self-determination about medical care can be restricted, for example, in order to prevent suicide or direct harm to other persons. "In most decisions to forgo life-sustaining treatment," however, the Commission found that the countervailing interests are "quite attenuated."[5] This is not the same as the balancing test that is required when the State attempts to mediate between conflicting interests, as in abortion. Rather, it recognizes that the decision not to initiate or not to continue treatment does not actually threaten interests which society defends on behalf of people who are unable to protect themselves. Were a patient's right of privacy to come into conflict with another interest, a balance would have to be struck, but both should be regarded as full and robust interests to be weighed against each other, not as variable matters that wax and wane according to the patient's prognosis.

In reversing the appellate court in *Conroy*,[6] the New Jersey Supreme Court went a long way toward removing certain of the confusions engendered by *Quinlan*, which concerned only patients in a persistent vegetative state. *Conroy* concerned severe dementia and multiple physical ailments and thus addressed a much broader group of affected patients. *Conroy* also clarified the notion of balancing that *Quinlan* had imported from the reproductive freedom cases. For competent nursing home patients, the court made clear, prognosis and present level of functioning are relevant in determining what course of treatment best serves the patient's interests, rather than in modulating constitutionally protected rights.

TWO MAJOR ISSUES FOR ANALYSIS

Quinlan explored such new territory that it is not surprising that it generated a certain amount of confusion. It also opened up the thinking of physicians and lawyers to a number of important questions. For the purposes of the present volume, the cases that came along after *Quinlan* can be sorted into two groups. The first—including cases such *Saikewicz*[7] and *Baby Doe*[8]—is concerned with the question, who decides? Thus, they involve initially the need to determine which patients lack the requisite decision-making capacity. Next, recognizing that this incapacity will frequently occur in patients near death, the question for the law becomes, where does one get guidance for life-and-death decisions?

The answer that seems to have emerged from these cases was underscored and elaborated in the recent *Conroy* opinion. First and preferably, directions on care should come from the views directly and clearly expressed by the patient while still competent. The *Conroy* court, following the President's Commission, recognized that such *substitute judgment* is subjective and may vary, according to individual values and goals, as much as the decisions of competent patients vary.[9]

Second, choice on behalf of an incompetent patient can be exercised by someone who, from personal knowledge of the patient's lifetime patterns, can choose as that person would have chosen. Since such knowledge may not be enough to leave a surrogate "clearly satisfied as to the patient's intent either to accept or reject the life-sustaining treatment,"[10] a more objective standard (of a "best interests" type) is appropriate, to prevent a spurious subjectivity from entering the decision-making. When there is "some trustworthy evidence," the New Jersey court recommends a "limited-objective" test, under which life-supporting treatment would be forgone only when "it is clear that the burdens of the patient's continued life with the treatment outweigh the benefits of that life for him."[11]

Finally—although one might be inclined to view this as a continuum, rather than as a separate category—there are cases in which the best-interests standard must be applied by itself because little or nothing is known of a patient's competent wishes vis-à-vis treatment continuation or termination. This the New Jersey opinion labels a "pure-objective test," which it restricted to situations in which "the recurring, unavoidable and severe pain of the patient's life with the treatment [is] such that the effect of administering life-sustaining treatment would be inhumane."[12]

In so holding, the New Jersey court placed itself directly at odds with the highest court of New York, which four years previously had held that surrogate decision-makers may never withhold life-support when acting under a best-interests rationale.[13] Plainly, then, the first issue (who decides?) blends into the second (what treatments may be withdrawn?). For example, may a patient who could be sustained indefinitely by a mechanical ventilator, despite a progressive disease, give it up? The *Perlmutter*[14] case addressed that issue for a patient with Lou Gehrig's disease; the recent *Bartling*[15] case in California posed it for a patient with a collection of life-threatening conditions rather than a single syndrome.

The furthest reaches of this substantive question—What treatments may be withdrawn?—carries us to the central topic of this volume: the contours of the ethical and legal obligation to provide food and water artificially, typically through nasogastric or gastrostomy tubes.

The resolution of this issue will undoubtedly depend heavily upon society's handling of two other important and recent issues: DNR (Do Not Resuscitate) and "Baby Doe." They are both reflections of concern over the uncontrolled use of technology, but at the moment they have very different outcomes.

What I think is the happier situation is the evolving picture of DNR cases. DNR policies arose because of the recognition that a procedure for resuscitation, developed initially for use in a few cases after surgery or heart attack, had come to be applied to all hospitalized patients. The initial concern in the development of DNR policies was, are they legal? Is it acceptable as a matter of law to put into a case record an order that a patient not be treated in a fashion that, for at least some of the patients, could predictably extend their life for at least some period, and, for a few patients, might actually lead to their recovery?

The initial concerns over this were laid to rest through a number of judicial decisions, and from the advice of some thoughtful (rather than overly anxious) lawyers to hospitals. Indeed, it became apparent that the failure to enter a DNR order—which leads instead to some form of subterranean DNR policy, perhaps disguised by such now-famous phrases as "light blue code" or "slow code"—is more likely to incur legal penalties. In the past two years, in part because the President's Commission and then the American Hospital Association strongly recommended that hospitals adopt such policies and that accrediting bodies review the existence of such policies in hospitals, many hospitals have adopted explicit DNR policies.

The cloud on the horizon in the DNR area is a widespread misinterpretation of the significance for patient care of entering a "no code." One example of this misunderstanding can be found in a 1981 statement from the reimbursement office of the California Department of Health.[16] Although later statements seem to have rescinded this guideline by omitting it, the Department originally stated that patients for whom DNR orders are written are not appropriate to be in acute care hospitals. Actually, it would be medically appropriate to enter a DNR order for some patients in extremis, who plainly need all the acute care that the most sophisticated hospital can provide. Sometimes in these situations, resuscitation would be predictably ineffective and therefore inappropriate. Some of those patients will not have a cardiac arrest and a few will get better, and resuscitation might again become appropriate. In the meantime, however, one may have both the vigorous effort to try to save them and a recognition that if the effort fails, resuscitation should be withheld. The message for public policy from the DNR experience is that careful decisions can be made, but everyone involved—including hospital administrators and reimbursement officials—needs to understand the underlying rationale for a policy if it is to be sensibly applied. Plainly, that is a lesson worth remembering as one thinks about policy on artificial feeding.

Less sanguine is the development in the area labeled "Baby Doe." The first concern in this area, and in all areas during the 1970s, was the growing recognition of overtreatment of babies and underinvolvement of their parents in life-and-death decisions.[17] But the "Baby Doe" case itself in Indiana in 1982 was catalytic in the opposite direction.[18] The federal government justified involvement through its interpretation of the 1973 Rehabilitation Act, to prevent discrimination against the handicapped, a category into which it cast all seriously ill newborns. This category included not only those—like the original "Baby Doe"—who suffer from both a permanent disability, like Down syndrome or other forms of mental retardation, and also a treatable, acute, life-threatening condition, but also newborns with multiple developmental problems or low birth weight due to prematurity. Rather than a single decision whether or not to operate, many complex treatment decisions have repeatedly to be made about the latter group.

In March 1983, what had begun as a reminder to hospitals about their obligation not to discriminate under the 1973 Rehabilitation Act was replaced by interim federal regulations establishing a hot line to Washington to dispatch "Baby Doe squads"; the hot line was announced by a notice, to be posted in every facility taking care of infants, that warned that discriminatory nontreatment was prohibited by federal law.[19] A month later Judge Gerhard Gesell threw out those regulations.[20] In July 1983, the regulations were reissued in essentially the same form as a proposal for comment.[21] The American Academy of Pediatrics, the National Association of Children's Hospitals and Related Institutions, and other medical groups, looking for a way to soften the effect of the regulations, seized upon the possibility of using institutional ethics committees (IECs) as discussed in a report of the President's Commission. The Commission tentatively endorsed such committees as one means for improving decision-making in hospitals, not only about newborns but also about other, particularly incapacitated, patients.[22]

In February 1984, the Department of Health and Human Services promulgated final regulations that combine IECs with the "Baby Doe squads" and the hot lines, backed up by threatened withdrawal of federal funds and state enforcement of child neglect and abuse laws.[23] Although the continuing validity of these regulations is in doubt,[24] as formulated the regulations pose the risk that the infant care committees will become institutionally committed to continue treatment (especially nutrition and hydration) in order to protect the hospital from a threat of on-site federal investigations and enforcement if the results are not up to the standards believed correct by government officials. Nor is this problem allayed by the subsequent grafting of Baby Doe requirements onto federal aid for state child protection agencies.[25]

The outcome of this second area of recent policy-making on life-and-death decisions is considerably less reassuring than developments in the DNR area. Federal intervention has cast parties concerned with institutional ethics committees into adversarial postures and has restricted the IECs' potential value. Some of this may be regained, if the committees are allowed to evolve in a way appropriate to each local environment. The President's Commission saw IECs as sources of compassion, of clarification, and of conviction, helping all concerned, especially in the case of seriously ill newborns, by providing insight into the ethical issues as well as improving the quality of information about the possibilities in each individual case. Properly functioning, they could provide the necessary resolve to go on with treatment when there is some cause for hope as well as the reassurance that forgoing treatment is morally and legally acceptable when the probable outcome seems too grim. Above all, an ethics committee offers one very good way to keep the best interests of the patient clearly in view as the goal that everyone should be striving to promote.

CONCLUSION

This recent experience with DNR orders (where the major initiatives have occurred among health care professionals and institutions, thereafter endorsed by courts and other public bodies) and with ethics committees (where local initiatives have been largely swamped by governmental intervention through so-called Baby Doe legislation, regulations, and litigation) sets the stage for the process of developing policy on providing nutrition and hydration by tubes to very sick patients. As in those other areas of policy, the difficulties include not only the establishment of substantive policies but also the identification of appropriate decision-makers and (as the Baby Doe developments illustrate) review mechanisms, at institutional, local, professional, and/or governmental levels.

By the time the New Jersey Supreme Court decided her case in January 1985 (nearly two years after her death), Claire Conroy had come to symbolize the issues on the public stage: Who decides and on what grounds, and with what review, about forgoing life-sustaining treatment? In particular, is the withdrawal of artificially provided food and water ever acceptable legally, or is it always tantamount to homicide? Beyond that, is it acceptable ethically or would it violate the trust and compassion that everyone should be able to expect? Are food and water always the necessary minimum expression of human caring? Does weighing the benefits and burdens of continued care—especially maintenance-type care, like food and fluids—amount to a "quality of life" decision? Is that acceptable in a society that proclaims human life to be a pearl beyond price? And who should make the judgment about "quality" if someone must?

These are momentous issues that were only dimly perceived a decade ago as the world watched the drama unfolding in Karen Quinlan's room in Newton Memorial Hospital and thereafter in the New Jersey courts. We may be less willing to address these questions and less engaged by the plight of elderly patients like Miss Conroy than we were by Miss Quinlan. But answers to these questions are urgently needed, especially as regrettable but seemingly inexorable economic pressures focus public attention on the medical maintenance of patients at the end of life.[26] We will need not only standards and decision-making mechanisms but also greater clarity about the underlying ethical precepts if good decisions are to be made about artificial feeding. As with all interventions, one must always be prepared to answer the basic question: *Why* is this being done for—and to—this patient?

NOTES

1. *In re* Quinlan, 70 N.J. 10, 355 A.2d 647, *cert. denied*, 429 U.S. 922 (1976).
2. 410 U.S. 113 (1973).
3. See e.g., President's Commission for the Study of Ethical Problems in Medicine and Biomedical and Behavioral Research, *Deciding to Forego Life-Sustaining Treatment*, Washington, D.C.: U.S. Government Printing Office (1983); President's Commission for the Study of Ethical Problems in Medicine and Biomedical and Behavioral Research, *Making Health Care Decisions*, Washington, D.C.: U.S. Government Printing Office (1982).
4. *In re* Conroy, 190 N.J. Super. 453, 464 A.2d 303 (App. Div. 1983).
5. *Deciding to Forego*, p. 32.
6. *In re* Conroy, 98 N.J. 321, 486 A.2d 1209 (1985).
7. Superintendent of Belchertown State School v. Saikewicz, 373 Mass. 728, 370 N.E.2d 417 (1977).

8. Weber v. Stony Brook Hospital, 60 N.Y.2d 208, 469 N.Y.S.2d 63, 456 N.E.2d 1186, *cert. denied*, 104 S.Ct. 560 (1983).

9. *In re* Conroy, 98 N.J. 321, 360, 486 A.2d 1209, 1229 (1985).

10. *Id.* at 364, 1231.

11. *Id.* at 365, 1232.

12. *Id.* at 367, 1232–1233.

13. *In re* Storar, 52 N.Y.2d 363, 438 N.Y.S.2d 266, 420 N.E.2d 64 (1981).

14. Satz v. Perlmutter, 379 So.2d 359 (Fla. 1978).

15. *In re* Bartling, 209 Cal. Rptr. 220 (1984).

16. California Department of Health Services, *Level of Care Determination on Acute Care Patients, and How It Relates to a Terminal Patient With a "No Code" Status* (Field Instruction Notice 5–81).

17. See e.g., Robert and Peggy Stinson, *The Long Dying of Baby Andrew* Boston: Little, Brown, and Co. (1983) (treatment continued despite parents' reluctance and outright objections); P. & M. Bridge, "The Brief Life and Death of Christopher Bridge," *Hastings Cent. Rep.* 11:17–19 (December 1981) (parents object to lack of information and to pressure for passive euthanasia).

18. *In re* Infant Doe, No. GU 8204–00 (Cir. Ct. Monroe County., Ind., April 12, 1982), *writ of mandamus dismissed sub nom.* State ex rel. Infant Doe v. Baker, No. 482-S-140 (Ind. Super. Ct., May 27, 1982).

19. 48 Fed. Reg. 9630 (1983).

20. American Academy of Pediatrics v. Heckler, 561 F. Supp. 395 (D.D.C. 1983).

21. 48 Fed. Reg. 30846 (1983).

22. *Deciding to Forego*, pp. 155–166 and 227–228.

23. 49 Fed. Reg. 1622 (1984).

24. United States v. University Hosp., 729 F.2d 144 (2d Cir. 1984) (Rehabilitation Act of 1973 does not provide adequate statutory basis for "Baby Doe" investigation by federal officials).

25. See Child Abuse Amendments of 1984, Pub.L. 98–457, and 49 Fed. Reg. 48170 (1984) (interim model guidelines for health care providers to comply with statutory expectations on protection of disabled infants).

26. Anne Scitovsky and Alexander M. Capron, "Medical Care at the End of Life: Interaction of Economics and Ethics," *Annual Rev. of Pub. Health* 7:(in press) (1986).

David Major, M.D.

2   The Medical Procedures for Providing Food and Water: Indications and Effects

Medical techniques for providing food and water are necessary for many patients who cannot maintain optimal nutrition or hydration by the usual oral route. A number of alternative means to improve nutrition and hydration are available. Conditions that give rise to the need for medical provision of food and/or water are diverse and common.

Short-term needs arise following many types of surgery when the patient cannot eat for a period of time. More prolonged requirements for nutritional support accompany such conditions as strokes, premature birth, severe neuromuscular diseases, severe dementing or psychiatric illness, anorexia associated with cancer or its treatment, and malabsorption syndromes.

Causes of inadequate nutrition and hydration can be categorized by the origin of the malfunction. Strokes, neuromuscular disorders, severe prematurity, and cancers of the mouth or throat can cause an inability to swallow. Various cancers, scarring, and other anatomical obstructions can block an otherwise functioning gastrointestinal tract. Toxic or neurologic processes can cause an anatomically normal gastrointestinal tract to fail to propel foodstuffs and therefore to fail to absorb them. Also, the enzymes and other factors necessary to absorb nutrients in the intestines may be inadequate, precluding optimal nutrition or hydration. Finally, the patient may have an anatomically and physiologically normal mouth, stomach, and intestinal tract but be averse to or uninterested in eating.

Medical techniques for nutrition and hydration[1] are of two major kinds: enteral (via the gut) and parenteral (via any route other than the gut). (See table 1 for a summary of the following techniques.) Parenteral techniques were developed earlier. Development of the hypodermic syringe is credited to a French surgeon named Pravez in 1851, a development that allowed fluids to be administered by a

Technique	Efficacy		Acceptability		Barriers	Cost*
	fluids & electrolytes	nutrition	patient	others		
hypodermoclysis	good	very poor	adequate	poor	infection inflammation anasarca	moderate
proctoclysis	good	poor	poor	poor	rectal irritation	lowest
intravenous	good	very poor	poor	adequate	hard to maintain	moderate
total parenteral nutrition	good	good	adequate	adequate	infection need for close monitoring	high
naso-gastric tube	excellent	excellent	poor	adequate	pneumonia enteral irritation patient restraint requires functioning GI tract	low
gastrostomy tube	excellent	excellent	good	good	initial surgery or endoscopy requires functioning GI tract	low

*Costs vary quite substantially; but, "low" implies cost similar to the costs of providing oral feedings ($5-$10 per day) and "high" costs are greater by an order of magnitude ($50-$100 per day or more).

Table 1
Comparison of Common Procedures to Supply Nutrition and/or Hydration

procedure known as hypodermoclysis.[2] A needle was simply inserted into the subcutaneous tissues and fluids were dripped into the tissue spaces, from which they were gradually absorbed. Patients often found this uncomfortable and it incurred some risk of infection or inflammation. Quite possibly because nonpyrogenic (without substances causing inflammation) and sterile solutions are now available, the medical complications may now be much less likely, though the technique is rarely used.[3] It is adequate for maintaining fluids and electrolytes, but not nutrition.

Another archaic method, which was very successful but not aesthetically pleasing, was Murphy's drip or proctoclysis. John B. Murphy (1857–1914) was a surgeon of great fame at Northwestern University.[4] Murphy's method involved the insertion of a rectal tube and administration of appropriate volumes of fluid and electrolytes as a constant drip enema.[5] Up to 24 liters a day of fluid could be administered, being absorbed readily through the mucosal surface of the large intestine. The fluids could contain glucose (sugar), salt, and soda (sodium bicarbonate), though it would ordinarily be difficult to maintain adequate caloric intake via this route.

The first of the "modern" techniques, gastrostomy (a surgical insertion of a tube through the abdominal wall into the stomach), was proposed in 1837, first attempted in human beings in 1849, and first successfully performed in a human being in 1875.[6] It uses an enteral route and remains very common.

Salt solutions (saline) were administered directly into the veins (intravenous or IV) in the 1890s.[7] The safety and efficacy of this approach have progressively improved since, but conventional intravenous procedures are adequate only for fluids and minerals, not for all nutritional needs.

Since World War II, medicine has developed a variety of effective methods for maintaining patients' total water and food requirements when the patient is no longer able either to ingest or to digest and absorb water and food adequately. Hypodermoclysis and proctoclysis have given way to intravenous methods for parenteral hydration and nutrition. Sharp, sterile, disposable needles have increased patient comfort in the insertion of peripheral intravenous access lines. The availability of prepackaged plastic catheters that are internal to the needle or that serve as sheaths to the needle allow the needle itself to be withdrawn from the vein, leaving only the plastic catheter in the vein. This allows longer retention of the catheter, since needles tend to penetrate the opposite wall of the vein, infiltrating the fluids into the tissues. Despite these advances the risks of infection or inflammation from a foreign body remain.[8] The risk of clotting (thrombosis) in these peripheral veins with relatively low flow rates is also significant.

A major advance in the 1960s was the introduction of a technique popularly known as the CVP. The CVP or central venous pressure line is simply the percutaneous insertion of a catheter through a needle into the subclavian vein. This is a very large central vein behind the clavicle (collarbone). These access lines were initially inserted for the primary purpose of measuring the pressure in this vein as a reflection of the pressure in the right side of the heart. However, as the technique became more widely used, it proved to be efficacious for the administration of large volumes of fluid, which can contain complete nutrition in solution.[9] The technique is not without hazards, including infection, bleeding, and puncture of the lung itself, all very substantial risks but relatively uncommon.

The availability of this access site led to TPN (total parenteral nutrition), one of the most rapidly growing fields in medicine. This technique provides complete nutrition, including water, electrolytes, amino acids, sugars, fats, minerals, vitamins, trace minerals, and so forth. In the 1970s it became clear that this process of total parenteral nutrition had become a mainstay for helping critically ill patients to survive acute illnesses where the prognosis had previously been nearly hopeless. Of course, the technique has also been applied in many situations where the benefits are doubtful.[10]

Widespread use precipitated a new problem—long-term maintenance of patients who had no functioning gastrointestinal tract. The major roadblock to long-term therapy was that the necessary catheter tended to become infected or clotted, both especially hazardous in a large central vein. The introduction of the "Hickman catheter" nearly eliminated these problems. The Hickman catheter is inserted by making an incision to provide direct access to the subclavian vein. The vein is cannulated with the Hickman catheter under direct observation and then the catheter is tunneled under the skin and brought to the surface at a site several centimeters away from the primary incision. This simple surgical technique removes the junction of the catheter and the skin surface from the area of the junction of the catheter and the vein, which nearly eliminates infections. The catheters can have either one or two lumens, the latter used when patients need to have fluids administered through one lumen and blood samples drawn through the other. These catheters can be used for long-term administration of antibiotics, chemotherapy, or pain-controlling drugs. They also allow for the administration of total parenteral nutrition for an unlimited time. The cost of the fluids is high because they must be prepared and administered under sterile conditions and because minor imperfections in designing or preparing the nutrient mix can have substantially detrimental health effects.

When the gut is available for nutrition, it is cheaper and often more effective to use the enteral route for hydration and nutrition. The most widely available, simple, and well-known technique using the gut is the nasogastric tube. Insertion of this simple plastic tube is uncomfortable and its retention is irritating. If awake and able to cooperate, the patient is asked to swallow water repetitively as the tube, which is lubricated with a tasteless jelly, is passed through the nose and pushed through the posterior pharynx and esophagus into the stomach. The tube is irritating to the nose and causes a gag reflex when it reaches the posterior pharynx, sometimes causing vomiting. The nasogastric tube continues to pose significant hazards while it is in place. It may cause vomiting and aspiration of the gastric contents, producing a serious aspiration pneumonia. It may irritate the mucosal surfaces, causing bleeding, sometimes severe. Many patients need to be restrained forcibly and their hands put into large mittens to prevent them from removing the tube, a thought which all patients with any degree of consciousness seem to have. These restrained patients may develop pneumonia and serious bedsores because of lack of activity and fixed positions. Patients with some insight are likely to become depressed or angry over being tied down.

Newer feeding tubes may have a smaller diameter, softer texture, and a tip weighted with mercury so that they may enter the beginning of the small bowel, lessening the chance of aspiration of gastric contents. However, these smaller diameter tubes require a constant drip mechanism for administration, rather than larger bolus feedings, and increases the cost of administration and the degree of restraint needed. In addition, because of their softness, they are packaged with a rigid inserter (wire or rigid plastic device), which is removed after the tube is in place. Often, these tubes cannot be reused if dislodged, adding to replacement cost as well as inconvenience.

An alternative to the nasogastric feeding tube is the gastrostomy feeding tube. This tube is inserted through the abdominal wall directly into the stomach by a simple surgical operation that can be performed under local anesthesia. The procedure has the advantage of eliminating the problems of nasal, pharyngeal, and esophageal irritation. The tube is quite comfortable for the patient once the incision for insertion is healed. The tube creates a track between the skin and the stomach in a fashion analogous to the track which forms after ordinary ear piercing. As with pierced ears, these tracks will usually close if the tube is removed subsequently. There are obvious possible complications from the surgical procedure, including infection of the peritoneal lining (peritonitis) and bleeding, but these complications are relatively uncommon. Formal informed consent from the patient or the patient's guardian is a necessary part of this surgical procedure. This often poses a serious practical problem in that many patients may not have a legally authorized representative.[11]

The percutaneous endoscopic insertion technique has recently been developed for the insertion of gastrostomy tubes.[12] The patient is sedated if necessary. A gastroscope (a long, flexible tube made for looking into the stomach) is passed through the mouth and esophagus into the stomach under direct observation. These flexible, fiberoptic instruments are relatively comfortable for the patient. A needle with attached thread is passed through the abdominal wall to the stomach. While being viewed from the inside of the stomach, this needle is grasped by forceps passed through the gastroscope. Then, the gastroscope, forceps, and needle are removed through the esophagus and mouth. This pulls the thread through these areas, leaving one end protruding from the abdominal wall and the other end from the mouth. A tube of the appropriate diameter is tied to the oral end of the thread. The thread is then pulled back from the abdominal side, pulling the tube through the esophagus into the stomach. With a very small incision where the string exits the abdomen, the tube is pulled through the abdominal wall, leaving only the tip of the tube in the stomach. This technique takes only a few minutes, avoids anesthesia and a larger surgical incision, and can be done by the medical gastroenterologist or the surgeon. The risk of insertion appears to be lower and the utility of the tube is comparable to that of the surgically inserted tube described previously. Formal informed consent will be required, posing the same problems as for gastrostomy.

Efficient provision of nutrition with any of these procedures requires skilled personnel and specialized techniques, often as special nutrition support teams in hospitals. The standards required are quite exacting, and substantial deviation from them greatly increases risks of infection or illness arising from erroneous nutritional balance. This summary of techniques for providing fluids and nutrition has shown parenteral routes of administration to be more hazardous and more expensive. However, enteral routes of administration (other than the normal oral route) are also invasive and have both risks and burdens to the patient. Over the long term, gastrostomy tubes are better accepted than nasogastric tubes, although they pose slightly increased risk when initially inserted. Prepackaged products for enteral feeding are readily available and relatively inexpensive. However, insurance coverage for any of these procedures is quite variable. The decision to use or discontinue the use of any of these techniques in an individual patient remains a continuing challenge in the practice of medicine today and in the future.

NOTES

1. See generally Canizaro, "Methods of Nutritional Support in the Surgical Patient," in Yarborough and Curreri (eds.), *Surgical Nutrition*, New York: Churchill-Livingstone (1981), 13; Silberman and Eisenberg, *Parenteral and Enteral Nutrition for the Hospitalized Patient*, Norwalk, Conn.: Appleton-Century-Crofts (1982); Luc Michel, Alfonso Serrano, and Ronald A. Malt, "Nutritional Support of Hospitalized Patients," *N. Engl. J. Med.* 304:1147–1152 (1981); and Faintauch and Deitel, "Complications of Intravenous Hyperalimentation: Technical and Metabolic Aspects," in Deitel (ed.), *Nutrition in Clinical Surgery*, Baltimore: Williams & Wilkins (1980); Nancy Nuwer Konstantinides and Eva Shronts, "Tube Feeding: Managing the Basics," *Am. J. Nursing* 1312–1320 (September 1983).

2. F. Christopher, *Minor Surgery*, Philadelphia: W. B. Saunders (1932), 846–849.

3. Rafael J. Schen and Maia Singer-Edelstein, "Subcutaneous Infusions in the Elderly," *J. Am. Geriatr. Soc.* 29:583–585 (1981); W. E. Abbot, S. Levey, R. C. Foreman, et al., "The Danger of Administering Parenteral Fluids by Hypodermoclysis," *Surgery* 32:305–315 (1952); Eugene Y. Berger, "Nutrition by Hypodermoclysis," *J. Am. Geriatri. Soc.* 32:199–203 (1984); Seymour M. Gluck, "Hypodermoclysis Revisited" (letter), *J.A.M.A.* 248:1310–1311 (1982).

4. J. Louri, *Medical Eponyms: Who Was Coudé?* London: Pitman (1982), 134–135.

5. W. W. Babcock, *A Textbook of Surgery*, Philadelphia: W. B. Saunders (1929), 504.

6. *Id.* at 1045.

7. Sporadic reports date from 1831, e.g., R. Lewins, "Injection of Saline Solutions in Extraordinary Quantities into the Veins in Cases of Malignant Cholera," *Lancet* 2:243–244 (1831).

8. R. J. Duma, "Thomas Latta, What Have We Done? The Hazards of Intravenous Therapy," *N. Engl. J. Med.* 294:1178–1180 (1976).

9. S. J. Dudrick, D. W. Wilmorc, H. M. Vars, et al., "Long-Term Parenteral Nutrition with Growth, Development, and Positive Nitrogen Balance," *Surgery* 64:134–142 (1968).

10. J. Thomas Goodgame, Jr., "A Critical Assessment of the Indications for Total Parenteral Nutrition," *Surg. Gynecol. Obstet.* 151:433–441 (1980).

11. Jeffrey L. Ponsky and Michael W. L. Gauderer, "Percutaneous Endoscopic Gastrostomy: A Non-Operative Technique for Feeding Gastrostomy," *Gastrointest. Endosc.* 27:9–11 (1981).

12. Select Committee on Standards of Professional Practice, Washington, D.C., American Society for Parenteral and Enteral Nutrition, "Standards for Nutrition Support: Hospitalized Patients" (January 1984).

Phyllis Schmitz, R.N., and Merry O'Brien, R.N.

3 Observations on Nutrition and Hydration in Dying Cancer Patients

BACKGROUND

Hospice is not a place, but rather a treatment modality based on professional assistance to the patient and family, who are encouraged to think and act according to their own values and priorities. Hospice providers try to affirm feelings of the patient and family in a non-judgmental fashion. In our hospice setting,[1] very few interventions are used "automatically"; instead, the attempt is made to individualize treatment. Since many of our patients have become unable to ingest "normal" amounts of fluid and nutrition, we have often had to confront the issues of whether or not to use artificial feeding. The following observations arise from experiences with these patients.

The progression of terminal illness commonly entails certain changes. In the earlier stages, there may be weight loss and weakness; later, increasing fluid deficit, reduced peripheral circulation, and possibly an increasing electrolyte imbalance and acidosis may occur. The blood volume and oxygen-carrying capacity may be lower. The patient's level of consciousness often declines toward somnolence and lethargy. Urinary output usually decreases. Skin turgor diminishes, both from dehydration and from depletion of the subcutaneous fat stores. There may be muscular irritability, restlessness, gastrointestinal bleeding, abnormal body temperature, and multiple organ failure.

EFFECTS OF DEHYDRATION

Our professional hospice team never unilaterally decides to withhold or withdraw nourishment from any patient, but we allow patients to choose what and when they will eat and drink. This includes those with gastrostomy tubes, nasogastric tubes, and intravenous fluids, although many patients coming to hospice have already chosen not to be fed artificially. As intake is spontaneously reduced by the patient, we have noted a reduction of nausea, vomiting, and abdominal pain, particularly where there is a bowel obstruction, liver disease, or malignant ascites. Lessened urinary output means fewer linen changes for incontinent patients and less frequent struggling with commode or bedpan for others.

Pulmonary secretions decrease as patients allow themselves to become dehydrated, resulting in less coughing, less congestion, and less shortness of breath. With the decrease in mucus, there is less gagging and choking for those with difficulty swallowing and/or extreme weakness. Frequently, the need for oral-pharyngeal suctioning is eliminated.

Dehydration can also lead to detrimental effects. Interestingly enough, our patients have not stated that they were thirsty but only that the mouth was dry, a symptom that can easily be relieved by local measures. However, sometimes the symptoms arising from electrolyte imbalances (especially hypercalcemia), such as twitching, muscle spasms, or altered levels of consciousness, require treatment. Sometimes these are best treated with rehydration, but often it is better to use antispasmodics or sedation. Of course, whenever possible, patients' options are made known to them and they are supported in their decisions.

Many patients experience relief and a renewed sense of autonomy from controlling their own intake. When they do not have to force themselves to eat under threat that otherwise tube feeding or intravenous fluids will be started, anxiety diminishes. Frequently, family members have a hard time with the patient's dwindling food intake, as eating represents recovery or at least continuation of life. We find it important to let patient and family move at their own pace in making decisions about nutrition and fluids so that they may come to terms with their impending loss. Among the issues that family members must address is the need to resolve for themselves the symbolic meaning of eating and drinking and of medical means to achieve nutrition and hydration.

GOALS OF THERAPY

Improving nutritional intake, when freely chosen by the patient, increases the patient's sense of well-being and improves morale.

However, success in developing a plan of care and achieving goals depends upon the ability of caregivers to acknowledge the patient's unique values and capabilities and to understand the interrelationship of the physical symptoms with the psychological and spiritual distress of dying.

An accurate evaluation of nutritional status depends on obtaining specific data in the context of a more general assessment. A diet history should disclose recent changes in intake, food preferences, dislikes, allergies, or intolerances. Specific cultural, socioeconomic, and religious factors might dictate diet modifications and explain particular attitudes toward food. Mechanical problems that affect chewing and swallowing, as well as chronic illnesses, recent surgery, or treatment protocols affecting nutrition, are revealed by a careful review of the patient's medical history.

At least weekly, members of the multidisciplinary team will need to update the care plan to reflect the patient's current condition. Our goals at the time of initial general assessment are (1) to appreciate the patient's and the family's understanding of the illness, (2) to explain the concept of hospice care and the capabilities of our program, (3) to focus on the symptoms most distressing to the patient, and (4) to determine the patient's priorities and goals. In this process, we begin to develop a bond of trust with the patient and family. This trusting and supportive relationship among staff, patient, and family members is centrally important in the management of nutrition, which we see to involve goals much more important than the normalization of food and fluid intake.

Whenever it might be advantageous to the patient, we discuss both oral and artificially provided food and fluid regimes with the patient and family. Education of patients and families is vital to developing a nutritional care plan that reflects both the patient's goals and his or her physical limitations.

CONTROL OF SYMPTOMS AFFECTING ORAL INTAKE

Decreasing unpleasant symptoms that interfere with nutritional intake is essential. Most of our patients have terminal cancer and chronic pain is frequent. The elimination of pain significantly decreases other symptoms such as fatigue, depression, fear, and anorexia.

Many of our patients have disturbances in patterns of elimination. Decreased activity, drug effects, and diminished intake contribute to constipation, which must be prevented with stool softeners and laxatives. Diarrhea is uncommon and usually results from the basic illness, from food/fluid intolerance, or from enzyme deficiency. A lactose-free diet sometimes corrects the food intolerance, while enzyme deficiency malabsorption syndromes respond well to enzyme replacement.

Nausea and vomiting are among the most distressing symptoms for the patient. Contributing factors are many, including disease, drugs, emotions, and environment, some of which may be remediable. Frequent small meals and the regular administration of antiemetics such as prochlorperazine (Compazine), either before meals or on an "every four to six hours" schedule, are often effective in relieving nausea. Metoclopramide (Reglan) is sometimes effective if the symptom is caused by decreased gastric and/or intestinal motility. The schedule of care, including treatments and meals, can be adjusted to avoid peak times of nausea and vomiting. Relaxation techniques can be helpful, but providing the patient with the appropriate environment in which to discuss fears and anxieties is most beneficial.

The most frequently neglected part of the alimentary tract is the oral cavity. Dry mouth, stomatitis, infection, and dysphagia are both particularly disturbing and usually readily remediable by cleansing the oral cavity and frequently lubricating the membranes. We rely on patient preference in regard to oral hygiene when appropriate. Many commercial preparations are available, but we have had best results with half-strength hydrogen peroxide, diluted with water or normal saline, or with baking soda and water. Chewing gum, drinking iced beverages, and sucking on hard candy or popsicles can relieve dry mouth. A room humidifier is also helpful when membranes are dry. Viscous lidocaine, offered before meals, will alleviate oral discomfort, but if often alters taste sensations undesirably. Recognition, treatment, and relief of these uncomfortable oral symptoms generally improve the patient's self-image as well as his or her intake.

The patient's nutritional status is affected by a number of other conditions, including metabolic disturbances (e.g., hypercalcemia, acidosis), hepatic failure, ascites, hypoxia, and changes in mental status. These conditions usually eventuate in death, but they are often temporarily reversible. The risks and benefits of available treatments are weighed, with primary consideration given to the quality of life expected as an outcome. The patient and family are included in the discussion of potential therapy, and treatment is initiated or deferred in accordance with the patient's needs and wishes whenever possible.

DIET MODIFICATIONS TO ENCOURAGE ADEQUATE ORAL INTAKE

When a satisfactory level of comfort is reached, many patients experience a renewed appetite for a few weeks or months. A patient's appetite and need for a particular kind of food change with time. Our dietician makes an initial assessment, usually within twenty-four hours of admission, and visits regularly throughout the patient's stay. Whatever help the patient may need in order to eat (setting up the tray, arranging the bed, spoon feeding, and so forth) is made available by the regular registered nurse staff or a volunteer, helping to make feeding times pleasant and social as well as free of time pressure.

A patient experiencing nausea and vomiting can generally tolerate a bland, nonfatty diet with small meals and snacks to supplement intake. Carbonated beverages, ice, and tea in small amounts can be offered even during periods of nausea.

Patients with sore or dry mouth respond favorably to a bland, nonirritating, high-caloric diet with popsicles and ice drinks between meals. Nectars, rather than citrus juices, appeal more to these patients and to patients with dysphagia.

Most dying patients have altered taste sensations. We find the best approach is to listen to the patient and try to provide the foods that are most appealing. Adding flavor enhancers, making extra sugar available, or incorporating bitter-tasting food in casseroles are often helpful modifications.

A regular diet, with a minimum of restrictions, is almost uniformly best for dying patients. We have never encountered serious problems allowing a patient free access to salt or fluids. Diabetic patients on regular diet often can be kept symptom-free with regular insulin as needed, with only an occasional fasting blood sugar determination to monitor serum glucose levels.

Diet modifications to accommodate the patient's preferences and capabilities are essential to maintaining or improving the patient's nutritional status. A diet that is planned to meet individual needs will contribute much to motivating the patient to enjoy remaining life.

ENHANCING PATIENT MOTIVATION

Our meals are delivered from a central kitchen, but the availability of a refrigerator and microwave oven on the unit permits us to serve patients at a time most comfortable for them. Patients thus can make decisions regarding time, amount, and kind of food. Small meals served more frequently are appreciated.

We have observed that a light meal served in the middle of the night is often therapeutic. Not only does the patient receive added nutritional benefits, but also she or he may be able to discuss concerns and fears with the staff member who joins in a "midnight meal." The late hours, with their absence of distractions, are very conducive to just such an exchange. This sort of approach, with each patient's individual concerns being central, usually results in increased interest in nutritional intake.

Occasionally the sight of food can precipitate a negative response. One of our patients, a woman with terminal cancer of the colon, was repulsed by the sight of a full meal. A staff member, having described the menu, would bring her selected small portions, usually one or two tablespoons, which she then consumed slowly and with great relish. Perhaps after enduring multiple surgical and treatment protocols to control her cancer, having this degree of control was important to restoring meaning to her life.

Caregivers should also be attentive to frequently overlooked environmental considerations such as noise, odor, and general appearance of the patient's room. Unemptied bedpans, dirty linens, or stale air can obviously have an adverse effect on appetite.

Food and water are certainly significant symbols, but the social experience associated with the giving and receiving of food and water may be equally important. The patient receiving intravenous fluids, lying alone in a hospital bed, is having a much less rewarding experience than the patient in a personalized room being given ice chips by a concerned caregiver. Both are receiving water, but there are few other similarities. Our policies encourage maximum family participation. The family is encouraged to be present during meals, to feed the patient, and to fill out menus. Not only do these practices stimulate patient interest at mealtime, they also help support relationships that are frequently disrupted by chronic illness.

Terminally ill patients may only be able to tolerate small meals. Our efforts are then focused on maximizing intake without significantly increasing the volume. Staff and volunteers exercise imagination to create high-caloric drinks for the patients, using a blender and a number of easily stored and readily accessible ingredients. Eggs, powdered milk, instant breakfast powders, malted milk mixes, fruit, and ice cream or sherbert can be blended into flavorful combinations that have wide appeal.

Food craving is a universal experience. Even patients who are not eating often fantasize about foods. A patient may request a particular food and, when it is presented, no longer desire it. Disease, drugs, or therapy have altered taste to make the item unpalatable, or it just isn't as perfect as it was imagined. Caregivers and loved ones might feel rejected if such reactions are not explained to them. Whether or not the food is eaten by the patient, nurturing and caring has taken place. The act of fulfilling the request demonstrates the responsiveness of the caregivers and family to the patient. Is this not nourishment in the broadest definition of the term? Often staff can explain this concept to family members who otherwise are often distraught at the patient's refusal to eat the "favorite foods" they have prepared.

We try to honor all requests and the responses have been very instructive. One patient with cancer of the colon and almost total obstruction was able to tolerate small amounts of ice chips and sips of water and ginger ale. When staff members ordered out for Chinese food on the July Fourth holiday, she became irritated, saying their action was "un-American." She asked for a hot dog and potato salad, and, while there was justifiable concern by the staff, the request was honored. Not only did she eat it with consummate pleasure, but she retained the meal, much to everyone's surprise and obvious delight. Being open to all possibilities and remaining nonjudgmental can clearly lead to unexpected outcomes.

Many people feel that "food is life." A strong emotional attachment to food is sometimes expressed by family members, either through words or actions. Our experience has shown that artificial feeding up until death generally increases patient discomfort, but caregivers need to be tactful and nonjudgmental when discussing this with the patient and family. Involving them in a discussion of the benefits and burdens can allow all involved to determine their real concerns about feeding. Frequently family members express their inability to cope with their impending loss by demanding force-feeding. Rather than disagreeing with their demand for feeding the patient, we offer suggestions as to what might be more appropriate and less disturbing for the patient.

WHEN DEATH IS IMMINENT

As the dying process continues, the patient usually becomes less acutely aware of his or her circumstances. The intake of food will no longer be a consideration, and hydration becomes the focus. Families may become anxious when they realize death is near. If intravenous feeding is mentioned, team members may need to discuss the risks of intravenous hydration for dying patients. Generally, family members are more concerned about patient comfort than length of life. What they need are reassurances that we know how to provide appropriate care. To provide reassurance and ensure understanding, we review with the family the comfort techniques and hydration measures we envision using. These include frequent mouth care and body lotioning. If the swallowing reflex is intact, we will administer small amounts of water, often using a small syringe. Vaseline will be applied liberally to keep lips moist and a room humidifier will be used. Encouraging family members to participate in this care is especially comforting for them.

We have not seen evidence that dehydration occurring at the termination of life results in any pain or distressing experience for the patient. To the contrary, even patients who remain quite alert and communicative become objectively dehydrated without substantial symptoms when treated for dry mouth.

ARTIFICIAL FEEDING

Our patients often forgo artificial feeding. However, especially when disruption of nutrition and hydration is abrupt and substantially in advance of death, gastrostomy, jejunostomy, nasogastric tubes, or intravenous lines can be employed to provide nutrition while avoiding substantial discomfort to the patient. This becomes a desirable option if the underlying disease would allow a substantial period with a desirable quality of life. The patient should be included in the discussion of the proposed therapy whenever possible.

We prefer to attach the same social significance to artificial feeding as we would to a meal consumed in the natural manner. For example, patients being artificially fed can retain control over their feeding schedule. Controlling "medical" feedings is usually a new and enjoyable experience for the patient. Our patients are surprised to learn that such "treats" as coffee, juice, or alcoholic drinks can be put through the enteral tubes, as well as the prescribed nourishment. One of our patients who had radical head and neck surgery described in writing her delight at receiving beer through her gastrostomy tube: "Gee, this is just like a bar, nice and slow."

One patient with pancreatic cancer and widespread liver metastases was admitted with pain, intractable vomiting, and diarrhea. He was receiving three thousand calories a day via a jejunostomy tube prior to admission. Decreasing this amount significantly reduced the vomiting and diarrhea, and proclorperizine and morphine sulfate administered on a regular schedule added to his comfort level. After a discussion with the patient, a feeding schedule was developed that would offer him nourishment by the feeding tube at times when nausea and diminished intestinal motility were least troublesome. He was encouraged to eat (orally) foods of his choice whenever he wished. He was able to eat small amounts several times a day without experiencing significant distress. Several weeks before he died, this patient said, "I feel in control of my life again."

In summary, nutrition and hydration are important and can often be improved, even for dying patients. However, caregivers must be willing to tailor care to the patient, which includes recognizing that force-feeding or artificial feeding can sometimes be harmful and may thus be contraindicated.

N O T E S

1. The Washington Home Hospice in Washington, D.C., is a six-bed in-patient unit for the care of terminally ill patients, primarily those with advanced cancer.

*Kenneth Micetich, M.D., Patricia Steinecker, M.D.,
and David Thomasma, Ph.D.*

4   An Empirical Study
of Physician Attitudes

American medicine is confronted with a serious problem: our technology has far outpaced our ability to alter the outcome of terminal diseases. The problem of providing nutrition and fluids for dying patients is actually but a footnote to the greater challenge medicine faces in gaining mastery over our technology.

Since the technology under examination in this book is epitomized by intravenous fluids (IVs), we report a study of the perceptions of a sample of physicians at one institution about use of IVs. We perceive these fluids as a therapy, analytically just like any other therapy, including open heart surgery, kidney transplants, cancer chemotherapy, and so on. We found it interesting that others perceived them differently.

The case that precipitated our study follows. About a year and a half ago, a patient was admitted to the care of one of us (K. M.) with advanced squamous-cell cancer of the tongue and spread of his disease to the bone. Chemotherapeutic agents were tried to no avail and, over the three months before admission, he had been experiencing worsening pain, now so severe that achieving adequate analgesia also caused significant obtundation and respiratory depression. In the same time span, his ability to walk had been lost and he had become completely bedridden. The patient had a cardiac arrest, was resuscitated, and was placed on a respirator. After three days, he was stable but remained in deep coma and was transferred out of intensive care to a general medicine ward, supported by a respirator and intravenous fluids. No real hope of any significant recovery remained. We posed the following question: Can we discontinue the IV and allow the patient to die of dehydration?

An informal hallway survey was taken of physicians, nurses, and social workers. Most objected to the withdrawal of the intravenous fluid support. Some respondents said that they would maintain the

IV at a "to-keep-open" rate, and they really wouldn't object if the IV were not restarted if it fell out. So our initial impression from these discussions was that giving intravenous solutions to a terminally ill comatose patient was a traditional, automatic response that served to appease the consciences of the treating staff.

We designed a formal survey with sequential management questions using the case just described.[1] The salient features of the case are important: the patient's cancer and anoxic brain damage were both incurable, the performance status of this patient had deteriorated substantially prior to hospitalization, and pain could not be adequately controlled without producing significant alterations in the physiology of the patient even before the resuscitation led to anoxic brain damage.

The survey was distributed to the medical staff and house officers. (See table 2.) We asked the medical-surgical house officers and attendings what initial IV orders they would write after the patient was resuscitated. They were to specify an IV rate and the type of solution. Seventy-three percent of all respondents wrote IV orders that provided physiologically correct amounts of salt and water. Twenty-seven percent of the respondents, however, wrote orders that could not sustain life, either requesting no IV or ordering an intravenous solution at a "to-keep-open" rate.

Table 2.
Outcomes of Physician Surveys Regarding Use of
Intravenous Fluids in an Unconscious, Dying Patient

Initial Fluid Orders	how many would restart IV?	how many would use surgery to restart IV?	how many would stop IV if no improvement in 3 days?	how many felt hydration was essential to quality care?
73% ordered adequate	84%	40%	21%	50%
27% ordered inadequate	28%	5%	64%	0

All subsequent questions were analyzed based upon whether the physicians initially wrote orders for adequate hydration or for deliberately inadequate hydration. The second question of the survey asked what the physician would do if the intravenous line became blocked, requiring reinsertion into a vein to continue administration of IVs. Of those physicians who initially felt strongly enough about hydration that they wrote physiologically adequate orders, eighty-four percent would restart the IV. Of those who wrote orders for inadequate hydration to begin with, seventy-two percent said that they would not restart it.

The third question asked about restarting an IV: If the IV fell out and you had to use more invasive procedures, such as a cutdown or a subclavian line, to start the IV, would you do so? Forty percent of the physicians who wrote adequate IV fluid orders would use an invasive means to restart the IV. Of the physicians who initially wrote orders for inadequate fluids, ninety-five percent would not use an invasive means to restart the IV.

Could the physician discontinue the IV in a patient who was showing no signs of neurological improvement or recovery of any kind after three days? Of those physicians who wrote adequate IV fluid orders, seventy-one percent of them would not stop. Of those who wrote inadequate IV fluid orders, sixty-four percent of them would discontinue the IV.

The final question of the survey asked about the standards of care for the terminally ill. Fifty percent of the doctors initially ordering adequate fluids said that hydration was the standard of care. Of those who wrote inadequate fluid orders, not a single person mentioned hydration as a standard of care.

The physicians surveyed were not giving IV fluids erratically. If a physician wrote an order for physiologically adequate IV fluids, he or she consistently sought to normalize hydration subsequently.

The decision made in this particular patient was that the IV fluids alone were discontinued. The patient died three days later, and permission for autopsy was granted. The autopsy showed that he had disseminated carcinoma and severe microscopic neuronal changes consistent with hypoxic encephalopathy.

Why did we decide to discontinue the IV fluids, knowing that death would occur? We discontinued the IV fluids for one reason only: the continued use of IV fluid therapy had no therapeutic.intent. It was impossible for this man to survive. Some would argue that perhaps the IV fluids served a palliative function. But our patient had no symptoms to relieve. Therefore the IV was not medically indicated, being a procedure devoid of therapeutic utility, and it could be discontinued.

It is not clear to us why seventy-five percent of respondents would not discontinue the IVs even when it was clear that the patient had no hope of survival. Perhaps the physicians were afraid of legal liability. Perhaps physicians viewed the IV as an "ordinary means" and felt obliged to continue the fluids. Perhaps the doctors felt that to stop the intravenous fluids would be seen as abandoning the patient, or perhaps they felt guilty that they just couldn't do any more for this patient.

In any case, IV fluids remain firmly entrenched as a standard of care, an automatic response to the serious illness which occasions no serious consideration of alternatives by most physicians.

Physicians should come to realize that there are choices to be made about initiating and continuing intravenous fluids. IV fluids as a form of therapy have indications and contraindications, and, just as with any other medical procedure, if the use of IV fluids cannot provide therapeutic results, then it need not be undertaken or continued. The indication for an application of a technology is not its mere availability. Rather, any therapy is indicated only if it has known therapeutic efficacy. Physicians should assess the merit and likelihood of achieving the goals of each therapy.

As others have pointed out,[2] "extraordinary" and "ordinary" as terms for categories of treatment are often used to reflect either the artificiality (vs. naturalness) or the relative frequency of use of a particular treatment. These categories are very often ambiguous and are certainly inadequate moral guidelines. It may be more clear to term all therapies as "medically indicated" or "medically contraindicated." The goal is to avoid contraindicated applications of therapy; a side effect is that we may thereby also avoid unnecessary "ethical dilemmas." Even the administration of IV fluids is sometimes contraindicated and should be forgone, but substantial reeducation of physicians will be necessary before that assessment is widely implemented.

NOTES

1. Kenneth Micetich, Patricia Steinecker, and David Thomasma, "Are Intravenous Fluids Morally Required for a Dying Patient?" *Arch. Intern. Med.* 143:975–978 (1983).
2. See,chapters 5, 7, 9, and 12 in this volume.

Part II Considerations in Formulating a Moral Response

Joanne Lynn, M.D., and James F. Childress, Ph.D.

5 Must Patients Always Be Given Food and Water?

Many people die from the lack of food or water. For some, this lack is the result of poverty or famine, but for others it is the result of disease or deliberate decision. In the past, malnutrition and dehydration must have accompanied nearly every death that followed an illness of more than a few days. Most dying patients do not eat much on their own, and nothing could be done for them until the first flexible tubing for instilling food or other liquid into the stomach was developed about a hundred years ago. Even then, the procedure was so scarce, so costly in physician and nursing time, and so poorly tolerated that it was used only for patients who clearly could benefit. With the advent of more reliable and efficient procedures in the past few decades, these conditions can be corrected or ameliorated in nearly every patient who would otherwise be malnourished or dehydrated. In fact, intravenous lines and nasogastric tubes have become common images of hospital care.

Providing adequate nutrition and fluids is a high priority for most patients, both because they suffer directly from inadequacies and because these deficiencies hinder their ability to overcome other diseases. But are there some patients who need not receive these treatments? This question has become a prominent public policy issue in a number of recent cases. In May 1981, in Danville, Illinois, the parents and the physician of newborn conjoined twins with shared abdominal organs decided not to feed these children. Feeding and other treatments were given after court intervention, though a grand jury refused to indict the parents.[1] Later that year, two physicians in Los Angeles discontinued intravenous nutrition to a patient who had severe brain damage after an episode involving loss of oxygen following routine surgery. Murder charges were brought, but the hearing judge dismissed the charges at a preliminary hearing. On appeal, the charges were reinstated and remanded for trial.[2]

Reprinted from the *Hastings Center Report* 13:17–21 (October 1983) by permission.

In April 1982, a Bloomington, Indiana, infant who had tracheo-esophageal fistula and Down Syndrome was not treated or fed, and he died after two courts ruled that the decision was proper but before all appeals could be heard.[3] When the federal government then moved to ensure that such infants would be fed in the future,[4] the Surgeon General, Dr. C. Everett Koop, initially stated that there is never adequate reason to deny nutrition and fluids to a newborn infant.

While these cases were before the public, the nephew of Claire Conroy, an elderly incompetent woman with several serious medical problems, petitioned a New Jersey court for authority to discontinue her nasogastric tube feedings. Although the intermediate appeals court has reversed the ruling,[5] the trial court held that he had this authority since the evidence indicated that the patient would not have wanted such treatment and that its value to her was doubtful.

In all these dramatic cases and in many more that go unnoticed, the decision is made to deliberately withhold food or fluid known to be necessary for the life of the patient. Such decisions are unsettling. There is now widespread consensus that sometimes a patient is best served by not undertaking or continuing certain treatments that would sustain life, especially if these entail substantial suffering.[6] But food and water are so central to an array of human emotions that it is almost impossible to consider them with the same emotional detachment that one might feel toward a respirator or a dialysis machine.

Nevertheless, the question remains: Should it ever be permissible to withhold or withdraw food and nutrition? The answer in any real case should acknowledge the psychological contiguity between feeding and loving and between nutritional satisfaction and emotional satisfaction. Yet this acknowledgment does not resolve the core question.

Some have held that it is intrinsically wrong not to feed another. The philosopher G. E. M. Anscombe contends: "For wilful starvation there can be no excuse. The same can't be said quite without qualification about failing to operate or to adopt some courses of treatment."[7] But the moral issues are more complex than Anscombe's comment suggests. Does correcting nutritional deficiencies always improve patients' well-being? What should be our reflective moral response to withholding or withdrawing nutrition? What moral principles are relevant to our reflections? What medical facts about ways of providing nutrition are relevant? And what policies should be adopted by the society, hospitals, and medical and other health care professionals?

In our effort to find answers to these questions, we will concentrate upon the care of patients who are incompetent to make choices for themselves. Patients who are competent to determine the course of their therapy may refuse any and all interventions proposed by others, as long as their refusals do not seriously harm or impose unfair burdens upon others.[8] A competent patient's decision regarding whether or not to accept the provision of food and water by medical means such as tube feeding or intravenous alimentation is unlikely to raise questions of harm or burden to others.

What then should guide those who must decide about nutrition for a patient who cannot decide? As a start, consider the standard by which other medical decisions are made: one should decide as the incompetent person would have if he or she were competent, when that is possible to determine, and advance that person's interests in a more generalized sense when individual preferences cannot be known.

THE MEDICAL PROCEDURES

There is no reason to apply a different standard to feeding and hydration. Surely, when one inserts a feeding tube, or creates a gastrostomy opening, or inserts a needle into a vein, one intends to benefit the patient. Ideally, one should provide what the patient believes to be of benefit, but at least the effect should be beneficial in the opinions of surrogates and caregivers.

Thus, the question becomes, is it ever in the patient's interest to become malnourished and dehydrated, rather than to receive treatment? Posing the question so starkly points to our need to know what is entailed in treating these conditions and what benefits the treatments offer.

The medical interventions that provide food and fluids are of two basic types. First, liquids can be delivered by a tube that is inserted into a functioning gastrointestinal tract, most commonly through

the nose and esophagus into the stomach or through a surgical incision in the abdominal wall and directly into the stomach. The
liquids used can be specially prepared solutions of nutrients or a
blenderized version of an ordinary diet. The nasogastric tube is
cheap; it may lead to pneumonia and often annoys the patient and
family, sometimes even requiring that the patient be restrained to
prevent its removal.

Creating a gastrostomy is usually a simple surgical procedure, and,
once the wound is healed, care is very simple. Since it is out of sight,
it is aesthetically more acceptable and restraints are needed less
often. Also, the gastrostomy creates no additional risk of pneumonia.
However, while elimination of a nasogastric tube requires only removing the tube, a gastrostomy is fairly permanent, and can be
closed only by surgery.

The second type of medical intervention is intravenous feeding
and hydration, which also has two major forms. The ordinary hospital or peripheral IV, in which fluid is delivered directly to the
bloodstream through a small needle, is useful only for temporary
efforts to improve hydration and electrolyte concentrations. One
cannot provide a balanced diet through the veins in the limbs: to
do that requires a central line, or a special catheter placed into one
of the major veins in the chest. The latter procedure is much more
risky and vulnerable to infections and technical errors, and it is
much more costly than any of the other procedures. Both forms of
intravenous nutrition and hydration commonly require restraining
the patient, cause minor infections and other ill effects, and are
costly, especially since they ordinarily require the patient to be in
a hospital.

None of these procedures, then, is ideal; each entails some distress,
some medical limitations, and some costs. When may a procedure
be forgone that might improve nutrition and hydration for a given
patient? Only when the procedure and the resulting improvement
in nutrition and hydration do not offer the patient a net benefit over
what he or she would otherwise have faced.

Are there such circumstances? We believe that there are; but they
are few and limited to the following three kinds of situations: (1)
the procedures that would be required are so unlikely to achieve
improved nutritional and fluid levels that they could be correctly
considered futile; (2) the improvement in nutritional and fluid bal-

ance, though achievable, could be of no benefit to the patient; (3) the burdens of receiving the treatment may outweigh the benefit.

WHEN FOOD AND WATER MAY BE WITHHELD

Futile Treatment. Sometimes even providing "food and water" to a patient becomes a monumental task. Consider a patient with a severe clotting deficiency and a nearly total body burn. Gaining access to the central veins is likely to cause hemorrhage or infection, nasogastric tube placement may be quite painful, and there may be no skin to which to suture the stomach for a gastrostomy tube. Or consider a patient with severe congestive heart failure who develops cancer of the stomach with a fistula that delivers food from the stomach to the colon without passing through the intestine and being absorbed. Feeding the patient may be possible, but little is absorbed. Intravenous feeding cannot be tolerated because the fluid would be too much for the weakened heart. Or consider the infant with infarction of all but a short segment of bowel. Again, the infant can be fed, but little if anything is absorbed. Intravenous methods can be used, but only for a short time (weeks or months) until their complications, including thrombosis, hemorrhage, infections, and malnutrition, cause death.

In these circumstances, the patient is going to die soon, no matter what is done. The ineffective efforts to provide nutrition and hydration may directly cause suffering that offers no counterbalancing benefit for the patient. Although the procedures might be tried, especially if the competent patient wanted them or the incompetent patient's surrogate had reason to believe that this incompetent patient would have wanted them, they cannot be considered obligatory. To hold that a patient must be subjected to this predictably futile sort of intervention just because protein balance is negative or the blood serum is concentrated is to lose sight of the moral warrant for medical care and to reduce the patient to an array of measurable variables.

No Possibility of Benefit. Some patients can be reliably diagnosed to have permanently lost consciousness. This unusual group of patients includes those with anencephaly, persistent vegetative state, and some preterminal comas. In these cases, it is very difficult to discern how any medical intervention can benefit or harm the patient. These patients cannot and never will be able to experience any of the events occurring in the world or in their bodies. When the diagnosis is exceedingly clear, we sustain their lives vigorously mainly for their loved ones and the community at large.

While these considerations probably indicate that continued artificial feeding is best in most cases, there may be some cases in which the family and the caregivers are convinced that artificial feeding is offensive and unreasonable. In such cases, there seems to be no adequate reason to claim that withholding food and water violates any obligations that these parties or the general society have with regard to permanently unconscious patients. Thus, if the parents of an anencephalic infant or of a patient like Karen Quinlan in a persistent vegetative state feel strongly that no medical procedures should be applied to provide nutrition and hydration, and the caregivers are willing to comply, there should be no barrier in law or public policy to thwart the plan.[9]

Disproportionate Burden. The most difficult cases are those in which normal nutritional status or fluid balance could be restored, but only with a severe burden for the patient. In these cases, the treatment is futile in a broader sense—the patient will not actually benefit from the improved nutrition and hydration. A patient who is competent can decide the relative merits of the treatment being provided, knowing the probable consequences, and weighing the merits of life under various sets of constrained circumstances. But a surrogate decision maker for a patient who is incompetent to decide will have a difficult task. When the situation is irremediably ambiguous, erring on the side of continued life and improved nutrition and hydration seems the less grievous error. But are there situations that would warrant a determination that this patient, whose nutrition and hydration could surely be improved, is not thereby well served?

Though they are rare, we believe there are such cases. The treatments entailed are not benign. Their effects are far short of ideal. Furthermore, many of the patients most likely to have inadequate food and fluid intake are also likely to suffer the most serious side effects of these therapies.

Patients who are allowed to die without artificial hydration and nutrition may well die more comfortably than patients who receive conventional amounts of intravenous hydration.[10] Terminal pulmonary edema, nausea, and mental confusion are more likely when patients have been treated to maintain fluid and nutrition until close to the time of death.

Thus, those patients whose "need" for artificial nutrition and hydration arises only near the time of death may be harmed by its provision. It is not at all clear that they receive any benefit in having a slightly prolonged life, and it does seem reasonable to allow a surrogate to decide that, for this patient at this time, slight prolongation of life is not warranted if it involves measures that will probably increase the patient's suffering as he or she dies.

Even patients who might live much longer might not be well served by artificial means to provide fluid and food. Such patients might include those with fairly severe dementia for whom the restraints required could be a constant source of fear, discomfort, and struggle. For such a patient, sedation to tolerate the feeding mechanisms might preclude any of the pleasant experiences that might otherwise have been available. Thus, a decision not to intervene, except perhaps briefly to ascertain that there are no treatable causes, might allow such a patient to live out a shorter life with fair freedom of movement and freedom from fear, while a decision to maintain artificial nutrition and hydration might consign the patient to end his or her life in unremitting anguish. If this were the case a surrogate decision-maker would seem to be well justified in refusing the treatment.

INAPPROPRIATE MORAL CONSTRAINTS

Four considerations are frequently proposed as moral constraints on forgoing medical feeding and hydration. We find none of these to dictate that artificial nutrition and hydration must always be provided.

The Obligation to Provide "Ordinary" Care. Debates about appropriate medical treatment are often couched in terms of "ordinary" and "extraordinary" means of treatment. Historically, this distinction emerged in the Roman Catholic tradition to differentiate optional treatment from treatment that was obligatory for medical professionals to offer and for patients to accept.[11] These terms also appear in many secular contexts, such as court decisions and medical codes. The recent debates about ordinary and extraordinary means of treatment have been interminable and often unfruitful, in part because of a lack of clarity about what the terms mean. Do they represent the premises of an argument or the conclusion, and what features of a situation are relevant to the categorization as "ordinary" or "extraordinary"?[12]

Several criteria have been implicit in debates about ordinary and extraordinary means of treatment; some of them may be relevant to determining whether and which treatments are obligatory and which are optional. Treatments have been distinguished according to their simplicity (simple/complex), their naturalness (natural/ artificial), their customariness (usual/unusual), their invasiveness (noninvasive/invasive), their chance of success (reasonable chance/ futile), their balance of benefits and burdens (proportionate/dispro- portionate), and their expense (inexpensive/costly). Each set of paired terms or phrases in the parentheses suggests a continuum: as the treatment moves from the first of the paired terms to the second, it is said to become less obligatory and more optional.

However, when these various criteria, widely used in discussions about medical treatment, are carefully examined, most of them are not morally relevant in distinguishing optional from obligatory medical treatments. For example, if a rare, complex, artificial, and invasive treatment offers a patient a reasonable chance of nearly painless cure, then one would have to offer a substantial justification not to provide that treatment to an incompetent patient.

What matters, then, in determining whether to provide a treat- ment to an incompetent patient is not a prior determination that this treatment is "ordinary" per se, but rather a determination that this treatment is likely to provide this patient benefits that are suf- ficient to make it worthwhile to endure the burdens that accompany the treatment. To this end, some of the considerations listed above are relevant: whether a treatment is likely to succeed is an obvious example. But such considerations taken in isolation are not conclu- sive. Rather, the surrogate decision-maker is obliged to assess the desirability to this patient of each of the options presented, including nontreatment. For most people at most times, this assessment would lead to a clear obligation to provide food and fluids.

But sometimes, as we have indicated, providing food and fluids through medical interventions may fail to benefit and may even harm some patients. Then the treatment cannot be said to be obligatory, no matter how usual and simple its provision may be. If "ordinary" and "extraordinary" are used to convey the conclusion about the obligation to treat, providing nutrition and fluids would have become, in these cases, "extraordinary." Since this phrasing is misleading, it is probably better to use "proportionate" and "disproportionate," as the Vatican now suggests,[13] or "obligatory" and "optional."

Obviously, providing nutrition and hydration may sometimes be necessary to keep patients comfortable while they are dying even though it may temporarily prolong their dying. In such cases, food and fluids constitute warranted palliative care. But in other cases, such as a patient in a deep and irreversible coma, nutrition and hydration do not appear to be needed or helpful, except perhaps to comfort the staff and family.[14] And sometimes the interventions needed for nutrition and hydration are so burdensome that they are harmful and best not utilized.

The Obligation to Continue Treatments Once Started. Once having started a mode of treatment, many caregivers find it very difficult to discontinue it. While this strongly felt difference between the ease of withholding a treatment and the difficulty of withdrawing it provides a psychological explanation of certain actions, it does not justify them. It sometimes even leads to a thoroughly irrational decision process. For example, in caring for a dying, comatose patient, many physicians apparently find it harder to stop a functioning peripheral IV than not to restart one that has infiltrated (that is, has broken through the blood vessel and is leaking fluid into surrounding tissue), especially if the only way to reestablish an IV would be to insert a central line into the heart or to do a cutdown (make an incision to gain access to the deep large blood vessels).[15]

What factors might make withdrawing medical treatment morally worse than withholding it? Withdrawing a treatment seems to be an action, which, when it is likely to end in death, initially seems more serious than an omission that ends in death. However, this view is fraught with errors. Withdrawing is not always an act: failing to put the next infusion into a tube could be correctly described as an omission, for example. Even when withdrawing is an act, it may well be morally correct and even morally obligatory. Discontinuing intravenous lines in a patient now permanently unconscious in accord with that patient's well-informed advance directive would certainly be such a case. Furthermore, the caregiver's obligation to serve the patient's interests through both acts and omissions rules out the exculpation that accompanies omissions in the usual course of social life. An omission that is not warranted by the patient's interests is culpable.

Sometimes initiating a treatment creates expectations in the minds of caregivers, patients, and family that the treatment will be continued indefinitely or until the patient is cured. Such expectations may provide a reason to continue the treatment as a way to keep a promise. However, as with all promises, caregivers could be very careful when initiating a treatment to explain the indications for its discontinuation, and they could modify preconceptions with continuing reevaluation and education during treatment. Though all patients are entitled to expect the continuation of care in the patient's best interests, they are not and should not be entitled to the continuation of a particular mode of care.

Accepting the distinction between withholding and withdrawing medical treatment as morally significant also has a very unfortunate implication: caregivers may become unduly reluctant to begin some treatments precisely because they fear that they will be locked into continuing treatments that are no longer of value to the patient. For example, the physician who had been unwilling to stop the respirator while the infant Andrew Stinson died over several months is reportedly "less eager to attach babies to respirators now."[16] But if it were easier to ignore malnutrition and dehydration and to withhold treatments for these problems than to discontinue the same treatments when they have become especially burdensome and insufficiently beneficial for the patient, then the incentives would be perverse. Once a treatment has been tried, it is often much clearer whether it is of value to the patient, and the decision to stop it can be made more reliably.

The same considerations should apply to starting as to stopping a treatment, and whatever assessment warrants withholding should also warrant withdrawing.

The Obligation to Avoid Being the Unambiguous Cause of Death.
Many physicians will agree with all that we have said and still refuse
to allow a choice to forgo food and fluid because such a course seems
to be a "death sentence." In this view death seems to be more certain
from malnutrition and dehydration than from forgoing other forms
of medical therapy. This implies that it is acceptable to act in ways
that are likely to cause death, as in not operating on a gangrenous
leg, only if there remains a chance that the patient will survive. This
is a comforting formulation for caregivers, to be sure, since they can
thereby avoid feeling the full weight of the responsibility for the
time and manner of a patient's death. However, it is not a persuasive
moral argument.

First, in appropriate cases discontinuing certain medical treatments is generally accepted despite the fact that death is as certain
as with nonfeeding. Dialysis in a patient without kidney function
or transfusions in a patient with severe aplastic anemia are obvious
examples. The dying that awaits such patients often is not greatly
different from dying of dehydration and malnutrition.

Second, the certainty of a generally undesirable outcome such as
death is always relevant to a decision, but it does not foreclose the
possibility that this course is better than others available to this
patient.[17] Ambiguity and uncertainty are so common in medical
decision-making that caregivers are tempted to use them in dis-
tancing themselves from direct responsibility. However, caregivers
are in fact responsible for the time and manner of death for many
patients. Their distaste for this fact should not constrain otherwise
morally justified decisions.

The Obligation to Provide Symbolically Significant Treatment.
One of the most common arguments for always providing nutrition
and hydration is that it symbolizes, expresses, or conveys the essence
of care and compassion. Some actions not only aim at goals, they
also express values. Such expressive actions should not simply be
viewed as means to ends; they should also be viewed in light of what
they communicate. From this perspective food and water are not
only goods that preserve life and provide comfort; they are also symbols of care and compassion. To withhold or withdraw them—to
"starve" a patient—can never express or convey care.

Why is providing food and water a central symbol of care and compassion? Feeding is the first response of the community to the needs of newborns and remains a central mode of nurture and comfort. Eating is associated with social interchange and community, and providing food for someone else is a way to create and maintain bonds of sharing and expressing concern. Furthermore, even the relatively low levels of hunger and thirst that most people have experienced are decidedly uncomfortable, and the common image of severe malnutrition or dehydration is one of unremitting agony. Thus, people are rightly eager to provide food and water. Such provision is essential to minimally tolerable existence and a powerful symbol of our concern for each other.

However, *medical* nutrition and hydration, we have argued, may not always provide net benefits to patients. Medical procedures to provide nutrition and hydration are more similar to other medical procedures than to typical human ways of providing nutrition and hydration, for example, a sip of water. It should be possible to evaluate their benefits and burdens, as we evaluate any other medical procedure. Of course, if family, friends, and caregivers feel that such procedures affirm important values even when they do not benefit the patient, their feelings should not be ignored. We do not contend that there is an obligation to withhold or to withdraw such procedures (unless consideration of the patient's advance directives or current best interest unambiguously dictates that conclusion); we only contend that nutrition and hydration may be forgone in some cases.

The symbolic connection between care and nutrition or hydration adds useful caution to decision making. If decision makers worry over withholding or withdrawing medical nutrition and hydration, they may inquire more seriously into the circumstances that putatively justify their decisions. This is generally salutary for health care decision making. The critical inquiry may well yield the sad but justified conclusion that the patient will be served best by not using medical procedures to provide food and fluids.

A LIMITED CONCLUSION

Our conclusion—that patients or their surrogates, in close collaboration with their physicians and other caregivers and with careful assessment of the relevant information, can correctly decide to forgo the provision of medical treatments intended to correct malnutrition and dehydration in some circumstances—is quite limited. Concentrating on incompetent patients, we have argued that in most cases such patients will be best served by providing nutrition and fluids. Thus, there should be a presumption in favor of providing nutrition and fluids as part of the broader presumption to provide means that prolong life. But this presumption may be rebutted in particular cases.

We do not have enough information to be able to determine with clarity and conviction whether withholding or withdrawing nutrition and hydration was justified in the cases that have occasioned public concern, though it seems likely that the Danville and Bloomington babies should have been fed and that Claire Conroy should not.

It is never sufficient to rule out "starvation" categorically. The question is whether the obligation to act in the patient's best interests was discharged by withholding or withdrawing particular medical treatments. All we have claimed is that nutrition and hydration by medical means need not always be provided. Sometimes they may not be in accord with the patient's wishes or interests. Medical nutrition and hydration do not appear to be distinguishable in any morally relevant way from other life-sustaining medical treatments that may on occasion be withheld or withdrawn.

NOTES

1. John A. Robertson, "Dilemma in Danville," *Hastings Cent. Rep.* 11: 5–8 (October 1981).

2. T. Rohrlich, "2 Doctors Face Murder Charges in Patient's Death," *L.A. Times*, August 19, 1982, A-1; Jonathan Kirsch, "A Death at Kaiser Hospital," *Calif. Mag.* (1982), 79ff; Magistrate's findings, California v. Barber and Nejdl, No. A 925586, Los Angeles Mun. Ct. Cal., (March 9, 1983); Superior Court of California, County of Los Angeles, California v. Barber and Nejdl, No. A0 25586k tentative decision May 5, 1983.

3. *In re* Infant Doe, No. GU 8204–00 (Cir. Ct. Monroe County, Ind., April 12, 1982), *writ of mandamus dismissed sub nom.* State ex rel. Infant Doe v. Baker, No. 482 S140 (Indiana Supreme Ct., May 27, 1982).

4. Office of the Secretary, Department of Health and Human Services, "Nondiscrimination on the Basis of Handicap," *Federal Register* 48 (1983), 9630–32. (Interim final rule modifying 45 C.F.R. #84.61.) See Judge Gerhard Gesell's decision, American Academy of Pediatrics v. Heckler, No. 83–0774, U.S. District Court, D.C., April 24, 1983; and also George J. Annas, "Disconnecting the Baby Doe Hotline," *Hastings Cent. Rep.* 13:14–16 (June 1983).

5. *In re* Conroy, 190 N.J. Super. 453, 464 A.2d 303 (App. Div. 1983).

6. President's Commission for the Study of Ethical Problems in Medicine and Biomedical and Behavioral Research, *Deciding to Forego Life-Sustaining Treatment*, Washington, D.C.: U.S. Government Printing Office (1982).

7. G. E. M. Anscombe, "Ethical Problems in the Management of Some Severely Handicapped Children: Commentary 2," *J. Med. Ethics* 7:117–124 (1981).

8. See, e.g., President's Commission for the Study of Ethical Problems in Medicine and Biomedical and Behavioral Research, *Making Health Care Decisions*, Washington, D.C.: U.S. Government Printing Office (1982).

9. President's Commission, *Deciding to Forego*, at 171–196.

10. Joyce V. Zerwekh, "The Dehydration Question," *Nursing83*, 47–51 (1983) with comments by Judith R. Brown and Marion B. Dolan. See also chapter 3.

11. James J. McCartney, "The Development of the Doctrine of Ordinary and Extraordinary Means of Preserving Life in Catholic Moral Theology before the Karen Quinlan Case," *Linacre Q.* 47:215 (1980).

12. President's Commission, *Deciding to Forego*, at 82–90. For an argument that fluids and electrolytes can be "extraordinary," see Carson Strong, "Can Fluids and Electrolytes be 'Extraordinary' Treatment?" *J. Med. Ethics* 7:83–85 (1981).

13. The Sacred Congregation for the Doctrine of the Faith, Declaration on Euthanasia, Vatican City, May 5, 1980.

14. Paul Ramsey, *The Patient as Person*, New Haven: Yale University Press (1970), 128–129; Paul Ramsey, *Ethics at the Edges of Life: Medical and Legal Intersections*, New Haven: Yale University Press (1978), 275; Bernard Towers, "Irreversible Coma and Withdrawal of Life Support: Is it Murder If the IV Line is Disconnected?" *J. Med. Ethics* 8:205 (1982).

15. See Kenneth C. Micetich, Patricia H. Steinecker, and David C. Thomasma, "Are Intravenous Fluids Morally Required for a Dying Patient?" *Arch. Intern. Med.* 143:975–978 (1983), also chapter 4.

16. Robert and Peggy Stinson, *The Long Dying of Baby Andrew*, Boston: Little, Brown and Co. (1983), 355.

17. See chapter 4.

Daniel Callahan, Ph.D.

6 Public Policy and the Cessation of Nutrition

Any movement toward a widespread acceptance of the cessation of nutrition for the dying ought to be a matter of public interest. For one thing, it would represent an escalation in the intensity of efforts to find effective ways of making certain that the dying do so promptly, something that cannot always be guaranteed by the stopping of medical treatment. For another, it would violate an inchoate though no less real repugnance felt by both medical personnel and lay people against the stopping of nutrition. James Childress and Joanne Lynn have effectively argued that such action is morally supportable in some circumstances,[1] and even the most conservative Roman Catholic moral theology presented similar arguments in an earlier era.[2] Nonetheless, since the morality of a society, which is expressed through its social practices, legitimately encompasses far more than the outcome of moral argumentation, it would be unwise to ignore the long-standing repugnance as nothing more than a vestigial prejudice.

An important function of a moral culture is to instill in its members deep feelings about the morality of various actions; and one of the most important in all cultures, save the most debased, is that the needy and the helpless must be fed. Few moral rules are more fundamental than that, at once of literal importance, because of the utter dependency of some on others for their very life, and of symbolic importance, as a sign of the interdependency of human life in any viable community. If the practice of ceasing to feed some dying patients would remain as rare, and as circumscribed, as called for by the Lynn-Childress standards, the matter need be of little public interest. But the enthusiasm that has greeted the opening up of the subject, the widespread frustration felt by many of those in charge of long-term or chronic care facilities in the face of the biological tenacity of their more vegetative charges, and the pressures to reduce or contain costs, are all reasons to guess that the practice may not remain rare and contained.

If those are all reasons for public interest, are they sufficiently strong to justify the development of a specific public policy toward the matter? But first, what do I mean by "public policy"? The term is widely and commonly used but is difficult to define with any great precision. For my purposes, let me define it as follows: some action or set of actions undertaken by government to bring about a systematic public presence and a set of standards to a matter of general social concern.

Broadly speaking, there are three possible stances that government can take toward matters of social concern. First, the government can consciously decide to stay out of the issues altogether. The 1973 Supreme Court decision in *Roe v. Wade* on abortion held that the government ought to stay out of the decision-making during the first two trimesters of pregnancy. That was a public policy decision, even though it was a decision to remove the government from a role in the decision-making. Second, at the other extreme, is what I think of as "hard policy." That is the positive devising of a law, or set of laws or regulations, or some set of formal oversight instruments or methods, to enable the government closely and directly to regulate. A hard policy encompasses the full panoply of means at the disposal of government for changing, modifying, controlling, or manipulating behavior. Third, policy might also be seen on occasion as a rather "soft" kind. There would be in those cases some oversight on the part of government, some encouragement by government of public discussion, and some watchful attitude on the part of government— but not necessarily the enactment of laws, the issuance regulations, or the establishment of formal oversight mechanisms.

Those are my preliminary definitions. My working premise is that this problem of cessation of nutrition for the dying is in general a legitimate area of public and governmental interest. It cannot be said to be a matter of private morality only, for it would ordinarily entail one or more persons doing or not doing something to another, where most commonly one of the parties will be incompetent. Since we customarily and correctly have public policies when the welfare of the incompetent is at stake, there seems to be no *a priori* reason why it should be omitted in this case. Moreover, some issues have to become matters of public policy if only because there is a certain degree of public agitation about them. The cessation of nutrition is such an issue; in some sense government must respond. So for at least two reasons there is a strong possibility that this is a legitimate area of public policy.

I think it only sensible also to ask why the issue has emerged for public discussion in the first place. Why do we care about it? Why has it emerged just within the last couple of years rather than earlier? On the surface, the most obvious reason would be a few recent cases that have attracted media and legal attention: the "Baby Doe" case in Indiana,[3] the Barber-Nejdl case,[4] the Claire Conroy case,[5] and others.

But the more important reason is probably that we know in our bones that we are going to be faced in the future with a growing number of cases of the biologically tenacious, those whom we think ought to be allowed to die but who simply will not die unless we apply the extra and exceedingly effective mode called forgoing life-sustaining food and water. The most important present case in that respect is that of Claire Conroy; its implications extend to a large number of people. What are we going to do about cases like that, particularly when we know demographically that the number of elderly people is increasing, the number of the chronically ill is increasing, and we have every empirical reason to believe that there is going to be a substantially larger number of people in the future who are going to be in a vegetative, semivegetative, or otherwise terribly debilitated state but simply will not die? Many, many lives will be at stake.

A few other factors make this a matter of legitimate public policy. We need to consider what has sometimes been called "the klutz factor." What happens to movements or practices when they are taken out of the hands of the first pioneers, who act carefully and thoughtfully after due deliberation, and are put in the hands of very large numbers of people who may not approach them with the same care? What happens when you turn something that was a minority movement into a mass movement? In this case, what if caregivers withhold food and water thoughtlessly, carelessly, and incorrectly, thereby causing much suffering and debasing a loyalty and duty to a large number of seriously ill people? That could well happen, as easily as other forms of abuse periodically reported in nursing and chronic care centers.

There is also reason to worry about what I would call "the scandal factor," that is, the way things look. I was recently asked to take part in a retrospective discussion on the appropriateness or inappropriateness of cessation of nutrition for a patient who, before becoming incompetent, had requested that nutrition be stopped. The patient happened to be black. Furthermore, this would have been that hospital's first case of stopping a patient's nutrition. I imagined a newspaper headline saying, "Black Man Starved to Death in Hospital." One has to worry about that kind of event in our society. What would it look like? What kind of impression would it make? There might be an effective defense against charges of discrimination, but the hospital's actions would be terribly difficult to explain.

Finally, in our society we have a solid history of seeing things that were initially introduced as possibilities for choice or discretion turned into matters of mandatory behavior. The reasonable argument now is that, on certain occasions, we ought to be allowed to stop nutrition with some patients. But it seems to me that under economic and other social pressure, that kind of choice might become mandatory and coerced. The way we usually change free choice into a coerced choice in our society is not by direct command. Instead, we just tell people what would count as the morally "responsible" choice, applying general social pressure in its behalf. Given the number of people who are a social burden, it is easy to imagine such pressure.

Those are some of my reasons for thinking that this is a legitimate area for public policy.

Should there, however, be "hard policy," as I defined it? Should we have specified laws, regulations, oversight procedures, and whatnot? In one sense, we are already beginning to get hard policy in that the courts are making decisions and court decisions are certainly one aspect of public policy. But a really systematic public policy would include such things as state statutes and regulations pertaining to the cessation of nutrition, and regulations applying to veterans' hospitals or federally supported programs. One could well imagine the Department of Health and Human Services trying to do such things as it did in the case of "Baby Jane Doe,"[6] that is to say, making administrative rulings that would very much have the power to modify and change behavior.

I do not think we have reached the point where "hard policy" is called for. I do not see, nor have I heard anything to suggest, that there are a large number of well-documented abuses, or that there is even a great deal of confusion in medicine, confusion of the kind for which one would want policy simply to help clarify the situation.

If there is to be hard policy, then there ought to be a strong case for it. Hard policy ought not to be enacted in matters of medical morality unless the situation is very bad and very desperate. The government should intervene with hard policy only as a last resort. It is quite possible, of course, that we will get hard policy whether it is needed or not, by virtue of capricious political action. Some case or isolated abuse will be taken up by some legislator or member of some executive branch and used as a catalyst for trying to establish hard policy, just as the "Baby Jane Doe" case was a catalyst for action on the part of the Reagan administration.

Ought there then, perhaps, be "soft" public policy? For example, there might be some informal oversight on the part of government, the encouragement of public discussion, and some prodding of the medical and hospital establishments to collect data, to publicize problems, and perhaps to devise informal guidelines—for instance, to stimulate the use of ethics committees to write policies for particular institutions. Such steps would fall short of actually establishing anything as hard and firm as statutory law. Government might, in short, focus continuing public and professional attention on the issues, but stop short of going any further. The way in which this subject was taken up by the President's Commission for the Study of Ethical Problems in Medicine and Biomedical and Behavorial Research represents an instance of what I have in mind as a soft policy response.

Even in the case of a soft policy response, however, one might well ask what the bias of government ought to be. One might argue that the bias of government ought to be toward a prudent and balanced approach: to encourage and support practices that neither force nutrition where it is morally sensible to stop it nor stop it when it is morally required to continue it.

I am, however, more concerned about the possibility—because of great mounting social and economic pressures—of precipitately and prematurely terminating nutrition than I am of the likelihood that it will be provided for too long and in too burdensome a way. Perhaps our main problem already is that too many people are being unnecessarily fed or given water and that this causes real problems. That is an empirical question, and I really don't know the answer. Nonetheless, if it were the case, then the arguments of James Childress and Joanne Lynn seem to be quite correct and to the point, and I will accept them. But I would prefer to see the burden of proof rest heavily with those who would discontinue rather than with those who would continue nutrition. We need to keep alive and active our moral and, to some extent, our esthetic, repugnance against deliberate starvation and hope that a bias against survival will not arise. If we want to avert the possibility that we will discontinue nutrition too precipitately, that we will too eagerly rush to forgo life-sustaining nutrition, then we need to take steps now to rest the burden of proof very, very heavily on those who would choose to so terminate nutrition.

There is every reason to think, given economic and social pressures, and particularly given an increasingly long average life span, that we are going to be faced with more and more such decisions. To curtail moral damage in the future, I think we must begin now to draw the lines very carefully.

Thus the force of a soft policy should be to continually alert us to the possibility of abuse—allowing the cessation of feeding in those circumstances where it is morally called for, but trying to guarantee that such cases remain few.

NOTES

1. Joanne Lynn and James F. Childress, "Must Patients Always Be Given Food and Water?" *Hastings Cent. Rep.* 13:17–21 (October 1983), reprinted as chapter 5 *supra*.
2. Gerald Kelly, S.J., "The Duty to Preserve Life," *Theological Stud.* 12:550–556 (December 1951).
3. See chapter 17.
4. Barber v. Superior Court, 147 Cal. App. 3d 1006, 195 Cal. Reptr. 484 (1983).
5. *In re* Conroy, 98 N.J. 321, 486 A.2d 1209 (1985).
6. Weber v. Stony Brook Hospital, 60 N.Y.2d 208, 469 N.Y.S.2d 63, 456 N.E.2d 1186, *cert. denied*, 104 S. Ct. 560 (1983).

James F. Childress, Ph.D.

7 When Is It Morally Justifiable to Discontinue Medical Nutrition and Hydration?

When, if ever, is it morally justifiable to withhold or to withdraw medical nutrition and hydration from patients? I want to raise this question in the context of two cases.

In the first case, Mrs. X, a seventy-nine-year-old widow, had been a resident of a nursing home for several years. In the past she had experienced repeated transient ischemic attacks. Because of progressive organic brain syndrome, she had lost most of her mental abilities and had become disoriented. She also had episodes of thrombophlebitis as well as congestive heart failure. Her daughter and grandchildren visited her frequently and obviously loved her deeply. One day she was found unconscious on the bathroom floor of the nursing home. She was hospitalized, and the diagnosis was a "massive stroke." She made no recovery, remaining obtunded and nonverbal, but she continued to manifest a withdrawal reaction to painful stimuli and some spontaneous purposeful behaviors. Mrs. X refused to allow a nasogastric tube to be placed in her stomach; at each attempt she thrashed about violently and pushed the tube away. After the tube was finally placed, Mrs. X pulled out of restraints and managed to remove it. After several days, her IV sites were exhausted. The question for the staff was whether to do further "extraordinary" or "heroic" measures to maintain fluid and nutritional intake for this elderly patient who had made no recovery from a massive stroke and who was largely unaware and unresponsive. After much mental anguish and discussion with the nurses on the floor and with the patient's family, the physicians in charge decided not to provide further IVs, cutdowns, or a feeding tube, and to allow Mrs. X to die. She took minimal oral intake and died quietly the following week.[1]

In the second case, Dr. David Hilfiker reports being called at 3:00 a.m. by the nurse at the nursing home where Mrs T, an eighty-three-year-old woman, has been confined since her stroke three years earlier.[2] Mrs. T is now bedridden and aphasic, weighs only 69 pounds, and has decubitus ulcers on her back and hip, but Dr. Hilfiker recalls her condition before her stroke—"her dislike and distrust of doctors and hospitals, her staunch pride and independence despite her severe scoliosis, her wry grin every time I suggested hospitalization for some problem." While talking to the nurse over the telephone and deciding what he should do, he also recalls admitting her to the hospital after her stroke, "one side completely paralyzed, globally aphasic, incontinent, and reduced to helplessness." And he recalls "aggressively" treating the pneumonia that developed, providing intravenous antibiotics despite her apparent desire to die. He rationalized that she was depressed and would get over it. Now the nurse reports that she has a fever (103.5°F), hasn't been eating much the last few days, and has a little cough. Dr. Hilfiker decides that he should not wait until the morning, and he goes to the nursing home to examine Mrs. T, who peers at him from behind her blank face. His tentative diagnosis is pneumonia, and he asks the nurse to call the technician out of bed for a chest X-ray and also orders a urine culture. As Dr. Hilfiker and the nurse discuss the case, they note that Mrs. T's only friend in the nursing home, who probably knows better than anyone else what Mrs. T would want, has said that she "hoped there wouldn't be any heroics if Mrs. T . . . got sick again." But the only relative (a distant niece who lives far away) had called to request that "everything possible" be done for her aunt. Dr. Hilfiker reflects:

> There in the middle of the night I consider "doing everything possible" for Mrs. T: transfer to the hospital, intravenous lines for hydration and antibiotics, thorough laboratory and x-ray evaluation, twice-daily rounds to be sure that she is recovering, more toxic antibiotics, and even transfer to our regional hospital for evaluation and care by a specialist. None of it is unreasonable, and another night I might choose just such a course. But tonight my human sympathies lie with Mrs. T and what I perceive as her desire to die. . . . In any event I decide against the heroics. But I can't just do nothing, either. My training and background are too strong. I do not allow myself to be consistent and just go home. Compromising (and ultimately making a decision that makes no medical or ethical sense at all), I write orders instructing the staff to administer liquid penicillin, to encourage fluid intake, and to make an appointment with my office so that I can reexamine Mrs. T in 36 hours.[3]

A FRAMEWORK OF ANALYSIS

In the first case, the staff decided to let Mrs. X die even though they could have prolonged her life for some time through medical nutrition and hydration. In the second case, Dr. Hilfiker decided to encourage fluid intake and to administer liquid penicillin but not to provide an intravenous line for hydration and antibiotics. He felt that his "compromise" made no "medical or ethical sense at all." Nevertheless, it represents one way to draw lines in withholding and withdrawing treatment. As both cases suggest, one major issue in drawing lines is whether all medical treatments, depending on the circumstances, can be construed as "heroic" or "extraordinary" rather than "ordinary." In particular, are medical nutrition and hydration by peripheral or central intravenous lines, nasogastric tubes, or gastrostomies morally similar to other medical and surgical procedures that are sometimes construed as "heroic" or "extraordinary?" Is it appropriate to view nutrition and hydration as "medical treatments" when they involve medical procedures or require surgery?

In accord with many commentators in the last several years, I believe that the language of ordinary and extraordinary or heroic means of treatment should be replaced because it is misleading.[4] It is misleading because it obscures the principles that should govern decisions about withholding or withdrawing medical treatments. If we replace "ordinary" with "obligatory," and "extraordinary" or "heroic" with "optional," we can then examine the principles by which to determine when a particular medical treatment is obligatory and when it is optional. Apart from constraints set by scarcity and principles of justice in the allocation of resources (to which I will return later), the fundamental moral principles for decisions about withholding or withdrawing medical treatments that prolong life are (1) beneficence, often stated in terms of patient benefit or the patient's best interests, and (2) respect for persons, often stated in terms of autonomy.[5] Because of these principles, health care professionals should always seek the best interests of their patients, subject to the constraints and limits set by the competent (or previously competent) patient's wishes, choices, and actions. In general, a competent patient should be free to refuse any medical treatment as long as that refusal does not violate the rights of others. Only limited or constrained paternalism—beneficence constrained and limited by respect for persons and their autonomy—is morally defensible.[6] More difficult and problematic are the sorts of cases presented at the outset, where the patient is incompetent (or not clearly competent) or where his or her wishes and preferences are unclear. In decisions about an incompetent patient who has not previously expressed his or her wishes, the relevant moral consideration, based on beneficence, is the patient's benefit or best interests.

This moral consideration establishes a presumption in favor of all medical treatments that prolong life. Such treatments may be presumed to be in the patient's interests (and even in accord with his or her wishes if they could be known). But this presumption is rebuttable. It can be rebutted, as I have noted, when a competent patient refuses treatment or a previously competent patient has refused treatment. But it can also be rebutted when the appropriate decision-makers for an incompetent patient determine (a) that the treatments are futile or useless, (b) that they provide no benefits to the patient, or (c) that their benefits are outweighed by their burdens to the patient. Thus, the same moral principles that establish a presumption in favor of treatment also indicate when the presumption may be rebutted. We may believe that this presumption should not be rebutted too quickly, easily, or lightly; we may even believe that decision-makers should experience anguish, as in our first two cases. But whatever burden of proof and whatever anguish is appropriate in such decisions, any medical treatment may be withheld or withdrawn as morally optional in some circumstances.

One response to this search for principles for decisions about life-sustaining medical treatment is to look at medical practice. This response is quite appropriate because we can expect to find the principles of beneficence and respect for persons at work in medical practice; to a greater or lesser extent, these principles are already embodied in medical practice. They are part of the ethos which ethics as critical reflection examines. But this response tends to fall into the same trap that has ensnared the language of ordinary and extraordinary or heroic means of treatment. That language is misleading because it directs attention toward customary medical practice and away from underlying principles. Thus, treatments are frequently viewed as "ordinary" if it is "usual" or "customary" for physicians to use them for certain diseases, such as pneumonia, or certain problems, such as malnutrition. Treatments are considered "extraordinary" or even "heroic" if it is "unusual" or "uncustomary" for physicians to use them for certain diseases or problems. The terms even become attached to technologies themselves. The patient tends to disappear from view, even though it is the patient's disease or problem that the physician treats with the technology in question. The criteria for distinguishing ordinary from extraordinary means of treatment tend to be located in the customary practice of medicine, which usually but not always reflects the patient's interests and preferences—the principles of beneficence and respect for persons.

Criteria other than usual and unusual, or customary and uncustomary, medical practice have also been proposed for determining which treatments are ordinary (obligatory) and extraordinary or heroic (optional). For example, some practitioners and commentators have considered whether the treatment is simple or complex, natural or artificial, noninvasive or invasive, inexpensive or costly. If a treatment is simple, natural, noninvasive, or inexpensive, it is more likely to be viewed as "ordinary" or "obligatory" than if it is complex, artificial, invasive, or costly. But if such criteria are relevant—and some may be relevant—it is only because they express other moral principles, particularly beneficence and respect for persons. For example, if a complex treatment is available and in accord with the patient's wishes and interests, it is difficult to see why morally it should be handled differently than a simple treatment also in accord with the patient's wishes and interests. To take another example, several oddities emerge when the criteria of natural and artificial are invoked. According to one study conducted after the Natural Death Act was implemented in California, physicians in that state generally viewed respirators, dialysis, and resuscitators as artificial, but split evenly on intravenous feeding, while two-thirds viewed insulin, antibiotics, and chemotherapy as natural.[7] In general, they viewed mechanical systems as more artificial than drugs and other treatments. Nevertheless, physicians' construals of some treatments as artificial and others as natural are not morally relevant to judgments about whether and when those treatments may be withheld or withdrawn, because they do not connect in any significant way with the moral considerations that should govern such decisions. Other criteria, such as the degree of invasiveness (noninvasive-invasive) and cost (inexpensive-costly), may be morally relevant in view of the patient's overall condition, interests, and preferences. But their relevance stems from their established connection with beneficence and respect for persons.

MAJOR ARGUMENTS AGAINST FORGOING MEDICAL NUTRITION AND HYDRATION

If this analysis is correct, then no medical treatment as such is always morally obligatory; whether it is morally obligatory depends on the patient's condition, interests, and wishes. Two main arguments have been presented to exempt medical nutrition and hydration from this general claim. In different ways, these arguments try to establish that medical nutrition and hydration are not relevantly similar to other medical treatments and that the formal principle of universalizability (treat similar cases in a similar way) does not require or even permit us to make the same judgments about medical nutrition and hydration that we make about other medical procedures.

The first argument holds that medical nutrition and hydration are always required because they are always necessary for comfort (patient benefit) and dignity (patient respect as well as benefit). Such an argument probably appears in the claim of the nurse whose actions led to the homicide indictment against Nejdl and Barber, the California physicians who discontinued intravenous nutrition to a patient who had severe brain damage after the loss of oxygen following a routine surgery: "Food is an ordinary means. And everyone has a right to ordinary treatment."[8] This argument clearly undergirds the rule proposed by the Department of Health and Human Services (July 5, 1983) for treatment of handicapped newborns: "the basic provision of nourishment, fluids, and routine nursing care is a fundamental matter of human dignity, not an option for medical judgment."[9] That rule includes medical as well as nonmedical means of providing nutrition and hydration. Whether this first argument appeals to beneficence or to respect for persons, to comfort or to dignity, it is difficult to defend an absolute requirement to provide nutrition and hydration by any possible means. For example, a central IV involves some risks.[10] There is also some evidence that patients who are allowed to die without artificial hydration may even die more comfortably than patients who receive intravenous hydration.[11] Whenever medical nutrition and hydration are required for the incompetent patient's comfort and dignity, they should be provided; the competent patient may, of course, decline them. But we should not suppose that the comfort and the dignity afforded by the relief of parched lips always necessitate the provision of medically adequate nutrition and hydration, which may not offer comfort and dignity in some circumstances.

A second argument that medical nutrition and hydration are always obligatory focuses on their symbolic significance: what they symbolize about caregivers and patients and their relationship. This argument from symbolic values stresses the similarities between *nonmedical* and *medical* acts of providing food and water, rather than the similarities between medical nutrition and hydration and other medical treatments. According to this line of argument, the medical provision of nutrition and hydration symbolizes, expresses, and conveys care and compassion. By contrast, "starvation" can never express care and compassion. The provision of food and water is a central symbol of care in both secular and religious contexts. We respond with care to the newborn by providing food and water, and we continue to extend care in this way. Daniel Callahan has noted that feeding the hungry is the most fundamental of all human relationships and "the perfect symbol of the fact that human life is inescapably social and communal."[12] Our interdependence combines with our actual experiences of thirst and hunger to make this symbol even more powerful: thirst and hunger are uncomfortable and we view severe malnutrition and dehydration as extreme agony. It is also important to note the religious rituals that involve sharing food and drink and the religious admonitions to feed the hungry and to give drink to the thirsty.

This argument from the symbolic value of medical nutrition and hydration hinges on assumptions about human interests and preferences for life and for the food and water essential to sustain life, about the net benefit of nutrition and hydration and particular means of providing them, and about the discomfort of thirst and hunger and of dehydration and malnutrition. Those assumptions are solid enough to establish a presumption in favor of the provision of medical nutrition and hydration, but, as I have argued, they do not hold in all cases. Indeed, sometimes medical nutrition and hydration may not be required by the patient's interests and preferences and may even violate those interests and preferences. In such cases, caregivers may be nourishing a symbol that has little or nothing to do with the interests and preferences of actual patients. Still there might be arguments for nourishing such a symbol.

One such argument appears in Daniel Callahan's brief statement, "On Feeding the Dying."[13] He admits ("cannot deny") "the moral licitness of the discontinuation of feeding under some circumstances (for example, those specified by Lynn and Childress . . .)".[14] But if withholding or withdrawing medical nutrition or hydration is not always morally wrong, it is always repulsive and repugnant. And we should continue to have revulsion, repugnance, and repulsion "at the stopping of feeding even under legitimate circumstances" and "even in those cases where it (stopping the feeding) might be for the patient's own good." Callahan does not use the moral language of guilt, which might be occasioned by the violation of moral duties or rights in a particular case. His major themes are the symbol of feeding and its attendant emotions or sentiments, particularly the ones evoked by not feeding. His main thesis is that it is a "dangerous business to tamper with, or adulterate, so enduring and central a moral emotion" as "repugnance against starving people to death."

It might be argued that the similarities among all acts of providing nutrition and hydration are so great as to make it impossible to differentiate their *recipients* (e.g., dying patients) or their *methods* (e.g., a gastrostomy). But Callahan cannot take this line of argument, because he admits that it is morally licit to discontinue medical nutrition under some circumstances. His argument can perhaps best be described as *symbol or sentiment utilitarianism*, by analogy with what is usually called rule utilitarianism. According to rule utilitarianism, certain *acts* should not be performed even when they appear to maximize welfare in particular circumstances, because over time and a wide range of circumstances the *rule* that prohibits those acts will maximize welfare. A rule utilitarian, for example, might defend a rule requiring that we provide nutrition and hydration by any means any time they will prolong life. If this rule would maximize welfare over time, it should be followed even if its violation might appear to maximize welfare in particular circumstances. (It may be difficult to imagine a utilitarian defense of this rule without any qualifications about the patient's interests and preferences, but the rule against "mercy killing" has been defended on utilitarian grounds.)[15] Callahan does not "rule out" acts of withholding or withdrawing medical nutrition in order to produce good consequences or to avoid bad consequences. But in order to avert "social disaster," it is essential that professionals and others respect the symbol of feeding even in their decisions not to provide medical nutrition and hydration. How can this symbol be respected? Callahan's answer is peculiarly Protestant for a philosopher in the Catholic tradition: respect for the symbol appears in the experience of revulsion even when not feeding is morally licit. Respect thus is a matter of emotions and sentiments of repugnance and repulsion. It is possible to avoid "social disaster" if there is widespread and "deep-seated revulsion at the stopping of feeding even under legitimate circumstances."

There are several weak links in Callahan's argument, including his image of "starvation," which, as I have suggested, may not be appropriate for the cases that concern us. But I want to concentrate on his sentiment or symbol utilitarianism, particularly his claim that we can avoid "social disaster" only by not educating people out of their emotion of revulsion, even in legitimate cases. Although we can morally differentiate acts, Callahan claims we cannot avoid "social disaster" if we try to differentiate the emotions regarding those acts, because of the centrality of the symbol of feeding.

Callahan fears a twofold disaster. First, subversion of the commitment to feed the hungry—for example, the poor who are hungry. Callahan may be right that repugnance against letting people starve to death is a "necessary social instinct." But he provides no evidence for supposing that the social commitment to feed the poor will decline or disappear if the society tolerates withholding or withdrawing medical nutrition without revulsion. Nor does he offer any evidence that caregivers will become callous to the hunger and malnutrition of the poor if they do not experience revulsion in stopping intravenous nutrition when it is morally licit to do so. The widespread phenomenon of compartmentalization of the moral life, which is frequently inappropriate and often has bad consequences, suggests that it is easier than Callahan supposes to direct our sentiments and emotions selectively. He underestimates what Joel Feinberg calls "human emotional flexibility"[16]—our capacity for selective expression of sentiments and emotions, for example, when it is obligatory to feed the poor who are hungry and also permissible to discontinue IV lines for some dying patients. Callahan also assumes that there is great interdependence among our emotions and sentiments; although he uses the language of a "cluster of sentiments and emotions," his argument presupposes another image, perhaps a web or a fabric. Finally, as Jonathan Glover notes about what he calls "utilitarian moral conservatism," Callahan assumes that "the reasons we have for the policies we choose are relatively unimportant to the reverberations of those policies in other parts of our system of attitudes."[17] These assumptions are very questionable.

If there is a moral presumption in favor of life-sustaining medical treatment, including nutrition and hydration, as in accord with the patient's interests and preferences, and if this moral presumption must be rebutted before treatment may be withheld or withdrawn, there is no need for the strong sentiments of revulsion, repugnance, and repulsion that Callahan affirms. Moral caution, hesitancy, and anxiety should be sufficient. In the early 1950s, the distinguished Catholic moral theologian Gerald Kelly, S.J., clarified the concepts and criteria of ordinary and extraordinary means of treatment, including intravenous nutrition, by a case: "A patient almost ninety years of age, suffering from cardiorenal disease, had been in a coma for two weeks, during which time he received an intravenous solution of glucose and some digitalis preparation. The coma was apparently terminal. A member of the family asked that the medication and intravenous feeding be discontinued. With the approval of a priest, the doctor and Sisters acceded to the request, but they did so with some disquietude and they continued to be disturbed for some time after the patient's death."[18] Their disquietude and disturbance were sufficient, despite Callahan's insistence on repugnance, revulsion, and repulsion.

Callahan's second major fear is the "social disaster" of moving from a right to a duty. He worries that in our society acceptance of a right to discontinue medical nutrition and hydration will eventually, if not immediately, become a duty to discontinue them. He worries about the slippery slope, the slide from "may" to "must" or from permissible to required, especially under the pressures of economic rationality, which is instrumental rationality rather than expressive rationality and which thus tends to ignore the sorts of symbols and sentiments that Callahan rightly emphasizes. According to the logic of hard economic rationality, if feeding does not benefit an irreversibly comatose patient, stopping it is not only permissible but obligatory. "The only impediment to the enactment of that kind of policy," Callahan claims, "is a cluster of sentiments and emotions that is repelled by the idea of starving someone to death, even in those cases where it might be for the patient's own good." In our article, to which Callahan responds, Joanne Lynn and I mainly focused on the moral rightness, justifiability, or permissibility of discontinuing medical nutrition and hydration in some cases, indicating that agents have a right to discontinue these and other medical treatments under some circumstances.[19] Before turning to the question of economic rationality—and broader questions of justice in the allocation of resources—I want to explore circumstances under which withholding or withdrawing medical nutrition and hydration might be obligatory.

Neither the traditional distinction between ordinary and extraordinary means of treatment nor my distinction between obligatory and optional treatments is sufficient, because they do not envision circumstances in which it may be wrong to treat and obligatory not to treat. The following indicates the range of judgments:

Categories of Moral Judgment about Treatment

    I.   Obligatory
    II. Optional
         A. Indifferent
         B. Heroic and praiseworthy
    III. Obligatory not to provide

Most ethical reflection has focused on I and II particularly in relation to incompetent patients; III has been developed mainly in relation to competent or previously competent patients. Even within the category of optional treatments, little attention has been paid to the different possibilities. A treatment might be optional in the sense that it is morally indifferent whether the agent provides it. However, it might be optional in the sense that providing it would be praiseworthy as a heroic act, although not providing it would not be morally blameworthy. Often the language of "extraordinary" and "heroic" suggests extra time, effort, and energy when there is limited chance of success.

Is it ever obligatory not to provide some treatments? If the principles of beneficence and respect for persons set the presumption in favor of treatment to prolong life and also the conditions for rebutting that presumption, the same principles may also dictate the conclusion that it is wrong to provide treatment in some cases and even obligatory not to do so. Perhaps the clearest example is the forcible

or deceptive use of life-sustaining treatment against the unambiva-
lent refusal of a competent patient, or previously competent patient,
when that decision does not violate anyone else's rights. Even if
such treatment is based on benevolence, it is a form of disrespect
and an insult to the patient as a person. Hence, it is appropriate to
say that it is morally obligatory not to provide life-sustaining treatment in such cases. Even if there is no record of a previously competent patient's preferences or even if the patient has never been
competent, life-sustaining treatment may sometimes violate that
patient's interests. The treatment may be against those interests as
well as not being required by them, for example, when the pain is
so severe and the restraints are so great as to outweigh the limited
anticipated benefits. It will often, perhaps even usually, be difficult
to determine the balance of benefits and burdens to the incompetent
patient, particularly where the patient has never had a life as a competent person expressing values, but, in principle, the burdens could
conceivably so outweigh the benefits to the patient as to make the
treatment not only optional but also wrong and thus obligatory not
to provide.

At this point we glimpse another potential danger of the argument
for providing medical nutrition and hydration because of their symbolic value. Such an argument may imply that it is permissible or
even obligatory to provide medical nutrition and hydration against
a patient's wishes and interests in order to maintain the symbol and
its associated emotions and sentiments. Parallel to rule utilitarianism, sentiment or symbol utilitarianism may justify overriding
the interests and preferences of individuals in particular circumstances because of the overall value of undifferentiated sentiments
and the symbol of feeding. It could justify forcing people, such as
Elizabeth Bouvia and Ross Henninger, to receive nutrition even
when they do not accept it or when its burdens outweigh its benefits
to them.[20] It may nourish the symbol at the expense of actual patients.

In general, then, it is appropriate to hold that it is morally wrong
to provide—and also morally obligatory not to provide—medical nutrition and hydration when it violates the principles of beneficence
and respect for persons. But to hold that there may be an obligation
or duty (these terms are here used interchangeably) not to treat in
some circumstances is not to repudiate obligations or duties to patients. It is important to distinguish an obligation to a person from

a particular obligation to do X, Y, or Z for that person. The physician may have an obligation to a patient to care for him or her, but the content of that obligation of care should be shaped by the patient's needs and preferences. Within the context of the obligation of care, medical treatments to sustain life are sometimes obligatory, sometimes optional (in both senses), and sometimes wrong. But even if it is appropriate to say that caregivers act wrongly when they provide life-sustaining treatment in some circumstances, it may not be morally appropriate for society to enforce that judgment.

Callahan is worried not only about the societal enforcement of a moral obligation not to provide treatment, but also about the grounds of that putative obligation, particularly the appeal to external factors, such as economic rationality, rather than to beneficence and respect for the patient. But it is appropriate to say with the utmost caution that in some circumstances, where a treatment is optional for the patient and also violates the interests of others, there may be a moral obligation or duty to stop (e.g., in order to avoid wasting resources that could benefit others). This is a matter of justice, which cannot be reduced to mere economic rationality. Earlier, it was important to protect the preferences and interests of patients against overtreatment; now it is important to protect them against the threats of external factors, including cost containment. Thus it is necessary to be as clear as possible about the nature and the centrality of the care of the patients, as defined by their interests and preferences. Then it may be possible to assess the justice of various policies of allocation of resources in health care. I agree with Callahan that we need strong barriers to prevent the triumph of a narrow and hard economic rationality, but the barriers themselves will not hold if we erect them hastily and in the wrong places.

DISTANCING DEVICES AND SELF-DECEPTION

Erecting barriers, drawing lines, or setting limits is a major issue in debates about withholding and withdrawing medical treatments. Obviously there would be few debates if physicians and other health care professionals, as well as family members, drew lines and set limits in the same places in their decisions about the use of various treatments, including medical nutrition and hydration. For example, some people feel comfortable withholding treatment they have not yet started, but do not feel comfortable withdrawing treatment they have already started.[21] Thus, they would not feel obligated to restart an IV if it became infiltrated and surgery was required to provide access, but they would feel obligated to continue an IV once it was started.

On one occasion an attending physician asked me, as an ethicist, to discuss a controversial case with the staff because of their disputes and discomfort about line-drawing. This case involved an elderly man who had numerous problems and could not be expected to survive long even with the most vigorous medical efforts. It was easy for all of the staff to accept an order not to resuscitate the patient in the event of cardiac arrest. Some of the staff also felt that the IV line providing fluids and antibiotics should be discontinued because it offered no reasonable chance of success, but others felt that the IV should be continued for the reasons given above. Yet many (but not all) in the latter group felt comfortable in not restarting the IV when it infiltrated. My task as an ethics consultant was not to provide the right answer, or to tell the caregivers what they ought to do, but to analyze and interpret categories and distinctions that have evolved in religious and humanistic traditions of ethical reflection to illuminate such controversies. The distinction between withholding (not starting) and withdrawing (stopping) is difficult to defend and may even be pernicious if it leads to decisions not to begin treatments that may be useful to reduce the risk of being locked into a treatment that cannot be terminated. And yet the psychological and symbolic significance of the distinction cannot be denied. Similarly, agents may find it easier to withhold or withdraw some treatments than others, usually for psychological and symbolic reasons, as was evident in my discussion of natural and artificial treatments.

Where people draw lines and set limits often depends, at least in part, on their sense of temporal, spatial, and moral distance. Sometimes they can easily dissociate themselves from their acts or from the consequences of their acts because of their sense of distance. Such dissociation appears when people discount remote future consequences. For example, a few professionals and commentators favor withdrawing the IV rather than the respirator because of the *immediacy* of death from the withdrawal of the respirator. They note that, in contrast to "letting patients die" of later dehydration, discontinuing the respirator "creates an immediate consequence of death for which we must take responsibility."[22] It is not clear, however, why the authors suppose that they can avoid moral responsibility for discontinuing the IV just because dehydration develops slowly as a delayed consequence of their actions.

Several of our categories create moral distance, often by invoking temporal or spatial distance. Clear examples include the rule of double effect, which contrasts direct and indirect courses of action, and the distinction between killing and letting die. Such distinctions may sometimes be important and defensible, but their function as psychological defense mechanisms should not be ignored. Thus, we should make sure that they are really rationally defensible, rather than matters of self-deception.

A clear but not uncommon instance of self-deception is to continue the IV but at a rate that will result in dehydration over time.[23] This action maintains the gesture and symbol of feeding, but at a rate that will not sustain the patient's life. It could conceivably serve as a compromise for those who want to respect the symbol and yet also act in accord with the patient's needs and wishes. But it necessarily involves self-deception, because an agent can carry it out only by failing to acknowledge that the patient will become malnourished and dehydrated while the IV line maintains the fiction and expresses the symbol of feeding. Otherwise the agent would have to take responsibility for the outcome. But moral responsibility requires that we face our actions and their consequences, looking clearly and critically at the lines we draw and the limits we set, particularly in decisions to withhold or to withdraw life-sustaining medical treatment, including medical nutrition and hydration.[24]

NOTES

1. This case has been adapted with permission from one presented by Dr. Martin P. Albert, Charlottesville, Virginia.

2. David Hilfiker, "Allowing the Debilitated to Die: Facing our Ethical Choices," *N. Engl. J. Med.* 308:716–719 (1983).

3. *Id.* at 717.

4. See Paul Ramsey, *Ethics at the Edges of Life*, New Haven: Yale University Press (1978), 153, and Robert M. Veatch, *Death, Dying and the Biological Revolution*, New Haven: Yale University Press (1976), chap. 3.

5. For a discussion of these principles, see James F. Childress, *Who Should Decide? Paternalism in Health Care*, New York: Oxford University

Press (1982). See also the chapters on "Autonomy" and "Beneficence" in Tom L. Beauchamp and James F. Childress, *Principles of Biomedical Ethics*, 2nd ed., New York: Oxford University Press (1983).

6. For a defense of this position, see Childress, *Who Should Decide?*

7. Diane L. Redleaf, Suzanne B. Schmitt, and William C. Thompson, "The California Natural Death Act: An Empirical Study of Physicians' Practices," Stanford L. Rev. 31:913–45 (May 1979).

8. Sandra Bardinella, quoted by John Paris, S.J., "Kaiser, Conroy, and the Withdrawal of IV Feeding: Killing or Letting Die," unpublished paper, p. 1.

9. Department of Health and Human Services, "Proposed Rules 45 CFR Part 84, Nondiscrimination on the Basis of Handicap Relating to Health Care for Handicapped Infants," *Federal Register*, 48:30846–30852 (July 5, 1983).

10. See, for example, the ruling by an intermediate appeals court in Massachusetts, *In the Matter of Mary Heir*, 18 Mass. App. 200 (June 4, 1984), which held that a ninety-two-year-old incompetent patient who had pulled out her gastrostomy tube several times did not have to undergo a surgical procedure to reinsert the tube. The Supreme Judicial Court of Massachusetts declined to review this case. See also *Barber v. Superior Court* 147 Cal. App. 3d 1006, 195 Cal. Rptr. 484 (1983), and chapter 2.

11. Joyce V. Zerwekh, "The Dehydration Question," *Nursing83* 47–51 (January 1983). See also chapter 3.

12. Daniel Callahan, "On Feeding the Dying," *Hastings Cent. Rep.* 13:22 (October 1983). All subsequent references to Callahan's position are to this article. (See also chapter 6.)

13. Id.

14. Joanne Lynn and James F. Childress, "Must Patients Always Be Given Food and Water?" *Hastings Cent. Rep.* 13:17–21 (October 1983), reprinted as chapter 5 *supra*.

15. See Beauchamp and Childress, *Principles of Biomedical Ethics*, chap. 4.

16. Joel Feinberg, "Sentiment and Sentimentality in Practical Ethics," *Proceedings and Addresses of the American Philosophical Association* 56(1):41–42 (September 1982).

17. Jonathan Glover, *Causing Death and Saving Lives*, New York: Penguin Books (1977), 296.

18. Gerald Kelly, S.J., "The Duty to Preserve Life," *Theological Stud.* 12:550–556 (December 1951).

19. Lynn and Childress, note 14 *supra*.

20. *Bouvia v. County of Riverside*, No. 159780 (Super. Ct., Dec. 16, 1983); *In re* Plaza Health and Rehabilitation Center (Super. Ct., Onandaga County, February 1, 1984) (elderly man allowed to starve himself to death in a nursing home). In mentioning both of these cases together I do not imply that there are no important differences between them. For example, in some of her claims, Elizabeth Bouvia appeared to assert a positive right to the assistance of others in her death rather than a negative right to noninterference.

21. See the survey by Kenneth C. Micetich, Patricia H. Steinecker, and David C. Thomasma, "Are Intravenous Fluids Morally Required for a Dying Patient?" *Arch. Intern. Med.* 143:975–980 (May 1983), reported in chapter 4 *supra*.

22. This position is taken by Micetich, Steinecker, and Thomasma, *id.*, p. 977.

23. Micetich et al. report that some physicians in an informal poll took this position. *Id.*, 975, and *supra*, chapter 4.

24. My ideas in this essay obviously reiterate and build on my article with Joanne Lynn (see note 14 *supra*), and I am indebted to her for fruitful discussions. In addition, some of the ideas and formulations in this essay have been drawn from "Caring for Symbols and Caring for Patients: Reflections on 'On Feeding the Dying,' " which I coauthored with Steven L. DalleMura (*The Bioethics Reporter*, forthcoming). I am also grateful to Mr. DalleMura for helpful discussions. They are, of course, not responsible for any of the flaws in this essay.

Ronald A. Carson, Ph.D.

8   The Symbolic Significance of Giving to Eat and Drink

A short dozen years ago, the question of the propriety of removing irreversibly ill and dying patients from the mechanical respirator (a machine that Paul Ramsey described as "a devilishly efficient instrument")[1] exercised the minds of doctors, lawyers, and moralists. Today, removing irreversibly comatose patients from respirators is common practice, and now we worry about withdrawing the seemingly more simple, but no less devilishly efficient, lines that infuse food and fluids into the moribund bodies of dying patients.

Is is ever permissible to withhold life-sustaining food and water in the treatment of irreversibly ill and dying persons? I think so, but only in ways that do not violate our sense of the fundamental importance and appropriateness of sustaining and protecting the sick and dying until they die—even protecting them on occasion from the suffering, or just plain nuisance, engendered by IV lines and nasogastric tubes. This question has risen to public consciousness and gained attention in the professional literature only in the last few years.

In a 1981 article in the *Journal of Medical Ethics*, Carson Strong asked, "Can Fluids or Electrolytes be 'Extraordinary' Treatment?"[2] answering with a qualified yes. A year later, reviewing the *Herbert* case in the same journal, Bernard Towers, referring to irreversibly comatose patients, asks, "Is it murder if the IV line is disconnected?" He replied, "If withdrawal of IV fluids from a deeply comatose patient is considered equivalent to denying food and water to a conscious patient and thereby 'starving him to death' . . . then we might as well be with Alice in Wonderland, playing crazy croquet with the Red Queen."[3] In a 1983 article, reported in chapter 4 above, Kenneth Micetich, Patricia Steinecker, and David Thomasma argue that when a comatose person is dying, when death is imminent and the family requests that no further medical procedures be done, IV fluids are not morally required.[4] Reviewing the "Infant Doe" regulations in *Law, Medicine and Health Care,* John Paris and Anne Fletcher concluded that traditions of medical ethics do not support the view that artificial feeding must be instituted for hopelessly ill children.[5] Joanne Lynn and James Childress have argued that "nutrition and hydration by medical means need not always be provided."[6] Bonnie Steinbock has pointed out that discontinuing intravenous feeding spurred the decision to prosecute in the *Herbert* case,[7] and George Annas, in a review of the *Herbert* and *Conroy* cases, reminded readers that withdrawing nutrition from incompetent patients was considered a lawful killing in California and an unlawful homicide by an appellate court in New Jersey.[8] A 1986 AMA statement on withholding or withdrawing life-prolonging treatment stipulated that with appropriate consent physicians may cease or not commence treatment of permanently unconscious or terminally ill patients. The statement expressly includes "artificially or technologically supplied . . . nutrition, or hydration."[9]

Although a body of reasoned opinion is building on this issue, much ambivalence remains. How are we to account for this ambivalence? The answer has less to do with the bare behavior of omitting to provide food and water to dying patients than it does with the meaning of this act. The symbolic meaning of an act is seldom obvious. Many events and experiences that we find meaningful are inexplicably so, or at least not self-consciously so. Symbolic significance is characteristically allusive. It cannot be gotten at directly. It tells us not how this thing is, but how things always are. Symbolic meaning is also elusive. It cannot be fabricated. Symbols emerge, evolve, change or not, and if not, they cease to resonate and thus cease to be.

The simple act of offering to allay hunger and to slake the thirst of a dying person is deemed, across time and cultures, to be not only right but good. In acting thus, one might give nutriments necessary to sustain the body. But beyond this, to nourish is to nurse, in the inclusive sense of harboring, as well as feeding. To offer food and water is to tend and to regard. This is perhaps the rudimentary healing gesture, the one that remains even when prospects for recovery are remote. In view of the weighty significance we ascribe to the act of giving to eat and drink, it is little wonder that the question of the propriety of leaving off that act prompts hesitation and ambivalence.

But is this merely squeamishness on our part? I noted earlier that we have come to accept the practice of removing from the respirator an irreversibly comatose patient with the consent of the family or guardian. This acceptance is, above all, an acknowledgment of the aimlessness of continuing a treatment that is ineffectual, that has no remedial value, and that may be harming the patient. Is it any different with alimentation and hydration? Not as far as I can see. By simple analogy, if it is permissible to withdraw the one, it is surely allowable to cease the other.

There is, of course, more to it than this. Removing a respirator feels different from disconnecting an IV line. We use the language of nurture when we speak of "weaning" someone from a respirator, but the same language employed in relation to feeding and giving drink yields nonsense. Such feelings, I suggest, should be taken seriously and should affect, but not dictate, our actions in these matters. Practically speaking, what might this mean?

Daniel Callahan, in a commentary "On Feeding the Dying,"[10] argued that "It is a most dangerous business to tamper with, or adulterate, so enduring and central a moral emotion, one in which the repugnance against starving people to death could be, on occasion, greater than that which a more straitened rationality would call for." Acknowledging the moral licitness of the discontinuation of feeding under some circumstances, Callahan urges the cultivation of "a deep-seated revulsion at the stopping of feeding even under legitimate circumstances." This seems to me sound advice in principle, although I wonder whether one need go quite so far as "deep-seated revulsion" to accomplish what Callahan (and I) want to encourage.

When past moralists spoke of repugnance in relation to medical treatments (potentially life-saving but definitely disfiguring surgical procedures, for example), they were referring to a sentiment that had to be reckoned with and overcome before such treatment could be considered morally imperative. But, to paraphrase Paul Ramsey, as medicine minimizes and eliminates the heretofore repugnant side effects and consequences of some treatments, these treatments, once morally elective (*because* repugnant), may become morally imperative. Conversely, when medicine has done all it can for a person and has no further useful treatment to offer, what is its warrant for continuing to treat that person? Might it not be offensive to treat, however minimally, in the face of the uselessness of treatment? (I am reminded of the eighty-five-year-old man who, because of his deteriorating health, starved himself to death in a Syracuse, New York, nursing home and who, during the course of his fast, told the physicians who tried to talk him out of his action to mind their own business.)[11]

I propose as an alternative to "stubborn emotional repugnance" and "deep-seated revulsion at the stopping of feeding [the dying] even under legitimate circumstances" the virtue of sadness—in both the customary connotation of that term and in the now obsolete but perhaps still serviceable old English sense of steadfastness, firmness, and constancy.

Feeding is a reciprocal act. Its symbolic significance resides in the mutuality of giving to eat and drink and of taking food and water. To ingest is to receive the food and drink offered. In the absence of this gesture of acceptance, the act of feeding is incomplete, useless, arguably elective. This is not to say that patients who have problems with taking food and drink are beyond care. It is, rather, an acknowledgment of the limits of usefulness of medical treatments, including intravenous hydration and tube feeding, in the care provided for dying persons. When these treatments become futile, different forms of care (which may already be in place but not prominent) may be appropriate—liquids for sipping, ice chips for dry mouth, analgesics, antiemetics, and backrubs are some of the supportive measures available. These activities involve attending, abiding, not abandoning, and providing safe haven and safe passage. The symbolic character of this kind of ritual is far removed from the symbolics of rescue. Instead of tubes there are small acts of considerateness that require no response. There is resignation and there is wonder.

Symbolic meanings are not sufficient for determining the rightness of actions, but they are as powerfully present at our dying as they are in our lives generally. The dying are imperiled and our care for them is poorer when this is ignored. I have tried to suggest that, while we may not be obligated always to feed the dying, new (old) forms of care can be fashioned that are both effective and an antidote to the personal suffering and social calamity that might well ensue were the lives of the dying to become cheap and expendable.

N O T E S

1. Paul Ramsey, *The Patient as Person* (New Haven: Yale University Press, 1970), 81.

2. Carson Strong, "Can Fluids and Electrolytes Be 'Extraordinary' Treatment?" *J. Med. Ethics* 7:83–85 (1981).

3. Bernard Towers, "Irreversible Coma and Withdrawal of Life Support: Is It Murder if the IV Line is Disconnected?" *J. Med. Ethics* 8:203–205 (1982).

4. Kenneth Micetich, Patricia Steinecker, and David Thomasma, "Are Intravenous Fluids Morally Required for a Dying Patient?" *Arch. Intern. Med.* 143:975–978 (1983).

5. John Paris and Anne Fletcher, "Infant Doe Regulations and the Absolute Requirement to Use Nourishment and Fluids for the Dying Infant." *Law, Med. and Health Care* 11:210–213 (October 1983).

6. Joanne Lynn and James Childress, "Must Patients Always Be Given Food and Water?" *Hastings Cent. Rep.* 13:17–21 (October 1983), reprinted as chapter 5 *supra*.

7. Bonnie Steinbock, "The Removal of Mr. Herbert's Feeding Tube," *Hastings Cent. Rep.* 13:13–16 (October 1983).

8. George Annas, "Nonfeeding: Lawful Killing in CA, Homicide in NJ," *Hastings Cent. Rep.* 13:19–20 (December 1983). The latter ruling was later overturned. See *In re* Claire Conroy, 98 N.J. 321, 486 A.2d 1209 (1985).

9. Current Opinions of the Council on Ethical and Judicial Affairs of the American Medical Association (Chicago: AMA, 1986), 13. See also Rebecca Dresser, "Discontinuing Nutrition Support: A Review of the Case Law," *Journal of the American Dietetic Association* 85:1289–1292 (October 1985); and Leslie Steven Rothenberg, "The Dissenting Opinions: Biting the Hands that Won't Feed," *Health Progress* (December 1986), 38–45, 99.

10. Daniel Callahan, "On Feeding the Dying," *Hastings Cent. Rep.* 13:22 (October 1983).

11. *In re* Plaza Health and Rehabilitation Center (Super. Ct., Onandaga County, Feb. 2, 1984).

Reverend Edward J. Bayer, S.T.D.

9   Perspectives from Catholic Theology

A dialogue on medical ethics has been going on among physicians, theologians, and the pastoral authorities of the Catholic Church for over nineteen hundred years. The first section of this chapter will address, out of this long dialogue within the Catholic community, some fundamental considerations that have considerable relevance even for our recent dilemmas. The second section will seek to express concretely the implication of these foundational considerations for both medical practice and public policy regarding the provision of nutrition and hydration.

I. FUNDAMENTAL CONSIDERATIONS

In her experience as a Church for over nineteen hundred years, Catholic Christianity has found that she has had to be on guard against three errors, some contradictory to one another and each, in its extreme, equally wrong.

A. ERROR: DISTINGUISHING THE BODY FROM THE PERSON

One error is the denial that the body is truly an aspect of the human person.[1] From the very beginning the Church met this error by persistently upholding as her own the doctrine of the ancient Jewish Scriptures regarding the body. Those scriptures, especially Genesis, tell us that God made man a *material* being. "God formed man from the clay of the earth."[2]

Moreover, Jesus confirms the Jewish Scriptures by teaching that when we serve a *bodily* need, we serve the *person*, and, indeed, vicariously Jesus Himself. "I was hungry and you fed me, I was thirsty and you gave me drink. . . . I assure you, as often as you did it for one of the least of my brothers, you did it to me."[3] Jesus is speaking here of things we do to the *bodies* of others. If you do it for the *body*, He says, you do it to the *person* and to Him. The body,

with the soul, *is* the person, and *not* simply something which happens to *belong* to the person, like a horse, or a wagon, or a house.

One cannot claim, then, that if one kills a person's body one is
somehow not killing that person.[4] The point is fundamental: to
prolong the physiological life of the person is to prolong the life of
that person as a totality. From this fundamental metaphysical truth,
then, follows a fundamental moral truth: there is an obligation—
limited, it is true, but for that no less real—to prolong the physiological dimension, the bodily life of every innocent person.[5] And
here we come to at least one point relevant to certain recent highly
publicized cases.

Regardless of where one stands on the issue of killing a non-
innocent person, no individual—as *individual*—has a right to judge
himself or herself (or another person) to be so guilty and worthless
that he or she may abandon the prolongation of physiological life.
It may be argued, and is, that *society*—and those who bear appropriate authority for society, i.e., jurors and judges—has the right to
make such a judgment; indeed this is the basis for any argument for
capital punishment. The *individual*, however, does not have such
a right regarding either his own basic guilt and worthlessness, or
that of another.[6]

Individuals do at times unfortunately take it upon themselves to
pass sentence of guilt or worthlessness on themselves.[7] This *self-*
conviction is often behind the efforts of patients to refuse rather
simple, unburdensome medical steps which promise to significantly
prolong life, or perhaps even significantly to relieve useless pain.[8]

St. Paul once wrote to one of his early Christian congregations:
"It matters little to me whether you or any human court pass judgment on me. I do not even pass judgment on myself."[9]

The same holds for the patient or for others who would second a
death judgment made by the patient's own private authority. Such
an act of self-condemnation to death may underlie a resolve to refuse
rather simple, relatively unburdensome, and clearly promising
means of prolonging life. Such a sentence of death is beyond the
right of any individual *qua* individual.

B. Error: Confusing the Ethically and Medically Ordinary[10]
Another error is to confuse the meaning of "ordinary" and "extraordinary" means of prolonging life. These terms have importantly

different meanings depending on whether one is using them in an *ethical* sense or in a *medical* sense.

On the one hand, "ethically ordinary" means "ethically obligatory" or, more simply put, "obligatory *on its own merits.*" On the other hand, "medically ordinary" means simply "medically standard." Accordingly, one should note that "obligatory on its own merits" could include both medically standard means and means which are unusual in medical practice.

A means of prolonging life is "obligatory on its own merits" when one must answer yes to all three of the following questions:

a) Is this means physiologically possible for the patient?
b) Will this means substantially prolong life or relieve useless pain?
c) Will this means, as a means, escape significantly adding to the burdens of the patient?

When the answer to any *one* of these questions is no, then the means in question is *not* "obligatory on its own merits." No one is bound to prolong life by means which are impossible, substantially useless, or unreasonably burdensome.

This does not mean that the particular means and the prolongation of life it will bring are ethically countermanded. The patient (or those who legitimately speak for him or her) may have other reasons which he or she considers compelling for choosing a means which, on its own merits, is quite unpromising. An aged woman might, for instance, want to be kept on a respirator that offers hope for at the most only four or five more days of conscious life because a long-absent son will have a good chance to reach her bedside before she dies. She may even be convinced that this is morally imperative for her, for instance, because it will contribute to reconciliation among family members alienated from one another. Her reasons for choosing these means would not, however, be based on the merits of the respirator for substantially prolonging life, but on considerations extraneous to such a means taken in itself.

Even connatural means of prolonging life can be nonobligatory. Connatural means are life-prolonging means that, unlike respirators, feeding tubes, and the like, are part of our very bodily *selves* (thus, "connatural," of our own nature). They include all natural capacities of the body for sustaining life. An example is the normal mastication and swallowing of food. Ordinarily, such functions are by their very connaturality more mandatory than artificial means of life support would be. A more serious reason would be required to exempt one from an obligation to use them. But if ingestion, for example, is extremely painful, produces nausea, sends the patient into spasms of coughing, or creates a danger of aspiration and suffocation, the patient would not be obliged to use this connatural function, despite the fact that it is part of his or her own physiological nature as a human being. Only normal ingestion is immediately and by its very nature obligatory if, in addition to being relatively unburdensome, it promises to prolong life substantially or relieve useless pain.

It is important to emphasize the purpose, then, of any life-prolonging means, connatural or artificial: not simply to prolong life, but to prolong it *substantially*.[11] Moralists have long recognized, for instance, that a condemned man on death row is not obliged to eat the customary "last meal," for it offers no substantial prolongation of life.

It should be noted that the phrase "terminally ill" is, as many Catholic moralists warn, dangerously vague. What it should really mean is "the *last phases* of terminal illness." In other words, the illness must be of such a nature that, no matter what one does medically or in any other way, the person is going to die within a rather short time.

The Special Case of the Irreversibly Unconscious Patient: A "Quality of Life" Consideration?

We have been considering up to this point the plight of patients dying in what might be termed a *chronological* sense. No matter what one does for them they have little *time* left. Many Catholic moralists today agree also that if a patient is irreversibly unconscious, his or her life need not be prolonged by artificial means, including artificial feeding and hydration. This would be true, they hold, even if such artificial means would considerably extend the unconscious patient's life span.[12]

It must be said right off, however, that this position is not based on any "quality of life" considerations.[13] Rather, it appeals to two basic facts about human nature, especially our bodily nature.

The irreversibly comatose patient has ceased to engage in the most typically human activity, the one which clearly identifies us as human beings, namely, human intercommunication. The person who is irreversibly comatose will, by definition, never again be *able* to give or receive communication.[14] He will never be able to see the hand of God in nature, nor really to receive or respond to the power and the plea of another human voice.

But precisely this *capacity*—rooted in the physiology of the brain—to recognize at least minimally the presence and workings of other personal beings, divine or human, marks one as a human being. This capacity is dead in the irreversibly comatose patient, even though the patient still lives. Therefore, in a true sense the *person* is *fast dying*, and we are not obliged to prolong the process by artificial means.

A second fact some moralists would rely upon is that the central organ necessary not only for interpersonal communication but also for all truly organic life of the body is dying: again, the brain. In irreversibly comatose patients, the person must be considered alive as long as even the brain stem is alive. Some kind of overall maintenance of organic functioning is still going on. Nonetheless, that person is dying, not chronologically perhaps, but anatomically, since the central coordinating organ is dying.

The Herbert case in California may well have been mishandled. As noted above, the problem is not that food and water, artificially administered, were withheld from someone in an irreversibly comatose state. It is rather that, at least according to reports generally available, the food and water were withheld days before the comatose state had been diagnosed as irreversible. The decision to withhold that food and water seems, then, to have been precipitous and thus ethically unjustified.[15]

C. Error: Usurping the Patient's Personal, Spiritual Responsibility to Discern and Decide

The considerations presented thus far center upon the Church's insistence that, to act morally, one must recognize and respect the bodily nature of the human person. It is essential also to recognize and respect each person's spiritual nature, his or her rational dimension.

The rational dimension of the human person is the power (1) to *discern* whether a particular life-prolonging means is "obligatory on its own merits" or not, and (2) if it is not such, but is optional, to *decide*, Do I want this nonobligatory means used to keep me alive or not? This discernment and decision is the patient's to make—no one else's. Indeed a proxy for an incompetent patient—be it an individual or society itself—acts legitimately only insofar as the proxy seeks to represent the *patient's discernment* and *decision*. It is a serious error for anyone to presume to substitute his or her own judgment or choice for that of the affected individual whenever the individual can make these decisions or has done so.

WITHDRAWING ARTIFICIAL FEEDING AND HYDRATION: AN ACT OF KILLING?

Before proceeding to the second section, on the implications of the fundamental considerations presented above, one further clarification seems advisable. The following question comes up regarding the withdrawal or the withholding of artificially supplied food and fluids: Is there any ethically significant difference between *actively* and *passively* contributing to someone's death? Are we not truly *killing* when we *withdraw* even nonobligatory means of sustaining life? If so, and if such withdrawing can in some circumstances be justified, then active euthanasia measures sometimes also might be justified.[16]

Catholic Christianity has faced these questions under the rubric of what is called the principle of double effect. The principle means that there indeed *can* be a significant ethical difference between (1) an act of killing and (2) an act of allowing a person to die as a partial result of not taking some action that would prolong life. It can be quite different, on the one hand, to withdraw a means of supporting life, and, on the other hand, to directly introduce an agent or procedure whose primary and intended effect is to bring about death.

It is not permitted to man to do evil (e.g., aim to take innocent human life, even when that life is handicapped) in order that good may come of it (e.g., the ending of an otherwise prolonged dying process). But we may do good (e.g., withdraw technological contrivances that are essentially useless and/or significantly burdensome) that results in one effect at which we have a *right* directly to aim (relief from burden which the contrivances are causing) and another effect at which we have *no right* directly to aim (the death of the patient).

The distinction between *actively* causing (aiming at) death and *passively* causing (allowing) death is really an attempt to express in intellectually coherent terms what the Catholic Church is convinced morally sensitive human beings can know spontaneously. For example, if parents decide to bring a child into the world, they are setting that baby up to die someday. If they did not conceive the child, it would never have to die. Yet most people would recognize that it would be foolish to conclude that the decision to *have* a child is a decision to *kill* the child. The parents choose to give something good to the child—human life—knowing that, unfortunately, the child will also share the fate of all of us—death. The principle of double effect says that what they commit themselves to when they bring a child into the world is one thing; what they tolerate as one of the consequences of that commitment is, morally, another thing.

A basic application of the principle of double effect, then, also carries through all Catholic considerations about prolonging life, and affirms that withdrawing or withholding nonobligatory means of life support is not in any valid ethical sense an act of killing. Morally justifiable instances of the former can never be used logically to justify the latter.

II. PRACTICAL APPLICATIONS FOR MEDICAL ETHICS AND PUBLIC POLICY

A. MEDICAL ETHICS

1) A *connatural means*, i.e., the taking of food and fluid by normally functioning ingestion, if it promises significantly to prolong basically conscious life or to relieve serious, useless pain, is "obligatory on its own merits." To refuse normal ingestion for one's self when it would significantly prolong conscious life is the moral equivalent of suicide.

If, however, such ingestion does not promise significantly to prolong basically conscious life or to relieve serious, useless pain, it is nonobligatory. There may be some other legitimate reason the person or the proxy of the patient would feel morally bound to take such a means, but not because the means itself is "obligatory on its own merits."

2) An *artificial means* of taking food and fluid is "obligatory on its own merits" if (1) it promises to prolong basically conscious life or to relieve serious, useless pain, and (2) at the same time, it does not add disproportionately, in itself or in its aftereffects, to the burden which the patient or others are already experiencing.

Should one force food and fluids against a patient's will? The recent Elizabeth Bouvia[17] case in California raises this question.

No one may licitly force a patient to accept food or fluid by artificial means *unless* the patient's refusal to accept it must be judged a cause of grave harm to another or society as a whole. This means that, *generally speaking*, society will not be justified in forcing a person to take artificially delivered food and fluid.

However, there may be exceptions to this general rule. Society does have an obligation to discourage suicide and must choose means to do this. Society has, therefore, the right (not necessarily the obligation) artificially to force food or fluids on someone who, with suicidal intent, refuses to use their own connatural powers of ingestion.[18] Society has also the obligation to protect the life of the unborn. It would follow, therefore, that society has a right to force food or fluids on a pregnant woman whose suicidal starvation would cause the death of a child who will otherwise survive. These examples are not, of course, intended as exhaustive, nor are they exempt from difficult discernment and even debate in practice.

Where only the patient's welfare is involved, however, the decision regarding artificial means must be left to the patient, even when the patient's refusal appears to onlookers to be the moral equivalent of suicide. Society simply cannot attempt to take over all responsibility for the individual. Nor is there any responsibility more intimately personal than that over one's own bodily and spiritual self. And, finally, what may appear to be a suicidal intent may actually be the patient's highly *personal* and *valid*, but *incommunicable*, understanding that the means is *de facto* not "obligatory on its own merits" for him or her. The amount of physical or emotional pain experienced from any given procedure will vary from individual to individual, and no norm for such burden is universally applicable.

B. Public Policy

Public policy, whether it be established legitimately through legislative action, judicial decision, or executive order, should both discourage suicide and cooperation in suicide (euthanasia) and support ethical decisions not to prolong the dying process.

This means that society must be open, where such action would seem not to cause more harm than good, to forcing food and fluids on someone who, in a suicidal enterprise, refuses to use their connatural powers of ingestion. This does not mean that such legal coercion can safely be brought to bear without due consideration to the precedents it might set for other areas of life where, unlike suicide or its moral equivalents, a true right to private responsibility and decision making needs to be respected. Nor are these and other prudential factors in issues of forced feeding or hydration always easy to evaluate in practice. Nonetheless, a society that is prepared simply to tolerate any and all suicidal ventures would do a grave disservice to its citizens, many of whom, especially the handicapped, need to be affirmed in their struggle to maintain a sense of worth for their lives.

For the same reason, though more important, society should be prepared to discourage with strong sanctions any incitement to or direct and positive collaboration with a patient's genuinely suicidal tendencies. Thus it should be clear to all that society will not tolerate actions designed by their very nature to bring on death, nor will it tolerate the withdrawal or withholding of food and hydration seemingly "obligatory on their own merits" without a clear mandate from the patient personally or through a legitimately functioning proxy. These proscriptions should be legally binding and are especially needed to counteract recent decisions involving handicapped neonates[19] and some recently published suggestions for nontreatment of the elderly in mental decline.[20]

Society must also be prepared to support legally the right of a patient to have food and hydration withdrawn when these are useless for substantially prolonging life or are, in a given patient's experience and circumstances, excessively burdensome. Legitimate proxies for the patient, and physicians and others who seek to implement as best as possible the honest discernment and true good of a patient in these matters, should be protected from civil or criminal liability.

Finally, society must be prepared *within reason* to allocate public funds to support a patient's decision to prolong life, even by artificial feeding and hydration which is "nonobligatory on its own merits." "Within reason" has all the imprecision lawyers love. It merely begins to point, not only to the claims of conscience as it makes inescapable demands on our collective and individual wealth, but also to the limits beyond which we need not and perhaps should not go in making *all* medical options effectively available to *all* persons under *all* circumstances. In discerning these issues, there are no mechanically easy answers, and Catholic moral dialogue across the centuries would caution us to seek a discernment which is both humane and godly.

NOTES

1. See *Handbook on Critical Life Issues,* Donald McCarthy and Edward Bayer (eds.), St. Louis: The Pope John Center (1982), chapter 1, "The Person as Known by Reason and Reflection" (hereafter *Handbook*).

2. Genesis 2:7. See *Handbook,* chapter 2, for a summary of other biblical teaching on the nature and unique sacredness of human life.

3. Matthew 25:35, 40.

4. See chapters 12 and 19.

5. The Sacred Congregation for the Doctrine of the Faith, *Declaration on Euthanasia,* May 5, 1980 (hereafter "*Declaration*"), in *Vatican Council II—More Post-Conciliar Documents,* Austin Flannery (ed.), Boston: St. Paul Editions (1982), 510.

6. *Summa Theologica,* Secunda Secundae, question 64, article 3, cited approvingly by Pope Pius XII in 1952 (AAS 47, 787).

7. E.g., Bouvia v. County of Riverside, No. 159780 (Super. Ct. Cal. 1984). See also the Second Vatican Council's condemnation of all crimes against life "such as murder, genocide, abortion, euthanasia or willful suicide." (*Gaudium et Spes*—"The Pastoral Constitution on the Church in the Modern World"—number 27).

8. On the importance of the distinction between useless and useful pain, see Edward Bayer, "Pain and the Principle of Totality," in *Ethics & Medics* (September 1983); and *Declaration,* 513–514.

9. 1 Corinthians 4:3.

10. *Declaration,* 515–516; Donald McCarthy and Albert Moraczewski (eds.), *Moral Responsibility in Prolonging Life Decisions* (hereafter *Moral Responsibility*), St. Louis: Pope John Center (1981); see also chapters 5, 7, and 12.

11. See also discussion of *goses* and *trefah* in chapter 10.

12. *Moral Responsibility, loc. cit.,* and *Handbook,* 179.

13. *Prolonging Life,* 129–130.

14. *Prolonging Life,* chapter 13: "Care of Persons in the Final Stages of Terminal Illness or Irreversible Coma."

15. Donald McCarthy, "Murder by Deprivation of Medical Treatment: Premature Withdrawal of Tube Feeding" in *Ethics & Medics* (October 1983).

16. Edward J. Bayer, "Allowing a Patient to Die: Is It an Act of Killing?" in *Ethics & Medics* (July 1984). See also chapter 12.

17. Bouvia v. County of Riverside, No. 159780 (Super. Ct. Cal. 1984).

18. Edward Bayer, "A Right Not to Eat? Refusal to Eat vs. Incapacity to Eat," in *Ethics & Medics* (January 1984).

19. See chapter 17.

20. Sidney H. Wanzer, S. James Adelstein, Ronald Cranford, et al., "The Physician's Responsibility Towards Hopelessly Ill Patients," *N. Engl. J. Med.,* 310:955–959 (1984).

Michael Nevins, M.D.

10 Perspectives of a Jewish Physician

A fourth-century writer, Ben Sidra, said, "Without experience there is little wisdom." Perhaps my sixteen years of practice as internist-cardiologist-geriatrician have given me some wisdom regarding care of the dying. Many of my patients reside in a nursing home near my office. When I audited my own practice in the past year, I was disturbed and surprised to learn that thirty-seven of the many patients in my charge at that nursing home last year had died. That is a large and sobering experience with death. For many, these deaths were sudden and unanticipated: for others, the decline was inexorable, and many decisions had to be made along the way.

Since I have so often been involved in making decisions for people who were at or near the end of life, I began to explore what the Jewish tradition might teach about a proper code of conduct in such situations. Medical practice is uniquely existential. Often there are no clear rules, but there are always choices. Many decisions must be made in a climate of uncertainty, and I wondered whether Judaism might offer any practical guideposts about what a physician ought and ought not to do when in doubt.

In a letter published in the *New York Times*, Orthodox Rabbi David Bleich of Yeshiva University argued that physicians should never be involved in making nonemergency life-and-death decisions.[1] He reasoned that in the case of a comatose patient who was dependent on a respirator, the real issues are theologic and moral, not scientific or semantic. Whereas doctors may be qualified to render diagnosis and treatment, he contended that the decision about whether or not they *should* treat is a value judgment better resolved by a rabbi. It is an instructive perspective, even though many persons might well disagree. However, it is clear that physicians *do* play a central role in clinical decision-making—a process which has both moral and scientific implications.

At this point, it is important that I state my religious convictions so that the reader can place my comments in context. Contemporary Judaism comprises a spectrum of attitudes and beliefs. I probably stand about midway between the strictly observant position on one extreme and a liberal and less observant persuasion on the other. I am fully aware of the mischief that can result from oversimplification and misapplication of labels, but it is necessary for the reader to appreciate that there is no single contemporary Jewish position on most ethical issues. However, a strong tide runs centrally throughout our history, as delineated in such classic religious texts as the Talmud.

This range of belief is important to an understanding and appreciation of the clinical and ethical issues of caring for a terminally ill Jewish patient. If the intent is to be consistent with that patient's own beliefs, there would very likely be vast differences in treatment. The personal preferences and values of a nonreligious, secular Jew might not coincide with those of another Jewish patient who was a Hasidic rabbi. Yet, the many dilemmas that arise from burgeoning technology are breaking new ground for all of us, and learning to apply the wisdom of the past to new situations is a universal challenge that the ancient scholars could not have foreseen.

JEWISH VALUES AND LAWS

Through the millennia, Judaism has been pro-life in the extreme, and it may be said that the Jews were the original right-to-life advocates, unequivocally opposed to suicide, infanticide, and euthanasia except in the most extenuating circumstances.

The duty to preserve life takes precedence over all other obligations except avoiding adultery, murder, and incest.[2] Since the value of every individual and every breath of life is considered to be equal, life cannot be discarded once it has begun. Quality of life is not an issue. Even noncognitive lives have value, if only for others as an object for caring. Our bodies are not our own—it is as if we are but tenants and have no absolute title. God is the source of health and sickness and alone decides when life is to end. In this sense, life is a gift which, when the time comes, must be returned. We are not to determine that time. Suicide, then, is regarded as a criminal act, no matter how tragic the circumstances or profound the individual's despair.[3] To take one's own life is equivalent to denial of divine ownership. Even willful neglect of one's own health is an act of partial self-murder. The Talmud and other early religious texts provide us with colorful illustrations of these basic principles.

It is written that if any man causes a single soul to perish, it is as if he caused a whole world to perish, and he who keeps alive a single soul, it is as if he has saved a whole world.[4] The Talmud elaborates on the idea and tells us that a person who kills a child who is falling from a roof is guilty of a capital offense even though his intention may be honorable and the child's certain death is hastened by only a few moments. The crucial element here was seen to be that the crime involves *active* killing.[5]

If a funeral cortege meets a bridal procession, the former must give way to the latter, since life takes precedence over death.

If on the Sabbath a person is buried under rubble from a falling building, the prohibition against performing work on the Sabbath is suspended so long as there is even a remote chance of life. However, once it has been established that the victim is no longer breathing and there is no remote chance of recovery, further labor must be suspended until after the Sabbath.

The Talmud states also that we may desecrate the Sabbath for a day-old infant if he is still alive, but if he already has died, we may not do so even for someone as great as David, King of Israel.[6]

One Talmudic tractate describes a prayer that patients should utter while undergoing therapeutic bloodletting; in the prayer, God is implored to permit healing to take place.[7] Only God has the ability to heal. The physician is merely God's instrument.

Prayer itself was considered to be therapeutic and an equivalent of medicine. Consider the death of the famous Rabbi Judah HaNasi. Many rabbis had gathered at Rabbi Judah's deathbed to pray for his recovery. The old scholar was suffering greatly until his handmaiden, a woman known for her great wisdom, had pity on him. She climbed up on the roof and from there threw a large earthenware jar down to the ground. The rabbis were startled by the crash and momentarily stopped their praying. As a result, Rabbi Judah died peacefully.[8] This charming story about the handmaiden's trick represents a fine example of termination of life support and was favorably viewed in the Talmud.

A variation on this same theme was written by an eighteenth-century rabbi in Smyrna. A woman was dying of some lingering disease and her husband and son were trying by every means, including prayers in the synagogue, to keep her alive. She called them to her bedside and said that she was grateful for their efforts, but asked that they please refrain from such prayers because her life was no longer bearable.[9] The rabbi was asked whether this would be permitted, and he answered that to refrain from praying is permitted, but that nothing positive could be done to shorten her life.

These accounts indicate that Jewish law does not categorically prohibit terminating artificial life support in all cases. It is permissible to allow death once the patient is, in fact, dying. Based on the famous line in Ecclesiastes, "There is a time to live and a time to die,"[10] man has a right to die. When a man is dying, we do not pray too hard that his soul return: in the same sense it is not incumbent upon the physician to force a truly terminally ill patient to live a little longer by virtue of active treatment. Although it is forbidden to perform a positive action which hastens death, not so an act of removing an impediment to death.[11] Regrettably, the fine distinctions between prolonging life and prolonging the act of dying, or between causing and allowing, are sometimes very elusive.

The sixteenth-century code of law known as the Shulchan Aruch[12] devotes an entire chapter to the laws of the dying and speaks of the concept of the *goses*. A *goses* is a person for whom natural death is imminent, literally, the "death-rattle" being in the throat.[13] The *goses* is the exception to the Jewish rule of total commitment to life. Even at life's terminus nothing direct can be done to hasten death. Here, life is fragile and the patient should not be moved or jostled. Even closing the eyelids or moving the pillow may upset a delicate balance. The matter was compared by one rabbi to a flickering flame: as soon as one touches it, the light is extinguished.[14] Yet there is a subtle difference in the moribund state, for now certain modifications are permissible.

As with the story of Judah HaNasi's death, where terminating prayer treatment was sanctioned, any artificial thing that hinders the soul's departure can be removed so long as it is done passively. Thus, if someone is chopping wood outside the window of a *goses* and the regular sound concentrated the mind of the patient or served as a stimulus, the chopping could be stopped because it was delaying a natural process.[15] Similarly, stimulants such as salt on the tongue can be very gently wiped away, although even here some Talmudists objected that this, too, might be rough and hasten death.[16] One thirteenth-century commentator forbade those attending the dying patient to cry, lest the noise revive the spirit,[17] and still another early rabbi suggested that even medicine must not be used, because it might delay the departure of the *goses* soul.

These early Talmudic statements clearly imply that, when life has become so fragile that even a mere touch is condemned, the modern act of inserting a nasogastric feeding tube or starting an intravenous infusion in a *goses* would be inappropriately active. The more difficult question arises when an artificial feeding tube already is in place; should it then be permissible not to replace the bag or bottle when it has run dry?

Rabbi Bleich has noted the parallel that Maimonides made between food and medicine.[18] As God created one to deal with hunger, he created the other to deal with illness, and as we are bound to use the one, so are we bound to use the other.

The Talmud did not distinguish between natural and artificial methods of feeding. To eschew the latter should not imply abandonment or neglecting patient care. Rather, in this situation there should be a heightened responsibility to provide comfort and to show respect by small considerate actions such as moistening the mouth.

How does one know whether or not a patient is a *goses* so that obstacles to death, be they woodchoppers, prayer, or feeding tubes, can be withdrawn? According to ancient rabbinic sources, death for a *goses* is expected within three days.[19] This may seem rather arbitrary. Modern Jews of a more liberal persuasion might be inclined to broaden the definition. After all, the moment of death cannot be predicted precisely. One might ask: Do the same rules apply for the less than terminally ill patient? When does a patient become terminal?

Some cynics have said that, once born, we all are terminal. Others suggest that one becomes "terminally ill" when an incurable disease is diagnosed or when treatment has failed. The Talmud makes clear that the *goses* is in the process of dying. My own interpretation of these traditional teachings is that prognosis dictates treatment. Technology and feeding tubes, per se, are neither moral nor immoral, but the context in which they are used determines appropriateness, extraordinariness, or what recently has been called "proportionateness."

A related concept in Jewish law is that of the *trefah*, defined by a rule in the *Mishnah*: "If an animal with a similar defect could not continue to live [for one year], it is *trefah*."[20] There is extensive discussion in the Talmud as to what physical impairments render animals *trefah*, and, by analogy, which apply to man. Although there are disagreements about particular injuries or illnesses, as Freehof notes, "by and large . . . [the rabbis] accept the standards set down for animals, namely that if a person . . . cannot be expected to live more than twelve months, such a person is considered to be in a dying condition."[21]

The difficulty in distinguishing between a *goses* and a *trefah* is in part reflected by the common English translation of both terms— "moribund" or "in a dying condition." According to law professor Alan Weisbard's review of these twin concepts as they apply to the case of Karen Ann Quinlan, "at the risk of some oversimplification, the *trefah* is one with an irreparable organic disease who 'will die'; the *goses* is anyone who 'is dying.' The death of a *trefah* is regarded as ultimately more certain, although perhaps less imminent, than that of the *goses*."[22]

APPLYING JEWISH LAW IN PRACTICE

Is it permissible for a Jew to take liberties and extrapolate or follow the spirit rather than the letter of the law? To answer this, one must understand that the major Jewish denominations have quite different attitudes about the law which is called *Halachah*.

About half of the nearly six million American Jews are unaffiliated, and probably most of those are not observant. Of the rest, about one million are members of the Reform movement, about one million are of the Conservative movement, and about half a million are Orthodox, who strictly follow the law of *Halachah*.

Although this is somewhat oversimplified, Reform Jews believe that it is best to let people make up their own minds while considering what God wants, what Jewish tradition teaches, and what others are doing. The Orthodox would object that Judaism is not a religion of personal convenience and equivocation but rather is a strict system of law. That law is immutable and complex, but by following it and doing the big and little things habitually, and in a specifically Jewish way, one follows the road to the perfection of man. Conservative Jews fall somewhere between these two poles. Like the Reform movement, they believe that Jewish law can and should change in time; but they also believe that such change should take place only within a strict framework and in a slow and thoughtful process directed by disciplined scholars who are knowledgeable about the law. Thus, there are three major contemporary attitudes about *Halachah*. There is little dispute about the foundation of the law, but there often is considerable disagreement about its implementation.

Rabbi Solomon Freehof, a modern Reform scholar, has noted that, although the spirit of the Jewish law does not allow death to be hastened, one may allow death to come under special circumstances of suffering and hopelessness.[23] Similarly, Conservative Rabbi Seymour Siegel has written, "We must not forget in our loyalty to tradition the welfare of the suffering patient who, when the giver of life has proclaimed the end of his earthly existence, should be allowed to die in spite of our machines."[24]

Traditional Jewish views do not cast these issues in terms of personal autonomy. The famous Jewish existentialist philosopher Franz Rosenzweig was afflicted with amyotrophic lateral sclerosis. As a deeply committed Jew, Rosenzweig claimed no right to free choice in hastening his own death. Instead he felt an obligation to preserve life, and so, clenching a pencil between his teeth to point to the typewriter keys which his wife would then push, Rosenzweig collaborated with Martin Buber on translating the Bible into German. The Jewish tradition would use Rosenzweig's example to teach that sometimes it is in the very struggle for life that man achieves dignity. In response to the familiar question "Whose life is it anyway?" traditional Judaism would answer, "It's not yours."

CONCLUSIONS

Judaism contains no absolute mandate to treat in order to extend life of patients who are dying. In a tight time frame, acts of omission are permissible at the very end of life. Acts of commission, if they would hasten death, are intolerable at any time. If a patient is *in extremis* and in pain and no treatment holds any hope for his or her recovery, it may be proper to withhold additional nonroutine or artificial medical care in order to permit the natural ebbing of life.

Sometimes it is difficult to reconcile the apparent contradictions between what Jews do and what their law allows, and disagreements over interpretation can be contentious. However, this very dynamism enriches the varied texture of modern Jewish thought.

If the traditional Orthodox Jewish attitude about caring for the dying seems a stern challenge for a contemporary society whose increasingly permissive values emphasize patient autonomy, it should be considered that Jewish *Halachah* has endured throughout history as a sensitive, responsible, effective, and consistent standard of behavior. The price that must be paid to preserve the principle of life's preciousness is high, but perhaps a society's willingness to pay that price is a moral litmus test of that society's humanity.

NOTES

1. J. David Bleich, "Life and Death Decisions Not for Doctors to Make," *New York Times*, January 22, 1984, p. 22.

2. *Mishnah Talmud* (ed. Romm, Vilna, 1911), Tractate Sanhedrin iv. 5.

3. *Babylonian Talmud* (ed. Romm, Vilna, 1895), Tractate Sanhedrin 78a; Maimonides Hil. Rotze'oh, ii. 7.

4. *Mishnah*, Tractate Sanhedrin iv. 5.

5. *Babylonian*, Tractate Sanhedrin 78a.

6. *Mishnah Yoma* 8:6–7.

7. Charles Green Cumston, *An Introduction to the History of Medicine from the Pharaohs to the XVIIIth Century*, London (1926), 24.

8. *Mishnah*, Tractate Ketuboth 104a.

9. Cited in Solomon B. Freehof, *Reform Responsa*, New York: Ktav (1973), 120.

10. Ecclesiastes, 3:2.

11. *Babylonian*, Tractate Shabbath 151b.

12. *Shulchan Aruch, Even haEzer* 121:7, cited in Teo Forcht Dagi, "The Paradox of Euthanasia," *Judaism* 23:157–168 (1975), at 164.

13. J. Rabinowitz, Notes to the Soncino Edition of Tractate *Semachoth*.

14. *Babylonian*, Tractate Shabbath 151b, and Tractate Semachoth i. 4.

15. R. Judah ben Samuel, *Sefer Chasidim*, Germany (1217), no. 723. See also Fred Rosner, *Modern Medicine and Jewish Law*, New York: Yeshiva University Press (1972).

16. *Sefer Chasidim*, nos. 315–318.

17. *Sefer Chasidim*, no. 347.

18. J. David Bleich, "Establishing Criteria of Death," *Tradition* 13:90–113 (1973) at 93.

19. Isaac Jakobovitz, *Jewish Medical Ethics*, New York: Bloch Publishing

Co. (1975), at 121, no. 18 citing Joshua Falk, *Perishah, Yoreh Deah* 339:5; cf. *Yoreh Deah* 339:2.

20. Freehof, *Reform Responsa*, 119–120.

21. *Id.*

22. Alan J. Weisbard, "On the Bioethics of Jewish Law: The Case of Karen Quinlan," *Israel L. Rev.* 14:337–368 (1979).

23. Freehof, *Reform Responsa*.

24. Seymour Siegel, "Updating the Criteria of Death," *Conservative Judaism* 30:34 (1976).

Alan J. Weisbard, J.D., and Mark Siegler, M.D.

11   On Killing Patients with Kindness: An Appeal for Caution

The powerful rhetoric of "death with dignity" has gained much intellectual currency and increasing practical import in recent years.[1] Beginning as a plea for more humane and individualized treatment in the face of the sometimes cold and impersonal technological imperatives of modern medicine, this rhetoric brought needed attention to the plight of dying patients not wishing to "endure the unendurable."[2] It has prompted legal and clinical changes empowering such patients (and sometimes their representatives) to assert some control over the manner, if not the fact, of their dying. The "death with dignity" movement has now advanced to a new frontier: the termination or withdrawal of fluids and nutritional support.

The increasing acceptability in respected forums of proposals to permit avoidable deaths by dehydration or malnutrition—proposals which, a few years ago, would almost certainly have been repudiated by the medical community as medically objectionable, legally untenable, and morally unthinkable—is evidenced by a slew of recent contributions to the medical and bioethics literature,[3] by a sprinkling of court decisions,[4] and, indeed, by the existence of the very conference that led to this volume. This new stream of emerging opinion, supporting the explicit ethical and legal legitimation of this practice, is typically couched in comforting language of caution and compassion, by persons of undoubted sincerity and good faith. But the underlying analysis is, we fear, unlikely to long remain within these cautious bounds.

Careful scrutiny suggests what is ultimately at stake in this controversy: that for an increasing number of incompetent patients, the benefits of continued life are perceived as insufficient to justify the burden and cost of care; that death is viewed as the desired outcome; and—critically—that the role of the health care professional is to participate in bringing this outcome about. Fearful that this development bodes ill for patients, health care professionals, the patient-physician relationship, and other vital societal values, we feel compelled to speak out against the all-too-rapid acceptance of withdrawal of fluids or nutritional supports as accepted or standard medical practice. While recognizing that particular health care professionals, for reasons of compassion and conscience and with full knowledge of the personal legal risks involved, may on occasion elect to discontinue fluids and nutritional support, we nonetheless believe that such actions should generally be proscribed, pending much fuller debate and discussion than has yet taken place.

QUALIFICATIONS

We do not intend to address here the deep philosophic issues posed by the moral status of the permanently unconscious. There is much philosophic dispute concerning whether the permanently unconscious are living persons who possess rights and interests, whether the obligation of care fully extends to such patients, and whether such patients should and eventually will be encompassed within a broadened understanding of brain death. The present authors take somewhat different views on these questions and present no joint position here on the withdrawal of fluids and nutritional support from patients reliably diagnosed as permanently unconscious.

Nor is our principal concern with decisions by competent, adult, terminally ill patients who contemporaneously or through advance directives (living wills, durable powers of attorney, or carefully considered, reliably witnessed, oral statements) direct that their process of dying not be prolonged through such techniques as those required to maintain life-sustaining nourishment and hydration. We encourage fuller discussion of these issues among patients, families and medical professionals at a time the patient is able to participate in an informed and thoughtful fashion. We caution only that patients should be made aware that some "artificial" techniques may be useful in making them more comfortable and in easing the dying process, and should not be rejected unthinkingly by those seeking a more "natural" death. Further, as the much publicized case of Elizabeth Bouvia[5] reminds us, neither physicians nor health care institutions may be compelled to assist in, or to preside over, the suicides of patients, especially those who are not terminally ill.

Nor, finally, do we mean to be understood as necessarily advocating the use of that modality of providing hydration or nutritional support considered most likely to extend survival time maximally without regard to other relevant factors, including the intrusiveness of the technology to the patient in comparison with plausible alternatives or the nature and likelihood of serious side effects. Our position is intended as neither vitalist nor absolutist, except with regard to our insistence on providing sufficient assistance to preclude painful hunger or thirst and to avoid directly causing death (as perceived by health care professionals and the wider society) by failing to provide food and water minimally necessary to preclude death by starvation or dehydration.

CRITIQUE

Our focus, then, is primarily on the withdrawal of fluids and nutrition from patients possessing the capacity for consciousness who have not competently rejected such support. While concerns may seem premature in light of the qualifications and thoughtful discussions of both substantive and procedural safeguards expressed in several recent contributions to the literature,[6] we remain troubled that the underlying analysis, once accepted by clinicians and courts, will not long be confined within the limits initially set forth.

What, then, is the underlying analysis, and why do we find it so potentially troubling? The argument rests on the dual propositions that, first, the provision of fluids and nutritional support by "artificial" means constitutes "medical interventions guided by considerations similar to those governing other treatment methods,"[7] and that, second, judgments regarding the withdrawal of such interventions should be based on calculations of the "burdens and benefits" associated with the treatment (sometimes also referred to as "proportionality"). These propositions are rooted in the work of the President's Commission for the Study of Ethical Problems in Medicine,[8] were adopted by the California appellate court in the *Barber* and *Nejdl*[9] case, and play a central role in the analyses set forth by several recent commentators.[10]

We do not dispute that the "benefits and burdens" formulation is useful in a number of contexts and marks a clear analytic improvement over unconsidered references to "extraordinary measures" or "artificial means," terms which have introduced much unnecessary confusion and provide little real assistance in decision-making. What we find troublesome is the assertion that physicians, families, courts, or other third parties can properly conclude that the "burdens" of withdrawal of fluids and nutrition—a generally unconvincing catalogue of potential "complications" or "side effects"—outweigh the benefit, sustaining life. (We recognize that, in rare cases, the provision of fluids and, particularly, nutritional support may be medically futile or counterproductive in sustaining life, and we do not here recommend that such futile or counterproductive steps be mandated.)

Advocates of withdrawing fluids and nutritional support that are effective in, and necessary for, sustaining life justify their position by arguing that a speedy and painless death is in the patient's "best interests" (a claim with little foundation in existing law, which has traditionally viewed the preservation of life, at least for noncomatose patients, as a core component of "best interests"). While the argument is compassionately made, and may be persuasive in certain cases, it fails to acknowledge explicitly that its objective may be attained more swiftly, more directly, more honestly, through the administration of lethal injections. Homicide is, in this setting, the ultimate analgesic. But to the extent active euthanasia is rejected— we think wisely—by existing law and medical ethics, we believe a similar conclusion is generally mandated for withdrawal of fluids and nutrition, and for much the same reasons.

If active euthanasia has found little support thus far in either medical or legal circles, the reasons are not confined to an exclusive concern with prolonging the life of the patient. The courts have made clear that respirators and dialysis machines are not legally mandated in all cases of respiratory or renal failure, even where their withdrawal is thought likely to result in death. In this sense, the withdrawal of fluids and nutrition is subject to a similar analysis. But in another and—we believe—more powerful sense, the result is quite different, at least in terms of our society's moral perceptions and self-image.

Withdrawal of respirators and dialysis machines can be seen, and *is* seen and emotionally understood, as the removal of artificial impediments to "letting nature take its course." Death can be understood in such cases as the natural result of the disease process. In cases where death may indeed be the desired (and ultimately unavoidable) outcome, it can be allowed to come without imposing a heavy burden of guilt and moral responsibility on physicians or family members for acting to bring it about, and without challenging important social barriers against killing.[11] And sometimes, as in the case of Karen Quinlan, nature can surprise us: the patient can survive despite some experts' predictions to the contrary.

The case of withdrawing fluids and nutritional supports is different in critical respects. Although the techniques for providing such supports may be medical, and thus logically associated with other medical interventions, the underlying obligations of providing food and drink to those who hunger or thirst transcend the medical context, summoning up deep human responses of caring, of nurturing, of human connectedness, and of human community. Social scientists and humanists have only begun to explore the deeper social meanings and ramifications of depriving patients of "food and water," of permitting deaths from starvation or dehydration. While sophisticated observers may argue that the image of "starvation" or "thirst" may be misleading in the cases of some patients, particularly the unconscious, or that limited nutritional intake may slow the progress of a cancer, it is far from clear that such explanations will be compelling to the public, or even, perhaps, to many members of the health professions, particularly if the practice of withholding fluids and nutritional supports takes root and is applied to an ever broader class of patients.

Further, unlike withdrawal of respirators or dialysis machines, withdrawal of fluids and nutrition cannot so readily be seen as "letting nature take its course." Dehydration or lack of nutrition become the direct cause of death for which moral responsibility cannot be avoided. The psychological and social ramifications of bringing death about in this fashion will, in our view, be difficult or impossible to distinguish from those accompanying lethal injections or other modes of active euthanasia. There will be no surprises: withdrawal of all food and water from helpless patients must necessarily result in their deaths.

Given the demographic trends in our society—the dramatically increasing pool of those characterized as the "superannuated, chronically ill, physically marginal elderly," those Daniel Callahan has labeled "the biologically tenacious"—denial of fluids and nutrition may well become "the nontreatment of choice."[12] The process is tellingly illustrated by two recent court cases. Clarence Herbert, the patient whose death gave rise to the homicide prosecution in *Barber*, was initially understood, at least by his wife, to be brain dead. In fact, Herbert was comatose but not brain dead, although the quickness of diagnosis and the subsequent nontreatment decisions led to some troubling questions of the adequacy of both diagnosis and prognosis. The sequence of decisions is instructive. First the respirator was removed. When Herbert failed to succumb as predicted, intravenous feeding was discontinued. Only then—a week later—did Herbert "comply" with the course desired, and expire.[13]

Similarly, in the *Conroy* case, the patient's nephew had previously refused to authorize surgery for his aunt's gangrene.[14] When that condition proved not to be terminal the nephew apparently expressed his disinclination to authorize other life-extending measures.[15] Only when this decision failed to bring about the desired result—death—did the nephew and physicians contemplate the next step: termination of fluids and nutrition supplied by nasogastric tube.

Both these cases illustrate a troubling dynamic, one much like a self-fulfilling prophecy. Once a determination has been reached—perhaps for understandable and humanitarian reasons—that death is the desired outcome, decision-makers become increasingly less troubled by the choice of means to be employed to achieve that outcome. The line between "allowing to die" and "actively killing" can be elusive, and we are skeptical that any logical or psychological distinction between "allowing to die" by starvation and actively killing, as by lethal injection, will prove viable. If we as a society are to retain the prohibition against active killing, the admittedly wavering line demarcating permissible "allowings to die" must exclude death by avoidable starvation. We frankly acknowledge that our concern here extends beyond a solicitude for the outcome for the patient to include our fears for the impact of decisions and actions on family members, health care professionals, and societal values, which will survive the death of the patient. If these separate and additional concerns are to be discounted, we are hard pressed to understand the remaining justifications for prohibition of active euthanasia in the perceived "best interests" of the incompetent patient.

We have witnessed too much history to disregard how easily society disvalues the lives of the "unproductive"—the retarded, the disabled, the senile, the institutionalized, the elderly—of those who in another time and place were referred to as "useless eaters."[16] The confluence of the emerging stream of medical and ethical opinion favoring legitimation of withholding fluids and nutrition with the torrent of public and governmental concern over the costs of medical care (and the looming imposition of cost-containment strategies which may well impose significant financial penalties on the prolonged care of the impaired elderly) powerfully reinforces our discomfort. In the current environment, it may well prove convenient—and all too easy—to move from recognition of an individual's "right to die" (to us, an unfortunate rephrasing of the legally more limited right to refuse medical treatment) to a climate enforcing a socially obligatory "duty to die," preferably quickly and cheaply.[17] The recent suggestions that all new applicants for Medicare be provided copies of "living wills" or similar documents illustrate how this process may unfold.[18] Our concern here is not with the encouragement of patient self-determination regarding medical care, including decisions about dying, which we vigorously support, but rather with the incorporation of such strategies *as a method of cost control*.

Finally, we would urge that efforts in this field be rechanneled from demonstrating that some patients' quality of life is too poor, too "meaningless," to justify the burdens of continued life, toward the challenge of finding better ways to improve the comfort and quality of life of such patients. In particular, we hope the current debate will stimulate further discussion of the comparative merits of different modalities of providing fluids and nutrition. For example, with the development of endoscopic placement techniques for gastrostomy tubes, this superficially more invasive "surgical" procedure may prove safer and more comfortable for many patients than the nonsurgical insertion of nasogastric tubes, which are sometimes a source of continuing discomfort for patients and are more likely to elicit the use of restraints to prevent the deliberate or accidental removal of the tubes. More attention must be paid to the clinical, institutional, economic, and legal implications of these and other alternatives.

CONCLUSION

When coupled with powerful economic forces and with the disturbing tendency, both among professionals and in the broader society, to disvalue the lives of the "unproductive," the compassionate call for withdrawing or withholding fluids and nutrition in a few, selected cases bears the seeds of great potential abuse. Little is to be lost, and much potentially gained, by slowing down the process of legitimation, taking stock of where we have come and where we are going, improving our methods of comforting and caring for the dying without necessarily hurrying to dispatch them on their way, and deferring any premature legal, ethical, or professional approval and legitimation of this new course. The movement for "death with dignity" arose in response to deficiencies on the caring side of medicine; it would be sadly ironic if this latest manifestation served to undercut the image of physician as caring and nurturing servant and to undermine deep human values of caring and nurturance throughout society.

NOTES

1. Portions of this paper appeared, in a somewhat different form, in Mark Siegler and Alan J. Weisbard, "Against the Emerging Stream: Should Fluids and Nutritional Support Be Discontinued?" *Arch. Intern. Med.* 145:129–132 (January 1985).

2. *In re Quinlan*, 70 N.J. 10, 355 A.2d 647, *cert. denied*, 429 U.S. 922, 97 S. Ct. 319, 50 L. Ed. 2d 289 (1976).

3. See, e.g., David W. Meyers, "Legal Aspects of Withdrawing Nourishment from an Incurably Ill Patient," *Arch. Intern. Med.* 145:125–128 (January 1985); Rebecca S. Dresser, and Eugene V. Boisaubin, Jr., "Ethics, Law and Nutritional Support," *Arch. Intern. Med.* 145:122–124 (January 1985); Joanne Lynn and James F. Childress, "Must Patients Always Be Given Food and Water?" *Hastings Cent. Rep.* 13:17–21 (October 1983) reprinted as chapter 5 *supra.*; S. H. Wanzer et. al., "The Physician's Responsibility Toward Hopelessly Ill Patients," *N. Engl. J. Med.* 310:955–959 (1984).

4. *Barber v. Superior Court of the State of California*, 195 Cal. Rptr. 484 (Cal. App. 2 Dist. 1983); *In re* Conroy, 98 N.J. 321, 486 A.2d 1209 (1985). *In the Matter of Mary Hier*, 18 Mass. App. 200, 464 N.E.2d 959, *app. den.*, 392 Mass. 1102 (1984).

5. *Bouvia v. County of Riverside*, Superior Ct. of St. of Calif., Riverside County, No. 159780 (1984).

6. See note 3, *supra*.

7. Lynn and Childress, *supra* note 3, at 18.

8. President's Commission for the Study of Ethical Problems in Medicine and Biomedical and Behavioral Research, *Deciding to Forego Life-Sustaining Treatment*, Washington, D.C.: U.S. Government Printing Office (1983).

9. See note 4, *supra*.

10. See note 3, *supra*.

11. See generally, Alan J. Weisbard, "On the Bioethics of Jewish Law: The Case of Karen Quinlan," *Israel L. Rev.* 14:337–368 (1979); Robert A. Burt, "Authorizing Death for Anomalous Newborns," in Aubrey Milunsky and George J. Annas (eds.), *Genetics and the Law* (1975); Robert A. Burt, "The Ideal of Community in the Work of the President's Commission," *Cardozo L. Rev.* 6:267–286 (1985).

12. Daniel Callahan, "On Feeding the Dying," *Hastings Cent. Rep.* 13:22 (October 1983).

13. See *Barber*, *supra* note 4, and Bonnie Steinbock, "The Removal of Mr. Herbert's Feeding Tube," *Hastings Cent. Rep.* 13:13–16 (October 1983).

14. *Conroy*, *supra* note 4.

15. Personal communications to author.

16. The reference is to the Nazi euthanasia program. While the authors have been unable to locate an explicit reference to "useless eaters," Nazi usage of the phrase "useless mouths" is documented by Nora Levin, *The Holocaust: The Destruction of European Jewry: 1933–1945* New York: Schocken (1968), 302.

17. Recent remarks on "the duty to die" attributed to Colorado Governor Richard Lamm are illustrative. *New York Times*, March 29, 1984 at A16, col. 5.

18. Proceedings of the House of Delegates, American Medical Association 133rd Annual Meeting, June 1984 at 177 (commenting on recommendations of Advisory Council on Social Security).

Dan W. Brock, Ph.D.

12 Forgoing Life-Sustaining Food and Water: Is It Killing?

The moral permissibility of patients forgoing life-sustaining medical treatment has come to be widely accepted. The issue of forgoing life-sustaining food and water, however, has only very recently gained attention in public policy discussions. One source of resistance to extending this acceptance of a general right to forgo life-sustaining treatment to the case of food and water has explicitly philosophical origins: for a physician to withhold food and water might seem to be not merely to allow the patient to die, but to kill the patient, and therefore wrong. A closely related moral worry is that for physicians to withhold food and water would be to make them the direct cause of their patients' deaths, which also would be wrong. And finally, many worry that providing food and water is ordinary care, not extraordinary or "heroic," and so must be obligatory.

In each case, a distinction is drawn—between killing and allowing to die, causing or not causing death, and withholding ordinary or extraordinary care—and in each case it is claimed that the former, though not the latter, is morally forbidden. I consider appeal to the intrinsic moral importance of these distinctions to be confused, both in general and as applied to food and water. In the hope of reducing the impact of these moral confusions in the policy debate about forgoing food and water, I will address here both the general meaning and the putative moral importance of these distinctions, as well as their specific application to the case of food and water. The upshot of my argument will be that forgoing food and water does not fall under any special moral prohibitions that would make it in itself morally different than the forgoing of other life-sustaining medical care. I believe that a competent patient has the moral right to forgo any life-sustaining treatment, including food and water. If the patient is incompetent, as is usually the case when forgoing food and water is seriously at issue, the surrogate's decision should reflect what the patient would have wanted if competent, or, in the absence of knowledge of the patient's preferences, reflect an assessment of the benefits and burdens to the patient.

I. KILLING AND ALLOWING TO DIE

Is it killing to forgo food and water? And why is that thought to be important? Since forgoing food and water is obviously behavior leading to death and is known to be such at the time it is done, why is it thought important to ask whether it is killing?

There is a common view, among physicians and much of the general public, that physicians can allow patients to die by stopping life-sustaining treatment, but they cannot kill patients. In this view, killing is wrong, and it occurs in the medical context only as a result of accident or negligence. This is to use the concept of killing normatively, to capture in the category of killings only wrongful actions leading to death. Physicians do, however, stop life-supporting treatments frequently in medical contexts, and rightly believe that they are generally justified in doing so. If they believe that killing is wrong, and occurs in medical contexts only as a result of accident or negligence, then they have a strong motive for interpreting what they do when they stop life support as allowing the patient to die, but not as killing.

I think this interpretation of all stopping of life support as allowing to die is problematic and leads in turn to worries about whether stopping life support is morally justified. Let me, therefore, address directly what the difference is between killing and allowing to die. I will offer two interpretations of that difference: on the first, most stopping of food and water—and of other life-sustaining treatments—will turn out to be killing; on the second, allowing to die.

In the first interpretation, the distinction between killing and allowing to die is the distinction between acts and omissions leading to or resulting in death. When I kill someone, I act in a way that causes that person to die when they would not otherwise have died in that way and at that time. When I allow someone to die, I omit to act in a way that I could have acted and that would have prevented that person dying then; that is, I have both the ability and the opportunity to act to prevent the death, but fail to do so.

Now suppose that the difference between killing and allowing to die is understood as we have just described it. Consider the case of ceasing respirator support: the respirator is turned off and the patient dies. Suppose this is done by a physician who believes it to be justified and who does it with the patient's consent. The patient may have asked to be allowed to die and may understand what is done as allowing him or her to die. But according to this first interpretation of the difference between killing and allowing to die, what the physician has done is to kill the patient, since in turning off the respirator he or she has acted in a way that causes the patient to die in that way and at that time. Now, is that mistaken? Is it mistaken to say that, by turning off the respirator, the physician killed the patient? Physicians, at least, do not commonly understand what they do when they turn off burdensome respirators with patients' consent as killing the patients.

To help see that this might be correctly construed as killing, consider the case of a nephew who, impatient for his uncle to die so that he can inherit the uncle's money, turns off the uncle's respirator. In this case, I think most would understand the nephew to have killed his uncle. We would take it as a piece of sophistry if the nephew defended himself by replying, "No, I merely allowed my uncle to die," or, "I didn't kill my uncle; it was the underlying disease requiring the use of a respirator that killed him."

The difference in the two cases, in my view, is not in *what* the physician as opposed to the nephew does. It is not a difference between killing and allowing to die. The difference is the presence of other morally important factors, most obviously the difference in motivations of the nephew and the physician, as well as whether the patient consented to the respirator being stopped. The difference is not that one and not the other kills, but that one and not the other kills justifiably.

Thus, if the difference between killing and allowing to die is interpreted in terms of the difference between acts and omissions resulting in death, it would seem that when one stops a life-sustaining treatment like a respirator expecting that a patient will die as a result, one thereby kills the patient. My examples also suggest that in some cases one does so with justification, in others not. But is this difference between killing and allowing to die of moral importance? Does the mere difference that one kills in one case, allows to die in the other, *in itself* make the one any more or less morally justified, or wrong, than the other?

Consider the following case:

A patient is dying from terminal cancer, undergoing great suffering that cannot be relieved without so sedating him that he is unable to relate in any way to others. This patient prepared an advance directive in an early stage of his disease indicating that in circumstances like this he wished to have his life ended either by direct means or by withdrawing life-sustaining treatment. In a recent lucid moment he reaffirmed the directive. The attending physician and the patient's family are in agreement that the patient's desire to die ought now to be granted.

Now consider two alternative conclusions to this case. In the first, while the patient is deeply sedated and not conscious, his wife places a pillow over his face and he dies peacefully from asphyxiation. In the second, while the patient is deeply sedated and not conscious, he develops severe respiratory difficulty requiring emergency professional intervention and use of a respirator if he is to live. His wife knows this, is present, and decides not to call the professional staff and thereby not to employ the respirator. Her goal is to allow him to die. The patient dies peacefully.

Suppose we still understand the difference between killing and allowing to die in terms of acts and omissions resulting in death. In the first outcome, the patient is killed by his spouse, while in the second outcome, the spouse decides not to treat or not to seek treatment and thereby allows him to die. Is there any reason why what the wife does in the first instance is morally (as opposed to legally) worse or different from what she does in the second instance? If not, then what one does if one kills is *in itself* no worse morally than if one allows to die. Of course a particular act of killing may be worse, when other features of the action are considered, than a particular allowing to die. But so also some allowings to die may be morally worse, all things considered, than some killings. And if the mere fact that in one case a person kills, in another allows to die, is not itself a difference of moral significance, then it is also not morally important whether stopping a respirator is interpreted as killing or as allowing to die. Some instances of killing and of allowing to die will be morally wrong; some of each will be morally justified. That what one does is to kill or to allow to die will usually count as a moral reason against doing it; which it is considered to be, however, will not make what one does more or less justified or wrong. Other factors, such as whether the patient consents, and what sort of life could otherwise be offered, will morally differentiate particular killings and allowings to die.[1]

The act/omission difference is the first interpretation of how killing differs from allowing to die, and on that interpretation, as I have briefly argued, killing is not morally worse in itself than allowing to die. There remains, nevertheless, strong resistance to accepting that physicians kill when they stop life-sustaining treatment, as follows on the act/omission interpretation. I have already noted one reason for this resistance: if killing is understood as a normative category, referring only to wrongful actions leading to death, then physicians quite justifiably do not want to understand what they do as killing and therefore wrongful when they stop life-sustaining treatment. They are quite correct that it need not be morally wrong.

There is a second reason for resistance to understanding stopping life-support treatment as killing, and that is a different interpretation of the difference between killing and allowing to die. Very loosely, the distinction is this. If you kill someone, what you do is to initiate a deadly causal process that leads to the person's death. If you allow someone to die, you allow a deadly causal process which you did not initiate to proceed to its result of a person's death.[2] One way to allow to die is simply to omit to act in a way that would have prevented the death. That is an allowing to die on the act/omission understanding of the killing/allowing to die distinction. But another way to allow to die is to *act* in a way that allows some deadly causal process, which at present is halted, to follow out its course so as to result in death.

Let me say a little bit more about this second way of allowing to die, since it is essential to the common understanding of stopping life support as allowing to die. Why does a physician who stops a respirator allow a patient to die in this account of allowing to die? There is a life-sustaining process in place—the respirator. There is a deadly disease process present which requires the use of a life-sustaining respirator, and which is, in effect, being held in abeyance by the use of the respirator. By the positive action of turning off the respirator, the physician then stops that life-sustaining process and allows the deadly disease process to proceed; the physician thereby allows the patient, as it is often put, to die of the underlying disease. Now, in this account of the killing/allowing to die distinction, the physician does allow the patient to die when there is an independent underlying disease process which is being held in abeyance and the physician takes positive action to remove the system which is holding that underlying disease process in abeyance.

But what about our earlier greedy nephew? In this account of allowing to die, doesn't he too, like the physician, allow to die? Doesn't he do the same as the physician does, though with different motives? He too merely allows the disease process to proceed to conclusion. Proponents of this second interpretation of the kill/allow to die distinction will be hard pressed to avoid accepting that the nephew allows to die, though they can add that he does so unjustifiably. Some will take this implication for the greedy nephew case to show that this second interpretation of the kill/allow to die difference is not preferable to the first act/omission interpretation after all.

There is not space here to argue that the difference between killing and allowing to die on this second interpretation of the distinction also lacks moral importance. I believe that is so, and that pairs of examples similar to the one cited above for the act/omission interpretation can be constructed to show that.

With these two interpretations of the killing/allowing to die distinction now before us, we are finally in a position to consider whether forgoing food and water is killing. Suppose that a decision has been made not to feed a patient and that the choice has been made according to sound procedures and in circumstances in which all concerned agree this course is morally justified. All further feedings are omitted and the patient dies of dehydration or malnutrition. But then the question is raised whether what was done killed the patient or allowed him to die. Since we have already noted more than one interpretation of that difference, we know the question is more complex than it might seem. On the act/omission interpretation of the difference, since we have said that feedings were omitted, it would seem that the patient was allowed to die. On the other hand, if, for example, IV's were in place and a physician had to take positive action to remove them, it would seem we then have an action leading to death, and so a killing. This shows the difficulty in practice of applying the kill/allow to die distinction in its act/omission interpretation. But it also displays the lack of any moral significance in this difference between killing and allowing to die. Suppose that just before the physician enters the patient's room to remove the IV, it falls out on its own, and upon seeing this the physician then deliberately omits to reinsert it so that the patient may die. Could there really be any moral importance attached to whether the physician removes the IV or fails to reinsert it in this case?

To think of omitting to feed the patient as allowing him to die is in keeping with common understandings of related cases. Suppose you consciously omit to send food to persons whom you know are starving in a famine in some distant land. The famine victims die. No one would say that you killed them by not sending food, but rather that you allowed them to die (whether or not you were morally wrong to have done so). Why do some persons, nevertheless, want to use the more active concept of killing and to say that one kills by denying food and water in the medical context? One reason lies in the confusion of thinking that one more strongly morally condemns what is done by calling it killing. If I am correct that killing is in itself no worse than allowing to die, but instead other factors morally differentiate actual killings and allowings to die, then withholding feeding is no worse morally for being killing instead of allowing to die.

There is a second reason why some persons might understand denying food and water to a patient as killing, and it reveals a further complexity in our moral thinking about this issue. I think the clue here is found in the naturalness of speaking of *denying* food and water to the patient. To speak in terms of denying food and water is implicitly to assume that giving food and water in a medical context of patient care is the expected course of events. It is seen as statistically expected, as what is standardly done, or, perhaps at least as important, as what is morally required. It is assumed that the statistically and morally expected course of events is that patients will be given the basic care of food and water, that this is part of the health care professional's moral obligation to care for the patient.

If so, then if some patient is not to receive food and water, someone must actively intervene to stop this normal course of events. The decision to omit to give food and water is seen as an active intervention in the normal caring process, making death occur when it would not otherwise have occurred. And so this positive decision not to feed, even if resulting in an omission to feed, is seen as killing. It is important to understand, however, that this line of reasoning gains its plausibility from standard cases in which the patient is able to eat and drink in normal ways and is clearly benefited by being provided with food and fluids. In those cases, providing food and fluids is both statistically and morally expected. In other cases, however, providing food and fluids requires sophisticated medical procedures, for example, total parenteral nutrition, and may not be of benefit to the patient; then, the assumption that feeding is either statistically or morally expected may be unwarranted. But without that assumption, omitting to feed should not be understood as an active denial of nutrition and therefore as killing.[3]

Some commentators have cited a further reason why stopping feeding, unlike stopping most other forms of life-sustaining treatment, is not allowing to die on the second interpretation I offered above of the killing/allowing to die difference.[4] In that interpretation, we allow to die when, by act or omission, we allow a deadly disease process that is being held in abeyance by a life-sustaining treatment to proceed to death. For example, when a respirator is withdrawn, the patient is allowed to die of the underlying disease requiring use of a respirator. But when food and water are withheld, it is said, we introduce a *new* process—that of dehydration or malnutrition—which will result in death. The patient dies from this new causal process we introduce, not from any already present fatal disease process that was being held in abeyance by a life-sustaining treatment. We thereby kill the patient. However, this line of reasoning appears to be mistaken.

Whenever a disease process attacks a patient's normal ability to eat and drink, and artificial means of providing nutrition are required, then feeding by artificial means can be seen as a form of life-sustaining treatment. Forgoing feeding when IV's, nasogastric tubes, and so forth, are required is then to forgo employment of a life-sustaining treatment—artificial provision of nutrition—and to allow the patient to die from a disease that has impaired his normal ability to eat and drink. It would seem to be only when the patient's normal human ability to take in nutrition is unimpaired, and a decision is then made not to sustain life and so to stop feeding, that a new fatal process is introduced as opposed to withdrawing a life-sustaining treatment and letting the disease process proceed to death. The vast majority of cases of forgoing food and fluids in the medical context are of the former sort, and so constitute allowing to die, not killing, on the second interpretation of that distinction.

Let me summarize my discussion up to here, since the analysis has become rather complicated. (In my defense, I believe that this complexity is not merely the result of philosophers making simple matters appear complex, but arises instead from existing complexities and confusions in common, nonphilosophical thinking on these issues.) Does one kill, or does one allow to die, by forgoing food and water? On the act/omission interpretation of the difference between killing and allowing to die, one kills if the forgoing involves a positive action to stop feeding, allows to die if one only omits to feed. In cases in which the expected course of events is feeding, any forgoing of feeding, even if it results in an omission to feed, can be seen as actively intervening to change that course of events, and so as killing; however, in many actual forgoings of food and fluids it cannot be assumed that feeding is either the statistically or the morally expected course of events. I have also argued that the difference between killing and allowing to die on its act/omission interpretation is of no moral importance, and so whether forgoing food and water is in any instance morally justified will turn entirely on other matters than whether it is killing as opposed to allowing to die.

In the second interpretation of the kill/allow to die difference, stopping a life-support system like a respirator is understood as allowing the patient to die from the underlying disease process held in abeyance by the respirator. But to forgo food and water is generally to stop the life-sustaining artificial provision of nutrition and to allow the patient to die of the underlying disease process that has impaired his normal human ability to eat and drink; thus, it too is usually to allow to die. However, I have also suggested, though not argued, that, on this second interpretation as well, whether any instance of forgoing food and water is morally justified turns entirely on other questions than whether it is killing as opposed to allowing to die.

II. CAUSE OF DEATH

I turn now to a related confusion in much discussion of forgoing
life-sustaining treatment that concerns a different aspect of the issue
about the cause of death than that discussed above. It is related
because many persons hold that to stop a life-support process such
as feeding is to kill, because one directly causes the patient's death;
whereas, when one allows to die, it is the underlying disease process,
not the physician, that causes the patient's death.

Questions of causality are exceedingly difficult and complex, but
I will try at least briefly to illuminate two important confusions
about causing death prominent in discussions about life-sustaining
treatment generally, and relevant to forgoing food and water in particular. Consider what can be called a "but-for" sense of causality:
but for this, that wouldn't have occurred; but for Jones poisoning
the food Smith later ate, Smith would not have died. Consider our
greedy nephew again. But for his turning off the respirator, his uncle
wouldn't have died: the nephew, therefore, causes the uncle's death.
As I suggested above, it would be absurd for the nephew to assert,
"No, not I but the underlying disease caused my uncle's death."
Now consider the physician who seemingly does the same thing and
stops the patient's respirator: he too satisfies the "but-for" condition
for the patient's death. But for the physician's stopping the respirator,
the patient would not have died; the physician causes the patient's
death. Finally, consider stopping feeding. But for that, the patient
would not have died; the physician's withholding food and water
causes the patient's death.

What I have called a "but-for" sense of causality is *not* by itself
an adequate account of ordinary attributions of causality. There, one
who kills another (e.g., by giving poisoned food) is considered the
cause of the other's death, whereas one who allows another to die
(e.g., by not providing food to a famine victim) is not generally said
to have caused the other's death. The point is that the broader "but
for" sense of causality seems to provide the necessary control over
the outcomes of what a person does ("does" interpreted broadly to
include both acts and omissions) to allow ascription of at least prima
facie moral responsibility to the person for the outcomes. And the
"but for" causality condition for the death is satisfied both when
one kills and when one allows to die, and equally by the greedy

nephew, the physician stopping the respirator, and the physician stopping feeding. Why then should we mark any moral difference in these cases because of supposed causal differences when the "but for" sense of causality is equally satisfied in all of them?

I will consider two responses to my claim that there is no morally important causal difference in these cases, each of which, I think, brings out something interesting about causing death, and about why causal talk is often confusing in this area. The first response is associated with talk of "merely prolonging the dying process," and goes like this: If a patient is terminally ill, then a physician who stops the patient's life-sustaining treatment neither kills nor allows him to die. The physician doesn't kill him; rather, the fatal disease does (more on this shortly). Nor does the physician allow him to die, because to allow someone to die it has to be possible for you to save the person; if the patient is terminally ill, you couldn't save him. So on this response, there's nothing the physician does that causes death, nothing that but for doing it the patient would live. There is more than one confusion in this response. Surely one *can* either kill or not save a terminally ill person. When one either kills or allows to die, what one does causes death in the "but-for" sense of causality. This can only mean that one causes a patient to die *at a particular time* (and, to avoid certain complications of causal overdetermination, in a particular way). No one ever prevents someone's death completely, without any qualifications to its being at a particular time (or in a particular way), because we can't make anyone immortal. What we do is to make or allow death to occur earlier than it otherwise would have done, and in that sense what we do does causally affect the person's death, whether or not the person was terminally ill.

It is worth noting that the claim that a physician is never a "but-for" cause of the patient's death would not help in some important cases of stopping food and water even if it was itself sound. I have in mind, especially, permanently unconscious patients who are usually not terminally ill in any plausible sense of "terminally ill." These patients can, and often do, survive for many years in that state. This ought to give some pause to the many commentators who seem prepared to agree that stopping food and water, or for that matter stopping other life-sustaining treatment, can only be justified if the patient is terminally ill.[5] If one believes, as I do, that stopping life-sustaining treatment, including food and water, can be morally permissible with permanently unconscious patients, then one should not endorse a restriction to stopping that treatment only with terminally ill patients.

Let me turn to a second response to my suggestions that it is a broad "but-for" sense of causality that is relevant to moral responsibility for outcomes, and that on this account physicians *do* cause death when they stop life-sustaining food and water or respirators. Consider the legal inquiry into the patient's cause of death. In the case of stopping a life-sustaining respirator, the cause of death would commonly be identified as the underlying disease which resulted in death once the patient was taken off the respirator. Doesn't this suggest that I am mistaken in identifying the physician and what he does as causing death? I think not, and that is because the inquiry into the cause of death is somewhat more complex than it may look at first. It is not simply an empirical inquiry into what conditions played a causal role in the death. It is in part an empirical or factual inquiry of this sort, but it is shaped as well by normative concerns; these are legal concerns when it is a legal inquiry, moral concerns when it is a moral inquiry.

The inquiry into the cause of death is, roughly, something like this: We take all the factors which are "but-for" causes, but for these factors the patient would not have died in that way and at that time. There will be a great many such factors, and we do not actually assemble them all, but rather restrict our selection of the cause from among them. On what basis do we select *the* cause of death from among all the "but-for" causes? We do not do it solely on empirical or factual grounds, we also consider normative grounds. We ask, for example, in the legal inquiry: Among the "but-for" causes, is there anyone who acted in a legally prohibited role with whom the law then wants to concern itself? And we can ask an analogous question in a moral inquiry: Among the "but-for" causes, is there anyone whose action was morally impermissible? This helps to explain "cause of death talk" in our earlier two cases in which respirators were stopped by a physician and by a greedy nephew. The action of each is a "but-for" cause of the patient's death. The physician's action, however, is within a legally protected role. He acts in accordance with a competent patient's right to refuse even life-sustaining treatment, and so the law does not single him out for further concern when he stops the respirator. The greedy nephew, on the other hand, acts in a legally prohibited role, since (among other things) he acted without the patient's consent, and so the law is concerned further with him. This difference is reflected in our holding the greedy nephew to be the cause of death, while in the case of the physician who also stopped a life-sustaining respirator, the patient's underlying disease is held to be the cause of death.[6]

If this is correct, then it should be no surprise that there is uncertainty and controversy about whether the physician who withholds food and water is the cause of the patient's death. That is a reflection of the uncertainty and controversy that exists about whether stopping food and water is legally and/or morally permissible. If we reach greater agreement on those questions, then it will become clearer whether the physician who stops food and water should be held to be *the* cause of the patient's death. But then it will be the legal and moral permissibility helping determine what or who is *the* cause of death, not whether the physician is the cause being a determinant of legal and moral permissibility.

III. "ORDINARY" AND "EXTRAORDINARY" TREATMENT

I turn finally to the distinction between ordinary and extraordinary or heroic treatment. Those who employ this distinction usually understand the provision of extraordinary treatment as optional and the provision of ordinary treatment as obligatory. This distinction is most often employed in the case of incompetent patients unable to decide for themselves about treatment. And it may seem especially important to the stopping of food and water, since if any care is ordinary, food and water would seem to be. But what is the ordinary/extraordinary difference? Some understand it to be the degree to which the treatment is (statistically) usual or unusual; others, the degree of invasiveness of treatment; others, the extent to which sophisticated, high technology or artificial treatment is employed; and so forth.

None of these differences, however, are in themselves morally important differences between treatments which could justify distinguishing some as morally obligatory, others as optional. If we understand extraordinary treatments instead as those excessively burdensome to the patient, then we do have a difference of obvious moral importance (and, I believe, the meaning the distinction had in its origin within Catholic moral theology). But to determine whether any treatment is excessively burdensome, those burdens must be weighed against the benefits of the treatment in order to judge whether the burdens are worth undergoing. In this interpretation, whether a treatment is ordinary or extraordinary is determined by an assessment of its benefits and burdens. And then, contrary to initial appearances, even providing food and water may be extraordinary care in those few cases in which the burdens of doing so exceed the benefits.

The point I want to press is that the classification of treatments as ordinary or extraordinary now is doing no work in the reasoning about whether the treatment may be withheld. What is doing all the work in the reasoning is the assessment of the benefits and burdens of the treatment. Only when that assessment has been made, and the burdens judged excessive given the benefits, do we label the treatment extraordinary. We put the label on after the analysis has been completed, and so the labeling of treatments as ordinary and extraordinary adds nothing to the analysis—except confusion. It adds confusion because the difference is so often understood not in terms of the benefits and burdens of treatment, but in one of the senses I noted earlier such as the usualness or artificiality of treatment. Given these multiple understandings, and the fact that the ordinary/extraordinary difference adds nothing of substance to the reasoning about forgoing life-sustaining treatment, I believe we do best to avoid its use.

CONCLUSIONS

I will conclude with two points. The first is that I believe the ordinary/extraordinary distinction in its "excessively burdensome" interpretation does at least point to the correct reasoning in decisions about forgoing food and water. It directs us to assess whether the benefits to a patient from continuing food and water outweigh the burdens, given that patient's particular circumstances. It is my view that there are at least some few cases where it may be that the burdens do outweigh the benefits.

Second, I want to emphasize that I have focused only on a few of the moral complexities and confusions about forgoing life-sustaining treatment in general and about forgoing life-sustaining food and water in particular. There are other difficult moral issues involved, such as the relevance of the economic cost and of the effects on persons other than the patient of feeding or forgoing feeding, which I have not addressed. Moreover, sound public policy should reflect additional considerations, such as slippery slope worries about abuse, the symbolic importance of providing food and water, and how authorization to deny it may affect our care of other potentially vulnerable populations. My concern here has been only with a few of the underlying moral considerations which ought to inform public policy in this area.

NOTES

1. I discuss and defend the assumptions in this argument from example further in "Taking Human Life," *Ethics* 95:851–865 (1985), from which my example is drawn. Other arguments to the same effect can be found in James Rachels, "Active and Passive Euthanasia," *N. Engl. J. Med.* 292:75–80 (1975); Michael Tooley, "Defense of Abortion and Infanticide," in *The Problem of Abortion,* Joel Feinberg, ed., Belmont, CA: Wadsworth Publishing Co. (1973), at 84–86; and Jonathan Bennett, "Morality and Consequences," in *The Tanner Lectures on Human Value II,* S. M. McMurrin, ed., Salt Lake City: University of Utah Press (1981), at 45–116.

2. The Appellate Court in *Conroy* tried to rely on such a distinction. *In re* Conroy, 464 A.2d 303, 315 (N.J. Super. A.D. 1983).

3. Whether tube feedings are part of expected care is an unsettled issue. See results of a survey of physicians in chapter 4 *supra.* See also an Australian perspective, W. J. Quilty, "Ethics of Extraordinary Nutritional Support," *J. Am. Geriatr. Soc.* 32:12–13 (1984).

4. See, e.g., *In re* Conroy, 90 N.J. Super. 453, 464 A.2d 303 (1983), *rev'd,* 98 N.J. 321, 486 A.2d 1209 (1985).

5. See, e.g., chapter 26.

6. *In re* Bartling, 209 Cal. Rptr. 220 (1984). *In re* Quinlan, 70 N.J. 10, 355 A.2d 647, *cert. denied,* 429 U.S. 922 (1976); and Superintendent of Belchertown State School v. Saikewicz, 373 Mass. 728, 370 N.E.2d 417 (1977).

Part III Perspectives on the Law

Ron M. Landsman, J.D.

13 Terminating Food and Water: Emerging Legal Rules

There is little "law"—that is, definitive determinations by courts or legislatures—on the narrow question of suspending artificial nutrition and hydration for a dying patient.

However, when mechanical nutrition and hydration may be suspended is logically a part of the larger question of when any kind of medical treatment can be withdrawn for a dying patient, which is part of the more general physician-patient relationship that determines who decides what shall be done. The doctrine of informed consent—the patient's right not to be treated without his or her knowing approval—goes a long way toward answering these questions for competent patients. For those who cannot voice their own choices, the resolutions are different but there is familiar legal terrain.

Termination of artificially provided nutrition and hydration may appear to be a new problem. It is not, once the following threshold question has been resolved: Are nutrition and hydration provided by medical means to be considered "medical treatment"? If so, decisions about initiating, withholding, or withdrawing treatment would then be subject to generally accepted rules requiring consent to medical treatment.[1]

MEDICALLY PROVIDED NUTRITION AND HYDRATION AS MEDICAL TREATMENT

Whether mechanical nutrition and hydration procedures constitute "medical care" subject to the rules respecting the provision or termination of care to the terminally ill is a mixed question of law and fact.[2] How are the methods ordinarily construed: Do they constitute the practice of medicine under health insurance policies and Medicare?[3] Are they the practice of medicine, performed by licensed personnel,[4] using medical methods and procedures?[5] Are they typically done in settings where medical care is commonly provided?

Medical interventions treat injuries or diseases and their effects. Malnutrition and dehydration are commonly associated with many diseases and may occasion various abnormal signs and symptoms.[6]

If mechanical hydration and nutrition were not considered medical treatment, would they be the same as eating and drinking? While both mechanical and natural means provide nutriments and fluids, mechanical means certainly may not provide comparable emotional satisfaction for the patient, for the supporting family members, or for the caregiving staff. While all of the means may relieve hunger and thirst, a comatose, severely demented, or dying person may not experience hunger and thirst. Thirst can also be satisfied by other means, means that are more intimate, more caring—by attending the patient, wetting the lips, and keeping the mouth moist.[7]

Such considerations may help resolve the legal question of whether mechanical nutrition and hydration should be deemed the same as other medical treatments or procedures, or, conversely, the same as simple feeding and drinking. Feeding or putting water to the lips of a helpless person is clearly much more than medical treatment. The invasive procedures used to normalize nutrition and hydration often have all the earmarks of being medical treatments. To equate the two would be profoundly misleading.

Administering mechanical nutrition and hydration is no picnic. It is not—like feeding and offering drink ordinarily are—close, intuitive, intimate nurturing, emotionally affecting for caregiver and recipient alike. It is not done by relatives or long-time friends or intimates. Moreover, for resistant patients who must be restrained, it really can be indistinguishable from torture.

The court decisions to date hold that mechanical nutrition and hydration are medical treatment. In *Conroy*,[8] the New Jersey Supreme Court held that mechanical nutrition should be treated like other medical treatments in deciding whether and when to terminate. It acknowledged that feeding has "emotional significance," even in "the realm of complex, high-technology medical care." But nasogastric tubes and other mechanical feeding techniques "are significantly different from bottle-feeding [an infant] or spoonfeeding. . . ."[9] Like other medical procedures, they carry risks and can have side effects and complications that can be "serious and distressing" for some patients. Like other medical procedures, they require the attention of skilled health care professionals. And they do what other medical procedures such as respirators do: "they prolong life through mechanical means when the body is no longer able to perform a vital bodily function of its own."[10]

The California appellate court came to the same conclusion more summarily in *Barber v. Superior Court*,[11] rejecting a proffered distinction between mechanical nutrition and mechanical respiration. Mechanical nutrition is like feeding only as a matter of "emotional symbolism."[12] Normal feeding is quite different from mechanical nutrition when one examines the actions taken and their effects. Still more summarily, a New York state trial court held in *Plaza Health*[13] that surgery to create a gastrostomy was medical treatment within the meaning of a state statute guaranteeing patients the right to decline treatment.

In *Hier*,[14] a Massachusetts appellate court refused to treat gastrostomy surgery as something other than "a major surgical procedure" that was "highly intrusive"; it considered medical factors—potential complications and risk to the patient—as it would for any other medical procedure. It said *Barber* and the subsequently reversed lower court decision in *Conroy* involved termination of "ongoing nutritional support." But it rejected the argument "that nutrition should be differentiated from treatment and the right of choice confined to the latter." The distinction was not between nutrition and treatment, "but between supplying nutritional support with only modest intrusiveness and supplying it through the use of highly intrusive surgical procedures."[15] Degree of intrusiveness has often been a factor in determining whether a medical procedure should be authorized for an incompetent person.

To conclude that the procedures for mechanical nutrition are medical goes far toward resolving many of the questions that concern when they may be terminated. For competent patients, for patients who expressed their wishes when competent, and for patients whose wishes can be determined from how they lived their lives, the right to control medical treatment means the right to refuse medical care of all types. For incompetent patients whose will cannot be known, the inquiry does not end with the conclusion that mechanical nutrition is medical. Not all medical treatments are the same, nor should all medical treatments be analyzed as a single, homogenous mass. Not only the intrusiveness of the treatment and the patient's prognosis—which is to say, what the effect of the treatment would be—but how common and familiar the treatment is, whether it is "ordinary" or "extraordinary," have all been considered important.

COMPETENT PATIENTS AND PATIENTS WHO HAVE EXPRESSED THEIR WISHES

In the past decade, courts and legislatures have required medical service providers to comply with the wishes of competent terminally ill patients to decline further treatment and have also outlined procedures for presently incompetent persons whose previous competent wishes are known.

(a) *Judicially-developed rights.* State courts have held that patients have a near-absolute right to decline unwanted medical treatment.[16] Even those courts which first said the patient's right was to be weighed against asserted state interests have come to conclude that state interests cannot overcome the will of a competent person where third-party rights or interests are not at issue.[17] The patient's right to bodily integrity and privacy generally prevails save in the special setting of prison.[18] This right to reject treatment rests on the common law right to be free from unconsented battery[19] and on the constitutional right to privacy.[20] Hospitals and nursing homes still often fail to comply, even where the law is well settled; and some instances of noncompliance are outrageous.[21]

A case whose reasoning is particularly apt to the mechanical nutrition question is *In re* Osborne.[22] There, an otherwise healthy man declined, for religious reasons, surgery believed to be necessary to repair injuries from a fall. While the treatment there was unquestionably "medical," the analogy to mechanical nutrition and hydration is appropriate given the common argument that maintaining artificial fluids and nutrition will maintain a life until (arguably unrelated) disease, illness, or injury brings death.[23] The court first considered whether the patient had "validly and knowingly chosen this course for his life. . . ." That was the first and foremost question, the *Osborne* court said, for it rejected the view[24]

> that the state [has] a compelling interest in sustaining life. The notion that the individual exists for the good of the state is, of course, quite

antithetical to our fundamental thesis that the role of the state is to ensure a maximum of individual freedom of choice and conduct.[25]

Even some courts acknowledging the primacy of individual freedom have said they require consideration of factors reflecting other state interests. Whatever the ongoing validity of these factors—preserving life, protecting the interests of minor children, preventing suicide, and promoting ethical medical practice[26]—they have no more bearing for the patient dying of malnutrition or dehydration than they have in situations where mechanical respiration or other medical treatment is at issue.

The courts have commonly discussed patients' rights in the context of terminal illness, and the bulk of the cases involve diseases labeled terminal.[27] But that would appear to be only to distinguish terminally ill patients from healthy individuals, not necessarily from patients suffering advanced chronic illness, and the broad sweep of recent decisions suggests that for competent patients, at least, any such distinctions should be of little significance.[28] While the distinction may be useful for some medical purposes,[29] the practical difference between a terminal illness and an advanced chronic illness would appear to be slight.

These principles of patient autonomy should control under the common law, whether or not a state has enacted patients' rights or natural death legislation, which typically save all existing rights.[30] But where there is legislative action, other questions arise.

(b) *Legislated rights.* More than thirty state legislatures have enacted "natural death" laws providing a mechanism by which patients anticipating possible incompetence can decline further care.[31] This mechanism is the health care declaration, popularly known as a "living will," and has precise legal effects under those laws where the statutory requirements are met.[32] State legislatures have also enacted various patients' rights laws further defining protections and the right to control treatment.[33] And durable power of attorney legislation, now almost universal, may provide a mechanism by which an individual can name the person to make his or her medical care decisions in the event of the patient's inability to act.[34] A recently amended Maryland statute combines these approaches in delineating the limited circumstances in which a person may be treated without his or her consent, and incorporating by reference the use of durable powers of attorney.[35]

Where the question arises under a patients' rights law or a living will, two related questions arise. The first is whether the legislature meant to include mechanical hydration and nutrition in the medical treatments covered by the law. The second is whether the patient who declared his or her wish not to be subjected to certain life-extending forms of medical care intended to bar medical procedures for mechanical hydration and nutrition.

Patients' rights laws and natural death laws apply to decisions respecting the provision, withholding, or termination of "medical" care.[36] Whether mechanical nutrition provided by doctors and nurses at medical institutions does or does not come within the term "medical treatment" as used in the statute is a question of legislative intent. Absent discussion of mechanical nutrition in the legislative reports or debates, that question would likely be resolved under general principles of statutory construction,[37] which would consider many of the factors detailed in the previous section.[38] The one court to address the precise question held that the right to reject medical treatment embodied in New York public health law entitled an ailing eighty-five-year-old man, a widower and stroke victim who elected not to eat, to decline surgery to implant a gastrostomy tube.[39]

Whether or not the patient with a living will meant to exclude the surgery or invasive procedures used for mechanical nutrition from the undesired medical treatment is a question of individual intent. When considered in the planning stage—when the patient is deciding whether to execute a living will—this problem is easily solved by expressly addressing whether the patient wants mechanical nutrition administered. Some model living wills now specifically refer to mechanical nutrition.[40] Natural death statutes often provide a form living will or "declaration," and some statutes provide that the model "may, but need not" be used, permitting variations "includ[ing] other specific directions." This invites patients to declare whether artificial hydration and nutrition are or are not to be used.[41] Even without such an invitation, a declaration reflecting such wishes should be dispositive as to the patient's wishes under the common law. An individual's declaration in a living will to forgo treatment should be respected by health care providers even in the absence of natural death legislation, and such respect has been judicially endorsed.[42]

Where the question arises only after the fact, without clear expression by the patient, intent will have to be inferred, as it often is, from circumstances and other limited available evidence.

INCOMPETENT PATIENTS WHOSE WISHES CANNOT BE KNOWN

Patients who are now incompetent but who expressed their views while they were able to do so should have those wishes honored. But for incompetent patients whose wishes cannot be known, courts are no longer effecting patient self-determination when they direct caregivers to follow one course of action or another. Whether medically provided nutrition and hydration are medical treatment may have substantial bearing on the rules to be applied. To conclude that mechanical hydration and nutrition are medical treatment suggests that the increasingly settled procedures for proxy decision making for incompetent individuals be followed. To conclude the contrary suggests that some other, likely less permissive, standard should be used to determine whether mechanical hydration and nutrition can or should be used.

If mechanical hydration and nutrition are medical care, then the case law and statutes on when care may be terminated provide guidance. For once-healthy adults now rendered incompetent, whether or not permanently comatose or vegetative, the substituted-judgment test requires a proxy or court to ascertain what the person would have elected for himself or herself.[43] For those who were never competent, the best-interests test may require a subtle and difficult weighing of the great imponderable: death versus an existence that can barely be called life.[44] Natural death acts in some states authorize family members or other proxies to terminate care (other than for comfort or palliation) where death is imminent and where further treatment will only "prolong the dying process."[45]

The decision to terminate life-sustaining care for another person should always be difficult. But many sane, competent, loved, and loving people have chosen death in the face of such life; this fact and the familiar procedural framework should render the task feasible.

Feasible but troubling. There is more than a touch of irony in the way our values lead to opposite results. Where the patient is least likely to be suffering in the present, where he or she is comatose or vegetative, the decision to terminate is, relatively, easy. But where the patient is conscious and aware, even if incompetent and uncommunicative, he or she may be suffering greatly. While that suffering might tend to encourage making choices that allow a shorter life, the decision to forgo treatments to sustain life will also curtail conscious life, something one should be reluctant to do. These decisions with conscious patients are therefore most difficult.

Three courts have dealt with these problems, and their decisions reflect three distinctive approaches.

In *Storar*,[46] a severely retarded man suffered from bladder cancer. The cancer was expected to kill him within six months in any event, but it also caused bleeding that would be fatal sooner if he did not undergo regular blood transfusions. Because the transfusions were painful and debilitating, the man resisted them and had to be restrained; his mother, unquestionably loving, opposed the transfusions because they terrified her son. Following a best-interests test, the court held that the transfusions should nonetheless be administered. It relied on an expert's argument that the "transfusions were analogous to food—they would not cure the cancer, but they would eliminate the risk of death from another treatable cause."[47] The result was to impose on health care providers a duty to treat in a wide variety of situations of doubtful wisdom, leaving little room for judgment or discretion in the treatment of incompetent patients.[48]

In *Hier*,[49] the patient had suffered severe mental illness for the last fifty-eight of her ninety-two years, and required a gastrostomy tube for nutrition because of other medical conditions not otherwise debilitating. She had pulled out gastrostomy tubes before and vigorously resisted surgery. She had no relatives, her court-appointed proxies favored treatment, and while the doctors were of different views as to the wisdom of surgery, the physicians opposing surgery did not do so on medical grounds.[50] Following earlier Massachusetts decisions[51] applying a substituted-judgment rather than best-interests test,[52] the court gave substantial weight to Mrs. Hier's opposition, notwithstanding her incompetence. It read her resistance to tubes and surgery as "a plea for privacy and personal dignity by a ninety-two-year-old person who is seriously ill and for whom life has little left to offer."[53]

In the most recent decision, *Conroy*,[54] the patient suffered from severe and permanent mental and physical infirmities—organic

brain syndrome, heart disease, diabetes, gangrene. She was not coma-
tose, but could not converse or move from her semifetal position; she was incontinent and, even if spoon-fed all day, was unable to take enough food and water by mouth to maintain herself. She followed people with her eyes, would moan occasionally or smile, and her facial expressions varied, but she was otherwise uncommuni-
cative. Her nephew, who was the court-appointed guardian and only living relative, sought permission to terminate mechanical tube-
feeding; medical opinion was divided. The New Jersey Supreme Court rejected as naive the use of a substituted-judgment test—
whose theoretical linchpin is self-determination—where a previ-
ously competent patient had failed to express his or her wishes in more than "general or casual terms."[55] It crafted a kind of inter-
mediate best-interests where there was trustworthy evidence the patient would have refused treatment. In that case, treatment could be terminated where the net burdens outweighed the benefits of continued life.[56] Absent such evidence, however, treatment could be terminated only where the burdens "clearly and markedly outweigh the benefits"; where treatment would probably engender such "recurring, unavoidable and severe pain ... that the effect of ad-
ministering life-sustaining treatment would be inhumane."[57]

All three courts view surgery or procedures to administer mechanical nutrition and hydration as they view other medical treat-
ments. The courts considered such factors as the burdens and benefits of each treatment, the risks and possible effect of compli-
cations, as well as the effects of not treating. The differences between the decisions concern not nutrition versus treatment, but each court's attitudes toward treatment.

The New Jersey Supreme Court in *Conroy* attempts to steer a middle ground between *Storar*, which imposes a rigid requirement of treatment, and the Massachusetts case, which follows a looser rule in relying heavily on incompetent patients' noncomprehending resistance to treatment.[58] It repudiates the lingering suggestion in earlier cases that competent patients may have to succumb to unwanted treatments for the good of the state or society. But in ex-
plaining when to apply its subjective substituted-judgment test, it says that a lifetime aversion to doctors and hospitals[59] is not ade-
quate to show that Miss Conroy "clearly" would have rejected mechanical feeding, and seems to require that the patient evidence something like a philosophical analysis of her wants and prefer-

ences.[60] To be sure, it is correct to treat lightly preferences stated only abstractly and casually; but a lifetime of active disregard of medical care is neither abstract, nor casual, nor general. And the court suggests that the principal medical fact to consider is pain. For the objective test, to be used where there is no evidence of the patient's preference respecting treatment, pain must be "recurring, unavoidable and severe," so much so that treatment is "inhumane." For the limited-objective test, to be used where there is "trust-worthy" but not compelling evidence of the patient's preference for no treatment, the court may be read to say that pain (alone) must "outweigh any physical pleasure, emotional enjoyment, or intellec-tual satisfaction that the patient may still be able to derive from life."[61]

Despite their differences, the courts are consistent on their view of mechanical hydration and nutrition as medical treatment. Faced with the hard facts of what the surgery or procedure required, none stepped away from the conclusion that surgery or procedures to sup-plant or compensate for inability to take fluids and food are medical treatment every bit as much as are procedures to supplant or com-pensate for inability to breathe or to dialyze blood.

To require mechanical nutrition and hydration in all circumstan-ces to the greatest extent medically possible and without regard to the benefits for the patient must rest largely on the symbolic sig-nificance of feeding.[62] To rely upon the symbolism of a treatment in requiring it is to acknowledge that the welfare of the individual being treated is irrelevant: it is a symbol not to the incompetent, likely comatose, or at least uncomprehending patient, but to others—perhaps other patients, perhaps healthy people who will someday be patients. Perhaps it is a symbol to caregivers that they should not come to accept death, not because that attitude will enable them yet to do this patient any good, but because it may affect how they respond to another patient in different conditions some time in the future.[63]

These are all reasonable arguments, but they turn on the interests of people other than the patient whose welfare is at issue; as such, a court which dismissed them as not addressing the real issue before it would, I think, be on solid ground. If the symbolic point is to honor the sanctity of life, then respecting self-determination, not subjecting it to medical institutions or state power, is the more powerful symbol. If self-determination is not at issue, as with incompetents, the problem remains that treatments conceived for one set of medical problems are being used in wholly new circumstances. It is perhaps too obvious to say that the difficulty derives from the severity as well as the finality of the choices: death as the only alternative to a life in pain and suffering, with few observable rewards. For some, this will be a terrible, tragic choice: withdraw mechanical hydration and nutrition and "kill" the patient, or impose it and "torture" her. That may sound harsh, yet the fact remains that much done in the name of medical care is hard to distinguish from torture.

We have created tools with immense potential for good. We must now decide when not to use them. The slope for making such decisions is, as they say, slippery. But that is the point of every slippery slope argument: the position at the summit is untenable. To maintain every person for as long as possible would be to cause suffering on a massive scale. We have no choice but to move along the slope, always testing our footing in the search for secure ground.

One feature of the cases is unmistakably clear. Competent patients and incompetent patients who have previously expressed their wishes are treated differently than are incompetent patients whose wants are unknown. This was presaged four years ago in the companion leading New York cases, *Storar* and *Brother Fox*.[64] The lesson is that advance planning for the aging and seriously ill is essential for those who want to control the course of their lives. Careful documentation is advisable—the courts in *Conroy*[65] and *Bludworth*[66] encourage the use of living wills—if not always required. Sometimes the courts will act on the strength of oral statements. But unless the patient is a Catholic priest and the proxy is another Catholic priest—as was the case in Brother Fox—it would be prudent, to say the least, for the patient's wishes to be expressed carefully and in writing, with appropriate documentation concerning competence.

N O T E S

1. I would like to acknowledge the thoughtful comments and criticisms of my partner, John Laster, and of Prof. Carol Sanger of the University of Santa Clara Law School. They contributed significantly to this discussion, although I remain responsible for errors and judgments in the final product.

2. See chapter 2; see also *In the Matter of Mary Hier*, 18 Mass. App. 200, 464 N.E.2d 959, 961–962, *app. den.*, 392 Mass. 1102 (1984) (methods for mechanical nutrition discussed), and Joanne Lynn and James Childress, "Must Patients Always Be Given Food and Water?" *Hastings Cent. Rep.* 13:17–21 (October 1983) reprinted as chapter 5 *supra* (description of the different methods of treatment and some of the medical indications relating their use).

3. They are typically treated as medical services under medical and health and accident policies, 10 *Couch on Insurance* 2d 41:452 (1984 Supp.), save where specific policy language warrants exclusion; 10 *Couch on Insurance* 2d (rev. ed.) 41A:56 (1982). Earlier Medicare regulations defined the provision of mechanical nutrition as skilled nursing care. 42 C.F.R. 405.127 (c) (2) (i) and (ii) (skilled nursing care includes "hypodermoclysis or intravenous feeding . . . Levin [large NG] tube and gastrostomy feedings . . .") (1982). Current regulations are less precise, but I understand the practice to be to cover all procedures to insert NG (nasogastric) tubes and IV (intravenous) lines and all surgical procedures to introduce mechanical nutrition into the body.

4. The question would likely come up if at all in an enforcement proceeding involving someone who had provided mechanical nutrition without a license and not under the supervision of a physician or nurse. The practicalities of mechanical nutrition are such that it would always be provided under a physician's supervision, so that a narrow licensing decision would be unlikely.

5. See chapter 2 and the authorities cited in note 2 above on the techniques and requirements for mechanical nutrition.

6. See Lynn and Childress, note 2 above ("In the past, malnutrition and dehydration must have accompanied nearly every death that followed an illness of more than a few days.").

7. See chapter 3.

8. *In re* Conroy, 98 N.J. 321, 486 A.2d 1209 (1985).

9. *Id.* at 1236.

10. *Id.*

11. Barber v. Superior Court, 195 Cal. Rptr. 484 (Cal. App. 2 Dist. 1983).

12. Id. at 488.

13. *In re* Plaza Health and Rehabilitation Center, (N.Y. Super. Ct., Onandaga County, February 2, 1984).

14. *In the Matter of Mary Hier*, 18 Mass. App. 200, 464 N.E.2d 959, *app. den.*, 392 Mass. 1102 (1984).

15. *Id.* at 964.

16. *In re* Conroy, 98 N.J. 321, 486 A.2d 1209, 1221–1226 (1985), Eichner v. Dillon (Brother Fox), 52 N.Y.2d 363, 420 N.E.2d 64 (1981).

17. Compare *Conroy*, note 8 *supra*, with *In re* Quinlan, 70 N.J. 10, 335 A.2d 647 (1976), *cert. denied*, 429 U.S. 922 (1976).

18. Superintendent of Belchertown State School v. Saikewicz, 373 Mass. 728, 370 N.E.2d 417 (1977); Satz v. Perlmutter, 362 So.2d 160 (Fla. App. 1978), *aff'd*, 379 So.2d 359 (Fla. 1980). The exceptions are for patients who are prisoners in state penal institutions, *e.g.*, Hall v. Myers, 399 N.E.2d 452 (Mass. App. 1979) (the state interest in orderly prison administration must also be considered), and where the patient is the parent of a minor child who might otherwise become a ward of the state, Application of President & Directors of Georgetown College, 331 F.2d 1000 (D.C. Cir.), *cert. denied*,

377 U.S. 978 (1964), *but cf. In re* Osborne, 294 A.2d 372 (D.C. 1972) (surgery would not be required where minor children were financially provided for).

19. Eichner v. Dillon, note 16 *supra*; Foody v. Manchester Memorial Hospital, 40 Conn. Supp. 127, 482 A.2d 713 (1984); *In re* Bartling, 209 Cal. Rptr. 220 (1984); Barber v. Superior Court, 195 Cal. Rptr. 484 (Cal. App. 2 Dist 1983).

20. Superintendent of Belchertown State School v. Saikewicz, 373 Mass. 728, 370 N.E.2d 417 (1977); *In re* Quinlan, 70 N.J. 10, 355 A.2d 647, *cert. denied*, 429 U.S. 922 (1976); *In re* Colyer, 99 Wash.2d 114, 660 P. 2d 738 (1983); Severns v. Wilmington Medical Center, 421 A.2d 1334 (Del. 1980); *In re* Bartling, 209 Cal. Rptr. 220 (1984); *In re* Guardianship of Barry, Memorial Hospital, 40 Conn. Supp. 127, 482 A.2d 713 (1984); *In re* L.H.R.,—Ga.—(No. 41065, decided October 16, 1984).

21. Leach v. Shapiro, 13 Ohio App.3d 393 (1984); In the Matter of Lydia E. Hall Hospital, 455 N.Y.S.2d 706 (1982).

22. 294 A.2d 372 (D.C. App. 1972).

23. See, e.g., *In re* Storar, 52 N.Y.2d 363, 420 N.E.2d 64 (1981), and the intermediate court opinion in *In re* Conroy, 190 N.J. Super. 453, 464 A.2d 303 (1983), *rev'd*, 98 N.J. 321, 486 A.2d 1209 (1985).

24. Reflected in John F. Kennedy Memorial Hospital v. Heston, 279 A.2d 670 (N.J. 1971).

25. 294 A.2d at 375, n. 5.

26. See Saikewicz, note 18 *supra*, 370 N.E.2d at 424–428.

27. The others are largely Jehovah's Witness cases. In the typical case, an otherwise healthy young person requires surgery because of injuries sustained in an accident but declines it because he or she reads the biblical proscription against "drinking blood" as proscribing blood transfusions. See, e.g., *In re* Estate of Brooks, 32 Ill.2d 361, 205 N.E.2d 435 (1965).

28. *Conroy*, note 8 *supra*; *Bartling*, note 19 *supra*.

29. Department of Health and Human Services, Health Care Financing Administration, "Medicare Program, Hospice Care, Final Rule," Federal Register 48:56008–56036.

30. West's Ann. Cal. Health & Safety Code 7193 (1984 Supp.); D.C. Code 6–2429 (a) (1981); Kan.Stat.Ann. 65–28, 108 (d); Nev.Rev.Stat. 449.680; N.M.Stat.Ann. 24–7–9; Ore.Rev.Stat. 97.085 (2); Tex.Rev. Civ.Stat.Ann. art. 4590h, 11, Va.Stat.Ann. 54–325.8:12.

31. The fifteen statutes enacted as of 1983 are reprinted in President's Commission for the Study of Ethical Problems in Medicine and Biomedical and Behavioral Research, *Deciding to Forego Life-Sustaining Treatment*, Appendix D, pp. 310–387 (1983). Florida, Georgia, Illinois, Louisiana, Maryland, Mississippi, West Virginia, Wisconsin, and Wyoming have since enacted statutes, and bills are pending in more than a dozen other states. See Society for the Right to Die, Newsletter, Fall, 1984, p. 8.

32. The most common requirement is that death be "imminent" and the effect of further care only to "prolong the dying process," but there are others, in addition to elaborate procedural requirements. They are summarized in Ron Landsman, "Legal Planning of Health Care for the Critically Ill," in Callahan, et al., *Estate and Financial Planning for the Aging and Incapacitated Client* (PLI 1984), pp. 149–152.

33. E.g., Minn.Stat.Ann. 144.651 (12) (1984 Supp.); Rev.Code Wash. 7.70.050 (1984 Supp.); Md.Stat.Ann. Health Gen., 19–344 (d) (1) (ii) and (iii) (1982); N.Y. Pub.H.Law 2803-c (3) (3) (1977).

34. All states have enacted or have pending durable power laws. Those enacted as of 1983 are reprinted in *Deciding to Forego Life-Sustaining Treatment*, note 31 *supra*, Appendix E, pp. 390–422.

35. Maryland Code Health-Gen. 20–107 (1984 Cum.Supp.).

36. E.g., "medical procedure or intervention," D.C. Code 6–2421 (3), and "medical procedure, treatment or intervention," Va.Stat.Ann. 54–325.8:2 (P3); but see also N.M.Stat.Ann. 24–7–2 (a), 24–7–3 (a) and *passim* ("maintenance medical treatment, defined as "medical treatment designed solely to sustain the life processes").

37. Among the guidelines for statutory construction are the rules that remedial social legislation—such as laws that confer or promote rights relating to health and safety—be liberally construed, Sands, 2 *Sutherland Statutory Construction* 60.01, 60.02 (1974). Such statutes do not derogate common law rights or natural or common right, for which there is a rule of strict construction, so that by negative implication a policy of liberal construction is again pointed to 2 *id.* 61.01, 61.06 (1981 Supp.).

38. See the text accompanying notes 1–7 *supra*.

39. See *In re* Plaza Health and Rehabilitation Center, note 13 *supra*, *citing* N.Y. Pub.H.Law 2803-c (3) (e).

40. Society for the Right to Die "Living Will Declaration" (no date).

41. Moreover, some laws provide that the invalidity of a specific direction "shall not affect the [validity of the] declaration," so that adding such specifics does not expose the patient to the risk that their entire effort might be undone. Va.Stat.Ann. 54–325.8:4. See also D.C.Code 6–2422 (c). But cf. Ore.Rev.Stat, 97.055 (1) ("The directive shall be in the following form . . ."); Nev.Rev.Stat. 449.610 ("The declaration shall be in substantially the following form . . .").

42. *Conroy*, note 8 *supra*; John F. Kennedy Memorial Hospital v. Bludworth, 452 So.2d 921 (Fla. 1984).

43. *Deciding to Forego Life-Sustaining Treatment*, note 31 *supra*, pp. 132–134; *In re* Spring, 380 Mass. 629, 405 N.E.2d 115 (1980).

44. *Deciding to Forego Life-Sustaining Treatment*, note 31 *supra*, pp. 134–136.

45. See note 32 *supra*.

46. See note 23 *supra*.

47. 420 N.E.2d at 73.

48. See chapter 14.

49. See note 2 *supra*.

50. See George J. Annas, "The Case of Mary Hier: When Substituted Judgment Becomes Sleight of Hand," *Hastings Cent. Rep.* 14:23–24 (August 1984).

51. *Saikewicz*, note 18 *supra*.

52. This was inappropriate. See Alexander M. Capron, "Ironies and Tensions in Feeding the Dying," *Hastings Cent. Rep.* 14:32–34 (October 1984); Annas, note 50 *supra*, at 25.

53. *In the Matter of Mary Hier*, 18 Mass. App. 200, 464 N.E.2d 959, 965, *app. den.* 392 Mass. 1102 (1984).

54. *In re* Conroy, 98 N.J. 321, 486 A.2d 1209 (1985).

55. *Id.* at 1231.

56. *Id.* at 1231–32.

57. *Id.* at 1232.

58. Capron, note 52 *supra*, p. 34 ("it seems questionable to equate Mrs.

Hier's removal of the feeding tubes with a competent choice to reject this form of treatment, . . . although [her actions] could not simply be ignored . . .").

59. *In re* Conroy, 98 N.J. 321, 339–40, 486 A.2d 1209, 1218 (1985).

60. *Id.* at 1242–43.

61. *Id.* at 1232. The concurring and dissenting opinions read the majority to "too narrowly define the interests of people like Miss Conroy [because] significant pain in effect becomes the sole measure of such a person's best interests." *Id.* at 1247.

62. Daniel Callahan, "On Feeding the Dying," *Hastings Cent. Rep.* 13:22 (October 1983); *cf.* chapters 19 and 8.

63. See chapter 8.

64. See notes 16, 23 *supra*.

65. See note 8 *supra*.

66. See note 42 *supra*.

Alan J. Weisbard, J.D.

14 Legal Perspectives on Withdrawing Fluids and Nutrition: The New York Experience

The starting point for any discussion of New York law regarding termination of treatment for dying and seriously ill patients is the decision of the New York Court of Appeals in the *Eichner* and *Storar* cases.[1] These cases were decided together in March of 1981, following earlier major decisions by the New Jersey Supreme Court in *Quinlan*[2] and the Massachusetts Supreme Judicial Court in *Saikewicz*.[3]

New York, unlike New Jersey and Massachusetts, viewed the critical legal issue as one involving a *common law* right of bodily self-determination, citing Justice Cardozo's famous opinion in the 1914 *Schloendorff* case, rather than as a matter implicating a *constitutional* right of privacy.[4] Under New York common law, the court found consistent support for the right of a competent adult to make his or her own decision, even when treatment is considered necessary to preserve the patient's life. Further, the court held that the patient's right to determine the course of his or her own medical treatment is paramount to what might otherwise be the doctor's obligation to provide "necessary" medical care. Thus, a doctor cannot be held to have violated his or her legal or professional responsibilities (including obligations under the criminal law) when he or she honors the right of a competent adult patient to decline medical treatment. (The court noted in a footnote that this analysis may be subject to modification in certain cases based on additional state interests in preventing suicide and protecting minor children or dependents.)[5] A competent adult patient's authority to decline medical treatment would likely extend to the artificial provision of fluids and nutrition.

The application of this principle to Brother Fox in the *Eichner* case was not entirely straightforward, since Brother Fox was respirator-dependent, in a vegetative state, and clearly incompetent at the time. The case was presented as if someone other than the patient could make a decision to discontinue life-sustaining treatment on behalf of the incompetent patient, much like the situation in *Quinlan*. But the Court resisted this way of seeing it, instead characterizing the choice as one made *by Brother Fox himself* before he became incompetent. The Court found "clear and convincing" evidence that Brother Fox had carefully reflected on *exactly* this situation in his previous discussion of church teaching regarding Karen Quinlan and had clearly expressed his own wishes regarding the limits on medical care in such situations.

The questions of third-party decision-making that the court could avoid in *Eichner* were unmistakably raised in *Storar*, involving a fifty-two-year-old patient with terminal bladder cancer who had been institutionalized for profound retardation for virtually his entire life. One effect of Mr. Storar's cancer was loss of blood, creating the need for repetitive blood transfusions, which Storar found unpleasant and which his seventy-seven-year-old mother felt should be discontinued.

The court sharply distinguished *Storar* from *Eichner*, saying it had to be decided from different principles. But the court *did not* take on the general issue of who should decide for incompetent patients. The court stressed the state's interest, as *parens patriae*, in protecting the health and welfare of the child. While parents can choose among reasonable medical alternatives (citing an earlier New York decision in the *Hofbauer* case),[6] a parent may not deny a child all treatment for a condition which threatens the child's life.

There were two threats to Storar's life—the incurable cancer, and the related loss of blood—and continuing the transfusions would not affect the cancer. The court, however, held that, because the transfusions would eliminate the risk of death from treatable cause, they could not be withheld. The court contended that the transfusions themselves did *not* involve excessive pain, and that a court should not allow an incompetent patient "to bleed to death."[7]

This aspect of *Storar* is puzzling and has created enormous controversy in New York regarding whether, absent the clarity and precision of Brother Fox's advance directive, withholding life-prolonging care from an incompetent patient is ever legal. Under

New York law, as opposed to that of New Jersey and Massachusetts, treatment might not have been discontinued for Karen Quinlan or Joseph Saikewicz. (These doubts were subsequently strengthened by language in the court of appeals decision in late 1984, accepting the concept of brain death in the *Eulo* and *Bonilla* cases.)[8]

The crucial passage in *Storar* is this:

> Thus, as one of the experts noted, the transfusions were analogous to food—they would not cure the cancer, but they could eliminate the risk of death from another treatable cause. Of course, John Storar did not like them as might be expected of one with an infant's mentality. But the evidence convincingly shows that the transfusions did not involve excessive pain and that without them his mental and physical ability would not be maintained at the usual level. With the transfusions on the other hand, he was essentially the same as he was before, except of course he had a fatal illness which would ultimately claim his life.
>
> . . . A court should not allow an incompetent patient to bleed to death because someone, even someone as close as a parent or sibling, feels that this is best for one with an incurable disease.[9]

Both in its direct reference to feeding and in the structure of its argument, the *Storar* court leaves little doubt as to its views on whether food and water could be stopped. Indeed, the court clearly thinks that cessation of feeding of incompetent patients is so evidently unacceptable that it serves as the unexamined starting point for the analysis of transfusions. The court also clearly rejects the proposition that bleeding to death—and, by analogy, starving to death—can be in the best interest of an incompetent patient. The strength and absoluteness of this position is evidenced by the context of the case: forgoing treatment was advocated by a close relative, clearly very knowledgeable, involved, and caring, who had no substantial conflict of interest, and for a patient who was close to death.

The New York court that decided *Storar* would clearly have decided against stopping Claire Conroy's feeding. Since *Storar*, though, three further developments have unfolded.

First was Baby Jane Doe.[10] Given its discussion in *Storar*, one might have predicted that the New York Court of Appeals would mandate surgery to correct Baby Jane's spina bifida and to shunt her hydrocephalus. That is not what happened. The court decided to view Baby Jane's parents' decision to reject the surgery as a choice of "more conservative" alternative treatment—even though this choice was considered likely to lead to early death. The court's decision was a bit mysterious, failing even to mention the *Storar* precedent, relying instead on a somewhat ill-defined and incompletely explained procedural point. This may be a signal that the court's commitment to *Storar* principles is uncertain, though those principles were subsequently reaffirmed in the *Eulo* and *Bonilla* cases.[11]

Second was the case of a nursing home patient in Syracuse, described as a former college president in his eighties, who fasted for seven weeks until he died.[12] The nursing home apparently did not object to the fast or the death but went to court on about the fortieth day of his fast, just to make sure that its acquiescence in the patient's impending death would not result in legal problems. The lower court upheld the competent patient's right to refuse food and did not mandate force-feeding or artificial nutrition. The decision would appear to follow from *Schloendorff* and *Eichner*. There may be some question whether the patient's fast might be deemed a suicide. Full evaluation of that question would depend upon unreported facts regarding the patient's medical condition.

Finally, a special grand jury has issued a report following a lengthy criminal investigation of "do not resuscitate" (DNR) practice at LaGuardia Hospital in New York City.[13] While the investigation did not result in any criminal indictment, it did include a scathing critique of procedural abuses, including the hospital's failure to enter DNR orders in medical records. New York's Governor Cuomo has now directed the State Commissioner of Health to explore this issue, which perhaps will break the logjam that has thus far inhibited the resolution of DNR policy under *Storar*.[14]

Thus, New York has broken its own path regarding withdrawal of life-prolonging therapies. New York law rejects a constitutional claim in favor of a common law analysis and sharply distinguishes between the clearly recognized right of competent adults to reject medical interventions and the impermissibility of third-party decisions to terminate or withhold life-prolonging treatments for an incompetent patient without clear and convincing evidence of the patient's own prior competent wishes. These general features of New York's approach would likely apply as well to the withdrawal of artificially provided fluids and nutrition.

N O T E S

1. *In re* Storar, 52 N.Y.2d 363, 420 N.E.2d 64, 438 N.Y.S.2d 266, *cert. denied*, 454 U.S. 858, 102 S. Ct. 309, 70 L.Ed.2d 153 (1981). (Consolidated with *In re* Eichner.)

2. *In re* Quinlan, 70 N.J. 10, 355 A.2d 647, *cert. denied*, 429 U.S. 922, 97 S. Ct. 319, 50 L.Ed.2d 289 (1976).

3. Superintendent of Belchertown State School v. Saikewicz, 373 Mass. 728, 370 N.E.2d 417 (1977).

4. *Storar, supra* note 1, 420 N.E.2d at 70, quoting Schloendorff v. Society of New York Hospital, 211 N.Y. 125, 129–130, 105 N.E. 92, 93 (1914).

5. *Id.* at 71, n. 6.

6. *In re* Hofbauer, 47 N.Y.2d 648, 419 N.Y.S. 936, 393 N.E.2d 1009 (1979).

7. Storar, *supra* note 1, 420 N.E.2d at 73.

8. People v. Eulo, 63 N.Y.2d 341, 482 N.Y.S.2d 436 (Consolidated with *People v. Bonilla.*)

9. Storar, *supra* note 1, 420 N.E.2d at 73.

10. Weber v. Stony Brook Hospital, 60 N.Y.2d 208, 456 N.E.2d 1186, 469 N.Y.S. 2d 63, 64 (Ct. App. 1983).

11. See note 8 *supra.*

12. *In re* Application of Plaza Health and Rehabilitation Center (N.Y. Sup. Ct., Onandaga County, February 2, 1984). See also *New York Times*, February 3, 1984, at A-1.

13. Deputy Attorney General for Medicaid Fraud Control (Edward J. Kuriansky), State of New York, Report of the Special January Third Additional 1983 Grand Jury Concerning "Do Not Resuscitate" Proceedings at a Certain Hospital in Queens County (February 8, 1984).

14. *New York Times*, September 17, 1984 at A-1.

Bernard L. Siegel, J.D.

15 Perspectives of a Criminal Prosecutor

To stop a treatment which provides the nutrition and fluids necessary to sustain life could well raise questions addressed by the criminal justice system. However, prosecutors have directed little attention to this subject. To paraphrase the California court that decided the case of Drs. Nejdl and Barber,[1] the criminal justice system is not, and should not be, in the business of designing ethical or moral codes for the medical profession. The purpose of our system of criminal law is to prosecute and penalize conduct which falls below the *minimum* that is deemed acceptable in a civilized society. Medical practice is usually more concerned with *maximums*.

What is this minimum level of conduct, the violation of which will cause the imposition of sanctions and punishment? The severity with which aberrant conduct is penalized indicates where the society's true concerns lie.

In this society, the welfare of individuals is most strongly protected. The penalties that are assessed for criminals vary and are based primarily upon the degree of physical harm suffered by individuals and only secondarily on the amount of property damage suffered. The scale ranges from lesser penalties for simple assault through more severe penalties for serious sexual assault crimes such as rape, to the most severe penalties for homicide. First-degree murder is uniformly penalized as the most serious crime that can be committed in the United States. In most jurisdictions that have the death penalty, first-degree murder is the *only* crime which may receive that harshest of penalties.

Similarly, any act that is destructive of human life receives the greatest scrutiny and draws the most attention from police departments and prosecuting attorneys. People who are willing to take the life of another person, those who in effect set themselves up as judges over who should live and who should die, are people whose potential danger to all of us is unquestioned and obvious.

The impact of this approach on medical treatment decisions occurs only in a very narrow range of cases. Obviously, physicians quite often make decisions that *might* lead to or contribute to loss of life. So long as these decisions are made in good faith, they do not ordinarily raise criminal justice concerns.

Sometimes, however, good-faith judgments are made by medical practitioners where, as a *necessary* consequence of that judgment, a human life will cease. The question is whether, in making that decision, such as the removal of nutrition and hydration, the practitioner violates the criminal law on homicide. In the case involving Drs. Nejdl and Barber, the doctors acted in apparent good faith, engaging in detailed medical consultations and receiving what seemed to be informed consents from relevant family members. In a case like this, the law of homicide *can* apply; neither the letter nor the spirit of the law exempts these kinds of cases, despite what the California courts held in the matter involving Drs. Nejdl and Barber.

In virtually every jurisdiction in America, murder is defined as the unlawful killing, with malice, of another human. The critical term *malice* is easily misunderstood by the general public. *Malice* does not mean that one is a calculating contract killer. While its precise legal definition is elusive and can vary in some respects from jurisdiction to jurisdiction, in general it means that the person has what might be called an "endangering state of mind"—a willingness, intent, and desire to bring about the result that actually flows from the person's conduct. In that respect, the legal term *malice* is a way of defining a person's *attitude* and intent toward the subject matter with which he or she is dealing. In the context of this issue, that subject matter is a patient and the attitude is one of intentionally and willingly taking action with the express understanding and hope that death is thereby hastened, if not directly caused.

Therefore, if a medical practitioner engages in conduct which is intentional and planned and which necessarily, deliberately, and intentionally causes someone to die, then that practitioner can be prosecuted for homicide, regardless of the good faith with which that conduct is undertaken. It is precisely that kind of ultimate decision-making that society quite clearly has stated is not to be made by *anyone* outside of the judicial system. Since the most fundamental concern of the criminal justice system is to protect society from people who would deliberately deprive other people of their lives, medical practitioners could be prosecuted for making judgments which may be quite valid in terms of pursuing the patient's interests and which may have the patient's valid consent. Depriving a patient of food and fluid may well make sense in a variety of medical cases. However, when that determination leads inevitably to death, as is the case with deprivation of nutrition and hydration, then the medical profession has crossed over into an area beyond medicine, an area that our society has determined should ultimately be dealt with by the judicial system or by the legislature.[2] If a practitioner chooses to arrogate to himself or herself the power to decide in that area, regardless of the precautions taken, then that practitioner *rightfully* runs the risk of scrutiny and penalty by the criminal justice system.

However, a relevant pragmatic question arises—What is the actual likelihood that a given prosecutor will bring a homicide prosecution against a doctor for making a good-faith decision to remove a patient from nutrition and hydration? After all, prosecutors, with their limited resources and tight budgets, have more than enough work to keep themselves busy just dealing with people who act in *bad* faith and who constitute far more constant and consistent threats to human health and happiness than do the limited number of medical practitioners involved in the issue under discussion.

The answer to the question is necessarily complex. Certainly, the track record of prosecutors in this and related areas does not indicate a great desire to press the matter. In all of the United States, only in one case has a prosecutor brought a homicide prosecution for the deliberate removal of someone from a nutritional system.[3] It would be naive to believe that the paucity of prosecutions is because these practices have never occurred until recently. As the New Jersey Supreme Court said, "Every day, and with limited legal guidance, families and doctors are making decisions for patients like Claire Conroy."[4] In the past, however, these decisions were not made into public issues: no complaints were brought to the authorities in the criminal justice system; and, therefore, there was no need to assess the impact of the criminal justice system on these decisions. With publicized cases such as those involving Karen Ann Quinlan,[5] and Claire Conroy,[6] and Drs. Barber and Nejdl,[7] and with the growing news media attention on the right to live or die, the criminal justice system is being forced to consider how to proceed when the issues arise.

A further disincentive to prosecutors' considering a case like this is the small handful of criminal cases dealing with active euthanasia. These prosecutions are so unsuccessful that one wonders why prosecutors bother to proceed.[8] With few exceptions, juries have simply nullified the law, essentially expressing the will of the community by acquitting the defendants, often finding temporary insanity.[9] If prosecutors have a difficult time securing convictions in euthanasia cases, where death-causing decisions by defendants are usually un-counseled and unchecked, then it would appear that the odds are overwhelmingly against prosecutions in the cases here discussed, where the putative defendants engage in constant counseling, dis-cussion, and reflection.

Were prosecution decisions based solely on the prospect of success in obtaining guilty verdicts, the probabilities are great that prose-cutors would opt not to proceed against health professionals who, in good faith, remove a patient from food and hydration. However, prosecutors are publicly accountable officials committed to enforce the law and answerable to the electorate. The obligation to enforce the law exists entirely apart from the question of whether a given prosecution is likely to yield a verdict of guilty. The obligation also is not dependent upon the personal opinion of the prosecutor as to whether the law is good or bad, wise or foolish, sound or shaky. Indeed, where the greatest uncertainty exists about the application of the law, sound prosecutorial discretion calls for the determination to be made by judge and jury. Until legislatures enact statutes which set out the conditions under which decisions can legitimately be made to take action which inevitably leads to a person's death, prose-cutors will have to prosecute, leaving the issue in the hands of juries.

Some progress could be made by educational interchange between prosecutors and health professionals. Education could point the way to alternatives to prosecution, for example, through civil litigation prior to discontinuing nutrition, or through legislation that creates reasonable procedures for the decision-making process. Perhaps this would create the institutional safeguards that will enable the medi-cal profession to pursue appropriate treatment while assuring that the citizenry is protected from potential arbitrary and misguided judgments with irrevocable consequences.

NOTES

1. *Barber v. Superior Court,* 147 Cal. App. 3d 1006, 195 Cal Rptr. 484 (1983).
2. The New Jersey Supreme Court suggests that the legislature is the appropriate body to formulate standards in this area for a variety of appropriate reasons. However, in the absence of legislative guidance, the court recognizes the obligation of the judicial system to shoulder the burden. Most prosecutors would agree with this analysis, that guidance should come first from the legislature, with interpretation following from the courts. *In re* Conroy, 98 N.J. 321, 343–345, 486 A.2d 1209, 1220–1221 (1985).
3. See note 1 *supra.*
4. *In re* Conroy, 98 N.J. 321, 345, 486 A.2d 1209, 1222 (1985).
5. *In re* Quinlan, 70 N.J. 10, 355 A.2d 647, *cert. denied sub nom. Garger v. New Jersey,* 429 U.S. 922, 97 S.Ct. 319, 50 L.Ed.2d 289 (1976).
6. See note 2 *supra.*
7. See note 1 *supra.*
8. See, e.g., Note, "Physician Liability for Failure to Resuscitate Terminally Ill Patients," *Indiana L. Rev.* 905-(1982); Ward, "Euthanasia: A Medical and Legal Overview," 15: *Kansas Bar J.* 49:317 (1980); Morris, "Voluntary Euthanasia." *Wash. L. Rev.* 45:239 (1970).
9. See Morris, "Voluntary Euthanasia," *supra,* note 8; Survey, "Euthanasia: Criminal, Tort, Constitutional and Legislative Considerations," *Notre Dame L. Rev.* 48:1202 (1973).

Part IV Special Considerations for Particular Populations

Joanne Lynn, M.D.

16 Elderly Residents of Long-Term Care Facilities

Many elderly people, about 1.3 million, now live in long-term care facilities, and these numbers are expected to double by 1990 and perhaps to double again by the end of the century.[1] For many of these, entering the facility is precipitated by serious deficits in self-care, often associated with cognitive deficits. Medical care decision-making in general, and decisions about nutritional support procedures in particular, pose special problems for long-term care residents, who frequently have reduced competence for decision-making, are isolated from the surrounding communities, have few concerned friends and relatives, are financially dependent upon public funds, and cannot readily move to a different facility. This is a typical situation:

> The resident is a moderately demented eighty-four-year-old woman who has been living in a nursing home since she developed incontinence and dangerous wandering five years ago. She has been unable to carry on a conversation or to walk for over a year, though she seems to enjoy sing-a-long parties and sensory stimulation with an occupational therapy group. She has lost 5 percent of her weight in the past five months for no apparent reason, and physical exam and laboratory tests done two months ago showed only a continued chronic anemia and a slightly reduced albumin content in the blood (both being consistent with mild chronic malnutrition and with a large number of chronic illnesses, including senile dementia).
>
> One day, she is found to have a slight fever and to be a little less responsive. Simultaneously, she has ceased to swallow food or water, though she clearly can swallow saliva (which shows that there is no obstruction or discrete problem with the nerves and muscles necessary for swallowing). The physician's examination discloses only mild dehydration and somewhat increased lethargy. The patient still responds to her name and is comforted by familiar caregivers, but has no energy to respond to usually pleasant pastimes.
>
> The patient has very little family and no friends still alive, and the family is emotionally distant. She has no estate and her care is financed by public funds. Her competence has never been the subject of a court

inquiry and she has no legally appointed guardian. Neither she nor the other residents in the facility have real alternatives to their present placement.

What special considerations should be weighed in deciding whether nutrition and hydration supports should be used? First, one must examine the range of options, their impact upon the patient and others, and their real availability. Second, one must establish a clear understanding of the standards and procedures that characterize good decision-making for this sort of person. Third, one must adjust these procedures so as to account for the particular problems and potentials of the setting of a long-term care facility. After considering these three conceptual issues, this chapter will return to an explicit examination of the case presented above.

THE OPTIONS FOR INTERVENTION

What futures can be made available for a nursing home resident who stops eating? (See figure 1.) I frame the question in terms of the "futures" that can be made available rather than the "treatments" that can be applied because one of the futures results from giving no specific treatment and because the relative desirability of the futures is more important than the mere technical availability of various treatments.

One possible outcome is that the patient will die of complications associated with dehydration, whether caused by ceasing efforts to feed, by the patient's inability or unwillingness to eat or drink, or by inadequate hydration despite using a medical procedure such as nasogastric feeding or intravenous fluids.[2] Early death could also result from complications of medical procedures aimed at improving intake (for example, aspiration associated with a nasogastric feeding tube).

A second possibility is that the patient will live a while longer, but in a state of reduced comfort and with fewer other satisfactions. This could result from partially successful efforts at oral feeding that served only to delay the effects of terminal dehydration, or from fully successful nutrition and hydration associated with an underlying illness that caused continuing discomfort (as, for example, if fever presaged pneumonia with pleuritis, which causes painful breathing), or from procedures for hydration and nutrition that were only partially successful, or allowed an uncomfortable illness to pro-

Figure 1.
Schematic diagram of the outcome of treatment options.

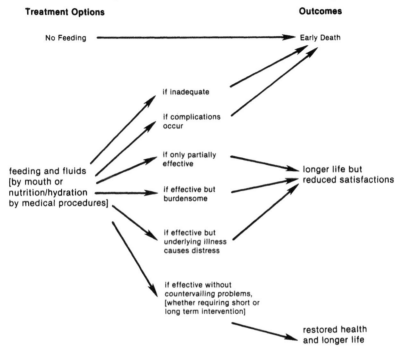

Treatment Options

No Feeding

feeding and fluids
[by mouth or
nutrition/hydration
by medical procedures]

if inadequate

if complications
occur

if only partially
effective

if effective but
burdensome

if effective but
underlying illness
causes distress

if effective without
countervailing problems,
[whether requiring short or
long term intervention]

Outcomes

Early Death

longer life but
reduced satisfactions

restored health
and longer life

ceed, or were directly onerous (as, for example, if intravenous or nasogastric tubes required distressing restraints).

Third, the patient might be restored to the same (or even to a better) state of health as before. Such an outcome might happen spontaneously with only the support of routine feeding; might require supplemental efforts to assure adequate oral intake; might be achieved with temporary use of nasogastric or intravenous tubes, hypodermoclysis, or other medical techniques; or even might be achieved with these medical procedures despite the need for prolonged or indefinite use.

With only one exception, any treatment modality might lead to any of the three major outcomes. The exception is that complete withdrawal of feeding guarantees early death, though it might not actually hasten death if the person's underlying illnesses are so grim that death is imminent in any case. With each of the other treatment modalities, some patients may experience any one of the potential outcomes—early death, later death with reduced satisfactions, and later death with somewhat restored satisfactions. What varies among patients is (1) the likelihood that any one option will lead to a specific result, (2) the desirability of the result, and (3) the availability of the treatments.

Generally, medical interventions are more likely to restore the prior state of health than is conventional oral feeding, since the patient will probably become less receptive to eating once dehydration has begun and, if untreated, will die. However, for some patients oral feedings may suffice if a different aide assists with feeding, if preferred foods are provided, or if feedings are administered by syringe. For some patients, physiologically effective procedures are contraindicated by the likelihood that there is a serious and distressing underlying illness or that the procedures necessary would themselves be distressing. Clearly, the likely outcomes of each potential intervention will need to be assessed for each patient who faces this situation.

Likewise, the desirability of the potential outcomes will need to be assessed for each treatment modality. Again, some generalization is possible—early death and reduced life satisfactions are usually less desirable than are partially restored health and longer life—but this is often misleading in any particular patient's case. An early death might be preferable to restoring the previous state of health if the life left behind were quite painful.

A prolonged life marked by continued distress and reduced satisfactions might be better than early death, or it might not. If one were committed to the infinite value of human life irrespective of the differences among life experiences, then one would certainly want life to be sustained in a case where oral or artificial feeding would probably do so. On the other hand, if some kinds of living are taken to be worse than 'being dead, is this one? If the resident's primary problem is a cognitive deficit, life itself may not be so bad, so far as others can tell, for the patient. Usually, some things remain pleasant for a demented resident of a nursing home; and, bereft of clear self-concept, memories, and aspirations, the patient is unaware of the aspects of human life now denied her. Yet, most mentally capable people, in my experience and in the experience of others working with older persons, would not want to have such a life sustained. Many people feel that a life without insight, aspirations, or achievement is not to be desired, even though such a life may be pleasant, and even though it is not expected to be painful or distressing to the patient.[3]

This conundrum admits no easy resolution. One cannot know which combinations of reduced life potential and increased suffering should be taken to be better or worse than being dead. Thus, when this is the central question, as it often is in difficult cases, there will have to be a procedural resolution that vests authority to decide in certain persons and constrains their choices only when clearly necessary.

The difference between ensuring that the resident receives adequate nutrition and hydration in physiological terms and ensuring that the resident is fed and cared for in human and symbolic terms deserves mention. Caring and concern might best be conveyed by hand feeding, even if it is physiologically inadequate.[4] And supplying physiologically adequate nutrition and fluids may well be dehumanizing and might even lead to diminished human contact.[5] Both the physiological effects upon the body and the social and psychological effects upon the person are ordinarily important in assessing the desirability of outcomes for the resident. However, to the extent that the two can be disengaged, "giving to eat and drink"[6] is the more powerful symbol. It may be a dishonesty to provide deliberately inadequate treatment in physiological terms, as more than half of the physicians would have done in the survey reported by Micetich, Steinecker, and Thomasma.[7] Nevertheless, doing so may also be a legitimate response to the need to evidence humanity, compassion, and steadfastness in tragic circumstances. Being able to separate the potential goals of treatment may encourage a careful examination of which ones are more central to the public policy concerns raised by Callahan[8] and by Weisbard and Siegler.[9] Since efforts to secure physiologically normal nutrition and hydration can be forgone while efforts to provide oral feedings are continued, and since the latter are more significant as expressions of human concern, allowing this course may reduce the likelihood of untoward effects on the society.

As a practical matter, the third consideration, that of the availability of various options, very commonly limits the choices realistically considered for any particular resident. Long-term care is shaped by a number of explicit requirements and policies, probably more than in acute care. The effects of these restrictions in the area of feeding are numerous and are often perverse to the patient's interests. For example, long-term care institutions are commonly licensed to care for certain categories of residents, with care needs of certain kinds. Often, this means that any one facility may be allowed to provide some of the treatment alternatives but not others. In my area, "intermediate" level of care implies that the resident may be fed by gastrostomy, but not by nasogastric tube or intravenously. While the staffing requirements may well justify such a distinction, having it also creates a barrier to using some procedures, since transferring the resident to another facility may be very difficult if the resident has no personal funds and may be harmful irrespective of funds.

Also, reimbursement for some procedures is seldom, if ever, denied—intravenous hyperalimentation, for example—while the necessary and substantial time required for occupational therapy to restore or maintain swallowing is frequently disallowed. Under Medicare, long-term technical procedures are sometimes covered, while the costs of long-term gastrostomy or nasogastric feedings are routinely disallowed. These barriers often make certain choices essentially unavailable. Although it is beyond the scope of this chapter to provide an ethical critique of these barriers, it seems likely that many of them were created for reasons having little to do with the desired life-span and life experience of residents in long-term care facilities. Indeed, these financial barriers often reduce access to beneficial care and enlarge gaps between the poor and the well-to-do in ways that would prove to be contrary to any reasonable theory of distributional justice and of efficient public policy.

The aggregate effect of these considerations is that some range of options can be made available to the patient, that any one option has a particular likelihood of eventuating in various outcomes,[10] and that the desirability of these outcomes, when taken together with the likelihood of achieving them, will determine the option to be chosen. If the resident is adequately competent, can be well informed, can act with adequate freedom from coercion, and wishes to make the choice, then the resident's choice among alternatives is binding (unless it violates conscientiously held commitments of the institution or its staff, whereupon the patient would have to be offered every realistic option of transfer).[11] However, most nursing home residents who face such a choice are incompetent to make their own choices, and certain characteristics of the nursing home setting justify more protective procedures than might be required for other settings such as out-patient or hospital care.

DECISION-MAKING FOR INCOMPETENT PERSONS

Many residents in long-term care facilities do not have the capacity to decide whether to use artificial support of nutrition and hydration. The intention here is to review the general standards and procedures for decision-making for incompetent patients, with attention to the problems that are especially prevalent for residents in long-term care.[12]

The choice made on behalf of an incompetent patient[13] should be the choice that the person would have made. Since that may prove very difficult to know, an alternate standard is often needed: when one cannot know what this person would have wanted, one should assume that the person would have pursued his or her best interests. Actually, there is a continuum between the two standards, since there are many people for whom some things are known about their preferences but not enough to determine precisely what they would have wanted. In such cases, what is known about the person might eliminate some options that would otherwise have been considered. From among those options remaining, the one which a surrogate decision-maker determines will advance the person's interests best should be chosen. The New Jersey Supreme Court in *Conroy*[14] has recognized these standards, calling the polar standards the "subjective" standard (when the patient's own preferences are known sufficiently accurately to be determinative) and the "pure-objective" standard (when the patient's own preferences are completely unknown and the decision must be based upon what would be in the best interests of the usual person in this condition). The middle positions on the continuum were said by the court to use a "limited-objective" standard, where some relevant things are known about the resident but not enough to determine the course of care.

Honoring the resident's past value commitments[15] provides a powerful instrument to ensure that elderly residents in nursing homes are treated as individuals. If, as is reasonable to assume, the sources of incompetence that frequently accompany aging do not themselves regularly alter value commitments or treatment preferences, then the value history of an elderly person can justify individualized decisions. However, applying this aid to decision-making requires knowing the value history of the resident. This aspect of history-taking is often ignored and, unless the resident is fortunate enough to have friends and family who can provide that history when it is needed, this deficiency may well unnecessarily handicap decision-making for many in long-term care.

The *Conroy* court,[16] the *Storar* court,[17] and the President's Commission[18] have emphasized the potential value of advance directives, which are made while a person is competent, to direct the care of that person during incompetence. Formal documents such as durable powers of attorney and living wills[19] are especially powerful, though they also take the most advance planning and certitude on the part of the person executing the document. More informal advance directives, including a value history recorded in the medical chart[20] or resulting from questioning upon admission to long-term care facilities,[21] offer the potential for more frequent expressions of preferences in advance, though the remoteness and informality of these statements may make them less reliable.

Assessing the contemporaneous evidence of the preferences of a presently incompetent resident may be of limited help. In the *Hier* case,[22] the judge made much, probably too much,[23] of the patient pulling out her gastrostomy tube. This patient was institutionalized because of a fifty-seven-year history of serious mental illness. It would be very hard to know whether her behaviors connoted a dislike for the tube or a rather random nervous activity. The justices in *Conroy* were more circumspect, taking note of the uncertainty that attended any interpretation of the fact that she moaned or smiled after various stimuli.[24] Sometimes the interpretation is clear—the patient who cries out and struggles to free herself from restraints. At other times, it is likely to be obscure, and sometimes it may be indicative without being quite clear. Certainly, it would be imprudent to require that one always rely upon the evidence from behaviors or statements of presently incompetent persons, and it would be just as imprudent to demand that this evidence be ignored. Judgment in such matters will require careful gathering of the evidence and careful reflection upon its significance.

Since the incompetent patient by definition cannot make binding decisions, a surrogate process must be instituted. It is a strong tradition in this country that decisions in such settings will be made by the physician and the next of kin.[25] Recently, there have been shifts toward requiring that the surrogate be appointed in a court process,[26] or designated by the attending physician with review by institutional processes and, only if necessary, by the courts.[27] These resolutions are difficult for many residents in long-term care facilities, for many have no family or personal friends—no one to serve as a "friend-surrogate."[28] Appointing a stranger to be surrogate, usually selected only because he or she is a lawyer, appears to protect the resident only against egregious error or abuse. Furthermore, guardianship proceedings are often very time-consuming and expensive,[29] and sometimes they are not even possible.[30]

Often, the resident's only real friends and advocates are members of the staff of the care facility. However, the history of abuse in these facilities and the conflicts of loyalties of the staff would make one hesitate before recommending that the caregiving staff routinely act as surrogate. In fact, even family and friends have frequent conflicts of interest, at least as to whether they will feel guilty or virtuous with a choice to allow death to come early for lack of artificial feeding techniques. What will be necessary will be to engineer a creative compromise that incorporates the special knowledge of the patient and the often quite sincere concern for his or her welfare by members of the staff and any remaining family and friends and to provide protection for the resident from any detrimental effects of self-interest on the part of any of these parties. The elements of that resolution are just now beginning to be developed.

EFFECTS OF BEING IN A
LONG-TERM CARE INSTITUTION

Long-term care institutions have a number of characteristics that require special considerations when applying decision-making models. First is the concern that this society is so prejudiced against the residents of such institutions that patterns of care that would be offensive in other settings might be allowed in this one. Certainly, society's lack of any truly positive role for the elderly has been well documented.[31] The history of abuse in nursing homes has sometimes led to a countervailing prejudice—that anything done there is contrary to residents' interests, and this assumption justifies circumscribing the behaviors of caregivers very conservatively.[32] Especially since residents are often powerless to defend themselves and since nursing homes are supported predominantly by public funds,[33] the public feels particularly responsible for maintaining acceptable standards.

The residents of long-term care facilities are predominantly elderly women with few concerned friends and family and with a high incidence of dementing illness. With few observers or activist residents, nursing home staffs are readily encouraged to take over the decision-making. In fact, allowing the residents to make decisions is likely to add substantially to the burdens of managing the facility, as any individual preferences are likely to cause more work and disrupt routines. In an "industry" where the standards are set by "for-profit" endeavors and where short staffing is the norm, vesting control of time expenditures in the staff has important effects. Prolonged efforts at oral feeding, where the resident can set the time frame and manipulate the staff, are likely to be intolerable. Artificial feeding actually diminishes time commitments to many residents and removes from them a significant source of control of their environment.

The residents of long-term care facilities are also often experiencing what they would themselves see as a very reduced quality of life. They are often very old, multiply handicapped, and socially isolated. It is not surprising to find that caregivers and the residents themselves may not find this to be a life worth a vigorous defense.

Residents of nursing homes are also physically fragile, often with borderline or substandard nutritional status at all times. This makes them particularly susceptible to rapid physical deterioration with malnutrition or dehydration, and forces the cessation of oral intake to be considered a major crisis.

These considerations have led to concerns that residents of nursing homes be given special procedural protections when life-sustaining treatments (or other substantially important treatments) might be withheld. The most expansive statement in this regard is to be found in the final ruling in *Conroy*,[34] in which the court establishes a cumbersome procedure to be followed before any life-sustaining procedure is forgone for a nursing home resident (who is additionally within a year of expected death and was previously competent). While the costs of the New Jersey procedure may prove to be overwhelming and the time required may be cruel, some special protections may prove to be warranted; otherwise, residents are at risk of recurrent abuse.

MANAGEMENT OF THE CASE

In the case that opened this chapter, what options are available to the physician? The first branch in the decision tree (see figure 2) is the choice between (1) attending to her comfort and making no further investigation or effort at definitive treatment, realizing that she is very likely to become more dehydrated and die with this course of action, or (2) investigating the possibility of a reversible cause for the recent worsening of condition.

"Supportive Care" in Anticipation of Death

What would happen if the first option were chosen? Dehydration and fever in an elderly person who refuses food and water are very likely to lead to death if no intervention is undertaken. What sort of dying results? This is probably the course that Osler had in mind when he said that pneumonia is the old man's friend. The patient is likely to become quite unresponsive early in the course of her decline and to evidence very little distress. Even if food and water continue to be offered, her fluid and nutritional status is likely to worsen. Uncomfortable symptoms are likely to be readily relieved by simple measures.

If nontreatment were the standard, older persons could be assured that their lives would not be mercilessly extended, that they would

Figure 2.
Decision tree for the case.

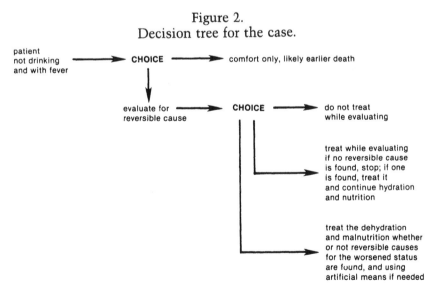

not suffer the indignities of dying reliant upon machinery, and that they would have to speak to the issue directly if they wished to have a different course of action taken in their case. Furthermore, the costs of treatment and of continued supportive care could be saved. However, such a plan could be applied in a sloppy and unreflective manner, leading to the tragedy of wrongful abbreviation of life. It could even lead to a general failure to cherish and honor the lives of profoundly dependent people, even when all they needed to survive and possibly to enjoy life was human compassion and warmth, shelter, and feeding in the normal way.

Deciding to Evaluate and Treat

The decision tree (figure 2) lists an option of evaluating the patient for a reversible cause of her acute problems but not treating during the evaluation. This is almost certainly an undesirable option, since the delay in treatment will ordinarily reduce the chances of successful treatment, thus also reducing the chances that the burdens of the evaluation will be counterbalanced by any benefits whatsoever. Thus, a choice for evaluation is almost certainly also a choice for initiating treatment.

What is the treatment like for the patient? A full description of the available treatments is given in chapter 2. It will suffice here to point out that the patient is very likely to have to be restrained in order to keep an intravenous or nasogastric tube in place, to find this frightening, even to develop skin sores or aspiration as a result of the treatment, to be uncomfortable from the tubes themselves, and, if she dies despite treatment, to die more uncomfortably than if she had died with substantial dehydration. Furthermore, she might have to be transferred to a hospital for evaluation and treatment, a maneuver which is itself a cause of fear, disorientation, aspiration pneumonia, restraints, and other medical complications.

From the start, the physician should decide whether the treatment providing hydration and nutrition is to continue regardless of other findings or whether it is to be stopped if no reversible etiology is found. Very often, treatment continues indefinitely because no attention was paid to the possibility of stopping. Physicians often feel that it is nearly impossible to stop a life-supporting treatment that has been started, even though they would not have felt obliged to start it if they had known its outcome. This is a thoroughly indefensible distinction and even creates an unwarranted threshold reducing the willingness to start a treatment that might later prove undesirable.

However, deciding to forgo the use of a treatment from the start is easier upon the emotions and much harder to trace or to hold anyone responsible for than is deciding to stop an ongoing treatment. To stop a feeding tube is certain to cause staff stress and to necessitate difficult discussions with staff and family; to fail to start one is likely to be overlooked. This creates an incentive for the physician to maintain what is actually a morally unjustified distinction that holds it less acceptable to stop than to fail to start.

Thus, if one is going to evaluate for treatable cause, feeling that if none is found the patient should not be sustained with artificial feeding, then one should decide from the start that the artificial feeding will be a time-limited commitment. Discussions with the family and the staff should reflect this decision, so that all involved know that, unless the situation improves or has reasonable prospects of improving, at some agreed time, the artificial feeding will be discontinued. The fact that such a choice must be public, documented, and discussed should provide some protection against its being done in an unreflective or haphazard manner. Of course, the same characteristics might make it difficult to exercise this option at all, if the discussions made necessary would be too difficult or would be expected to incur legal entanglements.

TREATMENT IRRESPECTIVE OF EVALUATION
Perhaps the physician should treat the malnutrition and dehydration irrespective of whether the patient has any prospects of improved life. This claim could be supported in three ways: it is a good thing to sustain the patient's life no matter what the nature of that life and the nature of the means needed to sustain life; or, it is a good thing to sustain life when doing so requires providing food and water through means that are not terribly difficult to obtain or to endure; or, it is a good thing to sustain the life of this patient using these means, even though it might not be for another patient (e.g., one near death or one who is suffering greatly). The first contention rests upon a conviction that any life is better than no life and usually relies upon a religious claim that sustaining life is an obligation to God. This claim can also be justified by a prudential assessment

that to do otherwise is to risk devaluing human life and thereby to allow all manner of unduly early deaths. If this particular patient held this religious belief, then life should usually be sustained. However, the prudential claim is weaker, for following such a claim requires that the patient be used as a means to protect the rest of the society, which is justifiable only if there were overwhelming evidence of serious harms if the patient were not used for others' benefit in this way. The available evidence does not support this claim.

Considering the burdensomeness and availability of the treatment makes a more acceptable standard. If a treatment is unduly painful, frightening, or otherwise troubling for the patient or too costly or difficult to obtain, there would be no imperative to use it. One could thereby avoid inflicting distress or necessitating bizarre budget priorities as one would have to have done with the unmodified proposal above. However, one would still have to save the life of a patient for whom the treatment itself poses no major travail even if the life saved would not have been one that the patient would have chosen to have sustained.

This, then, is the hard question: Is it to be expected, or even permitted, that decisions regarding life-sustaining treatment consider the nature of the life to be sustained? It is easier to forgo a treatment which directly imposes great burdens; it is harder to allow forgoings when the life of the patient is what imposes the burdens. Yet, the chronic illnesses and the growing dependency of elderly nursing home residents impose burdens upon the patients and upon all who care about them. Are those burdens ever to be seen as so great that they justify allowing the patient to die for lack of treatment that is not itself very burdensome? I believe that life can be too hard to require that anyone—patient or physician—expend efforts to sustain it. However, such a stance does entail risks of abuse, perhaps especially when the person dying is old and in a nursing home. Thus, procedures must be generated that limit the risks of abuse.

CONCLUSIONS

Elderly residents of nursing homes are not always best served by seeking to effectuate normal nutrition and hydration. The necessary treatments can be contrary to the patient's wishes or too burdensome, or can sustain a life that has itself become too burdensome.

While persons always should be offered food and drink (unless taking it would cause suffering), medical interventions can be too painful or restrictive to be warranted.

However, when the patient is resident in a long-term care facility, alternatives and advocates are likely to be in short supply. This creates the obligation to ensure exceptionally good decision-making practices in this setting. Forgoing food and water must not become a thoughtless choice aimed at ridding the society—or the patients' families—of burdensome, dependent elderly persons. Since the history of decision-making in long-term care facilities shows many deficiencies, procedures for deciding about nutrition and hydration should arise from a deliberate process and should be explicit and carefully evaluated in practice. However, these procedures should not be so onerous that they themselves make good decisions less likely. The chapters in this volume that address the *Conroy* decision by the New Jersey Supreme Court show that good decisions about life-sustaining treatments of all sorts may have become harder to achieve after that court required (1) appointment of a legal guardian, (2) an "abuse" investigation by the ombudsman, (3) consultations by two uninvolved physicians, and, generally, (4) consent by virtually all family. Since these decisions arise frequently, this procedure is too costly, too intrusive, and too time-consuming. There needs to be investigation and innovation to establish and evaluate alternative approaches, which might include institutional review committees, institutional programs to provide guardians or other surrogates, development and explanation of presumptions for treatment in each institution, and extensive use of advance directives.

The elderly residents of long-term care facilities need neither too much nor too little treatment. Neither error is truly more acceptable.

NOTES

1. Health and Public Policy Committee, American College of Physicians, "Long-Term Care of the Elderly," *Ann. Intern. Med.* 100:760–763 (1984).

2. For a description of these and other procedures for supplying nutrition and hydration to patients, see chapter 2.

3. *In re* Conroy, 98 N.J. 321, 486 A.2d 1209 (1985) (Handler, J., dissenting in part).

4. See chapter 3; also, Bernard Lo and Laurie Dornbrand, "Guiding the Hand that Feeds," *N. Engl. J. Med.* 311:402–404 (1984).

5. *Id.*

6. Chapter 5.

7. Chapter 4.

8. Chapter 6.

9. Chapter 11.

10. Each assessment of the likelihood of achieving each outcome is also attended by some degree of uncertainty, which does not change the decision-making theory involved but does make it more complex.

11. See chapter 21.

12. See also The President's Commission for the Study of Ethical Problems in Medicine and Biomedical and Behavioral Research, *Making Health Care Decisions*, Washington, D.C.: U.S. Government Printing Office (1982).

13. See chapter 20 for a discussion of the elements of competence, and thus of the determination that a resident is incompetent.

14. *In re* Conroy, 98 N.J. 321, 486 A.2d 1209 (1985).

15. Laurence McCullough, "Medical Care for Elderly Patients with Diminished Competence: An Ethical Analysis," *J. Am. Geriatr. Soc.* 32:150–153 (1984).

16. *In re* Conroy, 98 N.J. 321, 360–363, 486 A.2d 1209, 1229–1230 (1985).

17. *In re* Storar, 52 N.Y.2d 363, 438 N.Y.S.2d 266, 420 N.E.2d 64, *cert. denied* 454 U.S. 858 (1981).

18. The President's Commission for the Study of Ethical Problems in Medicine and Biomedical and Behavioral Research, *Deciding to Forego Life-Sustaining Treatment*, Washington, D.C.: U.S. Government Printing Office (1983).

19. *Id.* at 136–153.

20. McCullough, *supra* note 15.

21. Arnold Wagner, "Cardiopulmonary Resuscitation in the Aged: A Prospective Survey," *N. Engl. J. Med.* 310:1129–1130 (1984).

22. *In re* Hier, 18 Mass. App. Ct. 200 (1984).

23. George J. Annas, "The Case of Mary Hier: When Substituted Judgment Becomes Sleight of Hand," *Hastings Cent. Rep.* 14:23–25 (August 1984).

24. *In re* Conroy, 98 N.J. 321, 386–387, 486 A.2d 1209, 1243 (1985).

25. Alexander M. Capron, "Informed Consent in Catastrophic Disease Treatment and Research," *U. Pa. L. Rev.* 123:340, 424–425 (1974).

26. Superintendent of Belchertown State School v. Saikewicz, 370 N.E.2d 417 (Mass. 1977); *In re* Conroy, 98 N.J. 321, 486 A.2d 1209 (1985).

27. President's Commission, *Deciding to Forego*, *supra* note 18.

28. Robert Veatch, "An Ethical Framework for Terminal Care Decisions: A New Classification of Patients," *J. Am. Geriatr. Soc.* 32:665–669 (1984).

29. President's Commission, *Deciding to Forego*, *supra* note 18, 129–131.

30. In Washington, D.C., for example, guardianship proceedings for a person with a non-emergency problem who has no assets, a common situation, requires "creating" a somewhat dishonest claim that assets need to be managed.

31. See, e.g., Robert N. Butler, *Why Survive? Being Old in America*, New York: Harper & Row (1975); Sally Gadow, "A Philosophical Perspective," in Christine K. Cassel and John R. Walsh (eds.), *Geriatric Medicine*, New York: Springer-Verlag (1984).

32. Jane D. Hoyt and James M. Davies, "A Response to the Task Force on Supportive Care," *Law, Med. and Health Care* 12:103–105 (June 1984).

33. Robert L. Kane, "Long-Term Care: Policy and Reimbursement," in Christine K. Cassel and John R. Walsh (eds.), *Geriatric Medicine*, New York: Springer-Verlag (1984).

34. *In re* Conroy, 98 N.J. 321, 486 A.2d 1209 (1985).

Joel Frader, M.D.

17   Forgoing Life-Sustaining Food and Water: Newborns

ON FOOD AND WATER FOR INFANTS

Special considerations arise in choosing to forgo nutrition and hydration for babies. Assuming that one can find justifications for any death to occur by dehydration and/or malnutrition, those reasons should apply equally well to infants and older persons, even though feeding babies has special social significance. Historically, however, what has distinguished this issue in these times is the politicization of withholding food and water from infants. The government has not entered, in such a detailed way, into the control of many other medical practices.

Although the daily medico-moral problems of the neonatal intensive care setting far more often involve very premature infants, most of the public debate has centered upon two other paradigm cases—Down syndrome and spina bifida—and the role of nonfeeding has become a concern only in the case of the Down syndrome babies. Many newborns with Down syndrome suffer from associated congenital anomalies (such as duodenal atresia) which render normal feeding impossible without surgical repair. Unlike low birthweight infants, whose sometimes rocky course may present a series of complicated clinical options, the question for this group of Down syndrome newborns is stark and dichotomous: to operate or not. If there were no surgery, the infants would surely die for lack of ability to eat: with surgery, which is ordinarily done for similarly obstructed gastrointestinal tracts of infants with no Down syndrome, eating is often returned to normal.

The focus upon the possibility of starvation in this setting has arisen because of two public cases: first, a report by one respected medical center that a number of infants, including some of this sort, had died after deliberate decisions to withhold treatment[1] and, second, a film about such an incident at Johns Hopkins Hospital which was produced in 1971.[2]

These cases, along with the Bloomington, Indiana, Baby Doe, have achieved such widespread recognition that it is the image of the Down syndrome baby being starved to death that is most clearly in mind as policymakers designed their interventions. The language of the federal regulations throughout has applied most readily to these infants, and the effort to prevent their death by starvation has been applied, largely without reflection, to the preservation of the lives of all other ill and handicapped newborns.

Paris and Fletcher have pointed out that Health and Human Services (HHS) policies, in the pre-congressional phase of the Baby Doe phenomenon, led to troublesome contradictions and ironies.[3] Congress has fallen into the same trap with the Child Abuse Amendment of 1984. Without giving reasons, HHS and Congress distinguish medical treatment from hydration, nutrition, and medication. "All such disabled infants must under all circumstances receive appropriate nutrition, hydration, and medication."[4] Unless the word "appropriate" leaves room for maneuvering, federal law will now require exactly what some courts and many thinkers have been arguing may not be legally or morally necessary, at least when the patient is persistently vegetative. Therefore, physicians are required to provide food and water, even when "treatment" is regarded as futile. One can imagine circumstances where feeding and hydration would hasten death, say in cases of renal agenesis (congenital failure of the kidneys to develop) or irreversible renal failure. The law does not require in such cases that doctors provide dialysis. If dialysis is not used, "ordinary" food and water may be expected to speed the infant's demise. Such a result might or might not actually be in the child's best interests (however defined), but Congress or HHS surely did not have this outcome in mind.

A less confusing circumstance, as Paris and Fletcher suggested, is that of anencephaly. (Actually, hydranencephaly would be even clearer.) As in all cases of persistent vegetative state, the patient cannot perceive thirst or hunger, because the necessary brain tissue for those perceptions is absent. The primitive brainstem, however, can at times maintain cardiorespiratory function for extended periods. What point is made by requiring that such a child receive sustenance? The patient has and can have no interests. Continued life delays mourning and psychological healing for the family. Medical workers are frustrated by being forced to carry out utterly futile procedures. Substantial economic costs accrue as well.

If one agrees that supporting life sometimes will "merely prolong dying" or will "not be effective in ameliorating" disease, it must be the case that nutrition and hydration for some infants are at least morally optional. If medical measures can no longer control pain and suffering from an underlying illness, continuing to give food and water may be morally offensive. Good medical practice, that is, palliation, could require allowing dehydration and malnutrition. However, accurately predicting the outcome of any one baby is not possible, thus making it quite difficult to judge when to accept death in order to evade suffering.

As Macklin has argued, procedural solutions such as those employed by Congress and HHS may appeal in the absence of moral consensus. However, procedures do not settle substantive value questions.[5] Indeed, even if there were widespread agreement with Congress or HHS (and there may or may not be), the support would not make requiring fluids and nutrition morally correct.[6] When the provision of any medical treatment, including fluids and nutrition, will only prolong dying or extend suffering, it should be permissible to forgo them. This is true for the newly born, those in midlife, or the aged.

RESOLUTIONS?

Governmental intervention into the care of handicapped infants is not likely to help. Neither government investigators, such as state or federal Baby Doe squads, nor institutional infant care review committees (ICRCs) seem useful solutions. There probably are very few Baby Does like the one in Bloomington, Indiana, and the vast majority of them are transferred to tertiary care centers, if not actually born in them. Such centers are not likely to risk public censure or professional standing by failing to pursue treatment of such a disorder.

Routine governmental investigation would be even less personal than the blind technological imperative so chillingly described by the Stinsons.[7] Lacking adequate substantive criteria, governmental agencies, like courts, would move slowly and cautiously, while infants, families, and medical personnel suffer.

Internal hospital review committees are either unnecessary or functionally inadequate. While more likely to provide a rapid and perhaps more sensitive response, ICRCs seem to have little to add to ongoing consultation and discussion. If unbidden to begin with, the committee's probings and recommendations may well be rejected by physicians and/or families already bent on a particular course of action. ICRCs could even generate *sub rosa* processes whereby deliberations and decisions are dictated by institutional power and authority, by economic considerations (be they referral patterns or DRGs), and lack of moral expertise.

Skepticism about institutional review is not new. Questions have begun to appear about the scientific institutional review boards (IRBs) that oversee research on human subjects. Recently, Goldman and Katz in the *Journal of the American Medical Association* raised doubts about the consistency and quality of such review.[8] The President's Commission discussion of ethics committees pointed out a number of areas of concern, including medicolegal responsibility, liability, privacy, and access.[9] Youngner's study of hospital ethics committees for the President's Commission revealed the curious finding that chairpersons felt that their groups were effective.[10] However, their committees reviewed an average of only one case per year. It is difficult to imagine how such little activity could have much impact.

Greater public accountability in medical decision-making is essential. But families, doctors, and hospitals would have to invest substantial energy into the ICRC process. Committees must not persist if they are, in Annas's words, " . . . privately constituted groups with indeterminate membership, hazy mandates, undefined principles of decision-making, and nonexistent procedural requirements. . . ."[11] If families and providers make "bad" decisions, the states already have child protective mechanisms in place.[12] Judicial review and malpractice litigation are available. Professional quality review mechanisms exist now. New governmental or institutional processes may well be no better and might undermine the trust fundamental to the physician-patient relationship.

> Basic to the relationship between physician and patient is the expectation that life is worthy to be lived. If physicians will act on behalf of their patients towards this end and if acts of omission or commission lead to an earlier demise of a patient than might ordinarily have been expected, these decisions have to remain within the bounds of the expected compassionate and understanding relationship between patient and his doctor, the patient's family and the patient's doctor. The number of examples of this decision making is legend. It is unthinkable that the law would direct this decision making on the part of the physician,

because to do so would determine the fundamental principles in all the great field of health care."[13]

This observation, in 1976, by C. Everett Koop, might have been important to bear more prominently in mind when he, as Surgeon General, helped to draft the "Baby Doe" rules.

Two other important and interrelated issues have been largely disregarded in the discussions on the treatment of handicapped infants. The historic progress toward children's rights cannot justify dismissing the interests of parents, siblings, or the wider community. While families may not reject children because of sex, hair color, temperament, or the like, must families care for offspring come what may? Must parents and other relatives provide round-the-clock home nursing for the totally disabled? Some families may be enriched by caring for a severely handicapped child, but certainly not all. Surely families have some claims to make decisions that so profoundly affect their futures.

Furthermore, individual families often will not have the time, money, or skills necessary to provide optimum care. Families taking responsibility for multiply handicapped infants now face a tragic political irony. The very government that wants to mandate all manner of expensive, sophisticated treatment is dismantling much of our health and social welfare system. Goldstein, Freud, and Solnit have stated the contrary moral mandate for public policy: ". . . the state must take upon itself the burden of providing the special financial, physical, and psychological resources essential to making real the value it prefers for the child it 'saves.' "[14]

Finally, the merit of interventions to sustain life of a seriously ill newborn turns on the society's commitment to eliminate needless pain and suffering, which is now sorely lacking. Infants with life-threatening illnesses will often be subjected to prolonged hospitalization, often with many uncomfortable procedures. When the pain and suffering will be substantial and results of therapy dubious, perhaps treatment is worse than death. Sometimes the results of treatment could be, on balance, good. However, if society's allocation of resources allows only indifferent or altogether inadequate long-term care, aggressive treatment may well become inhumane and an indignity.

Pediatricians and pediatric surgeons have been in the business of saving lives, not wantonly ending life. But as in other areas of science and technology, we have begun to recognize unfortunate and unintended consequences of medical progress. Physicians and families need moral guidance regarding the proper application of our remarkable scientific tools. Unfortunately, narrow political considerations have determined the guidance that has thus far arisen from the political process and the public debate has lacked the insight necessary for the development of meaningful moral progress.

NOTES

1. Raymond S. Duff and A. G. M. Campbell, "Moral and Ethical Dilemmas in the Special Care Nursery," *N. Engl. J. Med.* 289:890–894 (1973).
2. "Who Shall Survive?" The Joseph P. Kennedy Foundation, Washington, D.C. (1971) (film).
3. John J. Paris and Anne B. Fletcher, "Infant Doe Regulations and the Absolute Requirement to Use Nourishment and Fluids for the Dying Infant," *Law, Medicine, and Health Care* 11:210–213 (1983).
4. Department of Health and Human Services, "Proposed Rules 45 CFR Part 1340, Child Abuse and Neglect Prevention and Treatment Program." *Federal Register* 49:48160–67 (Dec. 10, 1984).
5. Ruth Macklin, "Return to the Best Interests of the Child," in Willard Gaylin and Ruth Macklin (eds.), *Who Speaks for the Child?* New York: Plenum Press (1982), 269.
6. *Id.* at 271.
7. Robert and Peggy Stinson, *The Long Dying of Baby Andrew*, Boston: Little, Brown, and Co. (1983).
8. Jerry Goldman and Martin D. Katz, "Inconsistency and Institutional Review Boards," *J.A.M.A.* 248:197–202 (1982).
9. The President's Commission for the Study of Ethical Problems in Medicine and Biomedical and Behavioral Research, *Deciding to Forego Life-Sustaining Treatment*, Washington, D.C.: U.S. Govt. Printing Office (1983), 169–170.
10. Stuart Youngner and David C. Jackson, et al., "A National Survey of Hospital Ethics Committees," *Crit. Care Med.* 11:902–905 (1983).
11. George J. Annas, "Baby Doe Redux: Doctors as Child Abusers," *Hastings Cent. Rep.* 13:26–27 (October, 1983).
12. Angela R. Holder, "Parents, Courts, and Refusal of Treatment," *J. Pediatr.* 103:515–521 (1983).
13. C. Everett Koop, *The Right to Live; The Right to Die*, Wheaton, Illinois: Tyndale House Publishers (1976), 110–111.
14. Joseph Goldstein, Anna Freud, and Albert J. Solnit, *Before the Best Interests of the Child*, New York: Free Press (1979), 97.

Ronald E. Cranford, M.D.

18 Patients with Permanent Loss of Consciousness

One price of medical progress has been the growing number of patients with permanent loss of consciousness.

Along with the growing number of patients have come fundamental ethical and legal questions: Under what circumstances is it morally permissible to stop treatment, and what types of therapy may justifiably be discontinued in these patients? The simplicity of these questions belies the complexity of the issues, of which I shall address three here. First, where do we draw the line between consciousness and unconsciousness? Second, what is the meaning and moral relevance of the terms *terminally ill* and *imminently dying?* Finally, in dealing with these hopeless situations, can we consider fluids and nutrition "medical treatment," or are they something more?

PERMANENTLY UNCONSCIOUS VS. SEVERE DEMENTIA

In deciding when it is appropriate to forgo life-sustaining treatment, a major distinction has been drawn between those patients who are in a persistent vegetative state (Karen Quinlan)[1] vs. those who are severely demented but retain some degree of cognitive functioning (Claire Conroy).[2] The essence of the distinction rests on the presence or absence of consciousness.

In its report *Deciding to Forego Life-Sustaining Treatment*, the President's Commission for the Study of Ethical Problems in Medicine defined permanently unconscious patients as those in whom *all* possible components of mental life are absent—all thought, feeling, sensation, desire, emotion, and awareness of self or environment.[3] The Commission described five categories of patients: (1) patients in a persistent vegetative state; (2) those who are unresponsive after brain injury or hypoxia and who do not recover sufficient brainstem function to stabilize or to evolve into a vegetative state before dying (in other words, those who die still in a true coma); (3) end-stage victims of degenerative neurologic conditions such as Alzheimer's disease or other forms of extremely severe dementia (when there are *no* neocortical functions whatsoever); (4) comatose patients with intracranial mass lesions such as tumors or vascular lesions in whom consciousness is not regained before death; and (5) those with congenital hypoplasia of the central nervous system (e.g., anencephaly).

The persistent vegetative state is probably the most common, as well as the most widely discussed form of permanent unconsciousness. Such patients perceive neither themselves nor their environment. Neurological examination reveals no neocortical functions. Yet these patients do have sleep-wake cycles, and at times their eyes open. From a neurologic standpoint, they simply do not experience pain, suffering, or cognition.[4]

If a person is completely unaware of his or her surroundings and will never again experience consciousness, it becomes difficult to defend the premise that he or she has any interests at all.

> ... To be sure, Karen Quinlan was not "dead" in most of the increasingly multiple senses of that term, but the task of giving content to the notion that she had rights, in the face of the recognition that she could make no decisions about how to exercise any such rights remains a difficult one.[5]

Following this logic, one finds it nearly impossible to defend deciding about treatment based on the usual standard that treatments must be provided when the expected benefits are proportionate to the expected burdens.

Yet in trying to draw a line to separate awareness from unawareness, we cannot decide where exactly to place our pencil: from awareness to unawareness, or consciousness to unconsciousness, is a continuum. While it is very difficult to describe and diagnose many conditions on this continuum, the distinction between complete absence of consciousness and the retention of some slight awareness or thought can ordinarily be accomplished by careful examination by qualified specialists.

Claire Conroy certainly was not unconscious, although she was severely demented. The appellate court, in reversing the trial court, placed great ethical and legal weight on drawing lines between vegetative patients and those with some degree of cognitive functioning.

> The distinction between an "awake" but confused patient like Conroy and an "asleep", vegetative patient like Karen Quinlan is material and is determinative in this case. The Quinlan court held that the State's interest in preserving a patient's life depends upon whether the patient ever will return to cognitive sapient life. . . . Thus, it is plain that Quinlan applies only to noncognitive, vegetative patients. . . .[6]

In the case concerning Clarence Herbert, who was left permanently unconscious after a postoperative respiratory arrest, the appellate court in California ruled that Mr. Herbert's neurologic condition was crucial in deciding the propriety of withdrawing life-sustaining treatment, including fluids and nutrition. To a large degree, then, the court dismissed the homicide charges because of Mr. Herbert's permanent unconsciousness.[7]

The courts (and others) clearly are much more comfortable with stopping fluids and nutrition when a patient is permanently unconscious than if the patient is at all sentient.

TERMINALLY ILL, IMMINENTLY DYING VS. SEVERELY NEUROLOGICALLY IMPAIRED

Many patients with permanent unconsciousness have bodies that are capable of functioning for prolonged periods of time without artificial devices such as respirators. Is it ethical to discontinue all treatment on some of these patients, even when they are not terminally ill and imminently dying in the more traditional sense of these terms?[8]

A fairly recent consensus is that terminally ill, imminently dying patients deserve care and treatment whose overriding objective is not mainly to prolong life but to maintain comfort, hygiene, and dignity.

Patients who are in a persistent vegetative state or who are severely demented may no longer be considered "terminally ill" or "imminently dying," because medicine has developed ways of keeping them alive for long periods. These life-prolonging medical methods include artificial means of supplying fluids and nutrition. We now control more of the dying process and thus, to some degree, the moment and means of death. This misfortune is dramatically illustrated by the increasing numbers and longevity of patients in a persistent vegetative state, many of whom now live for years, with no hope of recovery. Karen Quinlan is only the most well-known patient of this kind: some estimate their numbers to be 5,000–10,000 in this country.

In the *Quinlan* case, the New Jersey Supreme Court put forth a general moral and legal standard in forgoing life-sustaining treatment: As the prognosis (for return of cognitive functions) dims, and the degree of bodily invasion (with artificial types of treatment such as respirators) increases, it is more justified to consider stopping treatment so as to exercise the right of self-determination of the patient, as expressed through the wishes of the parents. But once a vegetative state patient is stable, and once the respirator has been taken away, the degree of invasion is lessened. Perhaps all that is needed to sustain life is a nasogastric tube to deliver fluids and nutrition. Is it then justifiable to stop? In the *Conroy* case, the court held that artificial feeding is to be evaluated as a treatment, although a less intrusive one than a respirator.[9]

FLUIDS AND NUTRITION AS LIFE-SUSTAINING TREATMENT

Since stopping ventilators in permanently unconscious patients is justifiable,[10] is withdrawing artificial feeding also justified.? This question, along with the discussion just presented, alludes to perhaps the most fundamental question: Are fluids and nutrition "medical therapy," or are they different in some fundamental moral sense?[11]

The President's Commission defined life-sustaining treatment as encompassing *all* health interventions that increase the life-span of the patient. Among its examples of life-sustaining treatment, the Commission specifically mentioned special feeding procedures. In one of its major recommendations on patients with a permanent loss of consciousness, the Commission stated:

> The decisions of patients' families should determine what sort of medical care permanently unconscious patients receive. Other than requiring appropriate decisionmaking procedures for these patients, the law does not and should not require any particular therapies to be applied or

continued, with the exception of basic nursing care that is needed to ensure dignified and respectful treatment of the patient.[12]

The President's Commission, in discussing the goals of medical treatment in general, and specifically as they apply to permanently unconscious patients, focuses on this critical issue:

> The primary basis for medical treatment of patients is the prospect that each individual's interest (specifically, the interest in well-being) will be promoted. Thus, treatment ordinarily aims to benefit a patient through preserving life, relieving pain and suffering, protecting against disability, and returning maximally effective functioning. If a prognosis of permanent unconsciousness is correct, however, continued treatment cannot confer such benefits. Pain and suffering are absent, as are joy, satisfaction, and pleasure. Disability is total and no return to an even minimal social or human functioning is possible. . . . Any value to the patient from continued care and maintenance under such circumstances would seem to reside in a very small probability that the prognosis of permanence is incorrect.[13]

This was a major issue in the Barber-Nedjl case in California, and the appellate court addressed this question directly:

> Even though these life-support devices are, to a degree, "self-propelled", each pulsation of the respirator or each drop of fluid introduced into the patient's body by intravenous feeding devices is comparable to a manually administered injection or item of medication. Hence "disconnecting" of the mechanical devices is comparable to withholding the manually administered injection or medication.
>
> Further we view the use of an intravenous administration of nourishment and fluid, under these circumstances, as being the same as the use of respirator or other form of life-support equipment.
>
> The prosecution would have us draw a distinction between the use of mechanical breathing devices such as respirators and mechanical feeding devices such as intravenous tubes. The distinction urged seems to be based more on the emotional symbolism of providing food and water to those incapable of providing for themselves rather than on any rational difference in cases such as the one at bench.
>
> *Medical* nutrition and hydration may not always provide net benefits to patients. Medical procedures to provide nutrition and hydration are more similar to other medical procedures than to typical human ways of providing nutrition and hydration. Their benefits and burdens ought to be evaluated in the same manner as any other medical procedure.[14]

Thus, the courts which have addressed the matter have found that in permanently unconscious patients it is morally justifiable to withdraw life-sustaining treatment—including artifically adminis-tered fluids and nutrition.[15]

Yet the argument by Callahan and others that fluids and nutrition represent something deeper, more fundamental, to us as a society compels us to proceed in this unfamiliar area with great care. Four considerations might, in some situations, distinguish fluids and nu-trition from other traditional forms of medical treatment.

First, choices must be made with respect for the symbolic nature of feeding. Permanently unconscious patients are in some ways "helpless," as are newborns, children, the demented, and the re-tarded. The society is ennobled by a dedication to nurturing the helpless, whether near death or birth. In the case of newborns, no one doubts that nutrition is part of nurturing. With those near death, such automatic nurturance is more debatable.

Second, families sometimes face great emotional trauma in trying to decide whether to stop fluids and nutrition. They personally must decide what is nurturance. And, when a decision has been made to stop fluids and nutrition, each day may become more agonizing as the family watches the patient move toward the inevitable end.

That leads to the third consideration: If all fluids and nutrition are withdrawn from any patient, regardless of the condition, he or she will die—inevitably and invariably. Death may come in a few days or take up to two weeks. Rarely in medicine is an earlier death for the patient so certain. So, is stopping fluids to be considered an acceptable instance of allowing nature to take its course, or is it actually causing death? Perhaps there is no one answer; much de-pends on the patient's condition. Fluids and nutrition might be con-sidered to be like much conventional treatment when the patient is permanently unconscious and when the means of delivery is ar-tificial and invasive, such as with a nasogastric tube or gastrostomy. Some of the certainty can be reduced by continuing oral feedings whenever possible.

This raises a fourth consideration: the potential for abuse. As sug-gested by the Bouvia case, a policy of stopping fluids and nutrition in severely brain-damaged patients could have serious implications in the care of other patients, such as the severely retarded or those with cerebral palsy.[16] Thus, any form of public policy that permits the withdrawal of fluids and nutrition should be carefully articu-lated, and the potential for abuse recognized and minimized. Society must be reassured that all of the issues raised here have been evaluated and that the potential for abuse in all classes of patients has been addressed.

RECOMMENDATIONS

First, hospitals and other health care institutions ought to promulgate explicit policies regarding circumstances and procedures relating to forgoing life-sustaining fluids and nutrition, and these institutions should ensure that health care providers and patients' families substantially comply with the guidelines.

As recommended by the President's Commission, health care institutions are specially obligated to adopt clear, explicit, and publicly available policies regarding how and by whom these decisions are to be made for patients who lack adequate decision-making capacity. This recommendation would particularly apply to patients who are permanently unconscious and especially to the controversial measure of stopping artificially administered fluids and nutrition.

Such guidelines could require the following before forgoing life-sustaining treatment (of any kind): (1) that the patient is determined by appropriate specialists to be permanently unconscious; (2) that the family or other surrogate is acting in what is perceived to be the best interests of the patient, or is doing what the patient would have wanted; and (3) that the health care professionals attending the patient believe that further life-sustaining treatment of the sort envisioned, which might include artificially administered fluids and nutrition, would no longer benefit the patient.

Given the current lack of societal consensus on this issue and the lack of any clear-cut legal guidelines, when a decision is made to discontinue fluids and nutrition for a severely neurologically impaired patient who has the prospect of survival for long life otherwise, review by the institution's ethics committee is strongly recommended.

Finally, medical organizations at the local, state, and national level should take the lead in developing standards. Such neurological specialty societies as the American Academy of Neurology, the American Neurological Association, the Congress of Neurological Surgeons, and the American Association of Neurological Surgeons should begin to articulate specific diagnostic criteria and decision-making policies for use by neurological specialists and health care institutions on this issue.

CONCLUSION

The debate over whether and when to stop fluids and nutrition is in its infancy and some issues have undoubtedly gone unidentified, yet some arguments have been examined, and some consensus has emerged. For example, this society accepts many instances of forgoing life-sustaining treatment for those who are permanently unconscious or are terminally ill and imminently dying.

Fluids and nutrition can be considered medical treatment that falls within this consensus. But issues about feeding touch our sensibilities much more deeply than most other forms of medical treatment. Thus, health care providers and others ought to be cautious and sensitive in decision-making practices concerning nutritional support for permanently unconscious patients and to reflect carefully and deliberately before removing what may be the final barrier between life and death.

NOTES

1. *In re* Quinlan, 70 N.J. 10, 355 A.2d 647, *cert denied*, 429 U.S. 922 (1976).

2. *In re* Conroy, 98 N.J. 321, 486 A.2d 1209 (1985).

3. President's Commission for the Study of Ethical Problems in Medicine and Biomedical and Behavioral Research, *Deciding to Forego Life-Sustaining Treatment*, Washington, D.C.: U.S. Government Printing Office (1983), 180–181.

4. Ronald E. Cranford, "Termination of Treatment in the Persistent Vegetative State," *Semin. Neurol.* 4:36–44 (1984).

5. Laurence H. Tribe, *American Constitutional Law*, Mineola, N.Y.: Foundation Press (1978), 936.

6. *In re* Conroy, 90 N.J. Super 453, 464 A.2d 303, 310 (1983), *rev'd*, 98 N.J. 321, 486 A.2d 1209 (1985).

7. Barber v. Superior Court, 195 Cal. Rptr. 484, 147 Cal. App. 3d 1006 (1983); Bernard Lo, "The Death of Clarence Herbert: Withdrawing Care is Not Murder," *Ann, Intern. Med.* 101:248–251, (1984); George J. Annas, "Non-feeding: Lawful Killing in California, Homicide in New Jersey," *Hastings Cent. Rep.* 13:19–20 (1983).

8. John R. Connery, "The Clarence Herbert Case: Was Withdrawal of Treatment Justified?" *Hosp. Prog.* 65:32–35, 70 (February 1984).

9. *In re* Conroy, 98 N.J. 321, 486 A.2d 1209 (1985).

10. Kenneth C. Micetich, Patricia H. Steinecker, and David C. Thomasma, "Are Intravenous Fluids Morally Required for a Dying Patient?" *Arch. Intern. Med.* 43:975–978 (1983). Sidney H. Wanzer, Steven J. Adelstein, Ronald E. Cranford et al., "The Physician's Responsibility Toward Hopelessly Ill Patients," *N. Engl. J. Med.* 310:955–959, (1984); Bernard Lo and Laurie Dornbrand, "Guiding the Hand that Feeds: Caring for the Demented Elderly," *N. Engl. J. Med.* 311:402–404 (1984); John J. Paris and Anne B. Fletcher, "Infant Doe Regulations and the Absolute Requirement to Use Nourishment and Fluids for the Dying Infant," *Law, Medicine and Health Care* 11:210–213 (1983).

11. One poll of physicians showed that, for a patient with persistent vegetative state, 90 percent would discontinue a respirator, 80 percent would discontinue antibiotic treatment for pneumonia, and only 50 percent would stop nasogastric feedings. David W. Meyers, *Medico-Legal Implications of Death and Dying*, Rochester, N.Y.: The Lawyers Cooperative Publishing Co. (1985), 159–168.

12. President's Commission, *Deciding to Forego, supra,* note 3, at 6.

13. *Id.* at 181–182.

14. Barber v. Superior Court, 195 Cal. Rptr. 484, 147 Cal. App. 3d 1006 (1983).

15. Families have petitioned courts for authorization to stop feeding tubes in at least three additional cases, which are pending as this publication goes to press. Brophy v. New England Sinai Hospital, No. 85 E 000961 (Norfolk Probate Court, Massachusetts, 1985) (trial court ordered continued feeding; appeal filed); *In re* Jobes, Superior Court of N.J., Chancery Division, Morris County, No. C–4971–85E (trial court permitted discontinuation of artificial feeding); *In re* Helen Corbett, see Sandra Bower Ross, "Remove Tubes From Dying Wife, Husband Asks," *Fort Meyer News-Press* (February 23, 1985) at 12A (first appellate court permitted discontinuation of artificial feeding).

16. Bouvia v. County of Riverside, 159780 (Calif. Sup. Ct. 1984); George J. Annas, "When Suicide Prevention Becomes Brutality: The Case of Elizabeth Bouvia," *Hastings Cent. Rep.* 14:20–21, 46 (1984).

Gilbert Meilaender, Ph.D.

19   Caring for the Permanently Unconscious Patient

WHY FEEDING IS NOT MEDICAL CARE

The argument for ceasing to feed seems strongest in cases of people suffering from a "persistent vegetative state," those (like Karen Quinlan) who have suffered an irreversible loss of consciousness. Sidney Wanzer and his physician colleagues suggest that in such circumstances "it is morally justifiable to withhold antibiotics and artificial nutrition and hydration, as well as other forms of life-sustaining treatment, allowing the patient to die."[1] The President's Commission advises: "Since permanently unconscious patients will never be aware of nutrition, the only benefit to the patient of providing such increasingly burdensome interventions is sustaining the body to allow for a remote possibility of recovery. The sensitivities of the family and of care giving professionals ought to determine whether such interventions are made."[2] Joanne Lynn, a physician at George Washington University, and James Childress, a professor of religious studies at the University of Virginia, believe that "in these cases, it is very difficult to discern how any medical intervention can benefit or harm the patient."[3] But we need to ask whether the physicians are right to suggest that they seek only to allow the patient to die; whether the President's Commission has used language carefully enough in saying that nutrition and hydration of such persons is merely sustaining a *body*; whether Lynn and Childress may too readily have assumed that providing food and drink is *medical* treatment.

Should the provision of food and drink be regarded as *medical* care? It seems, rather, to be the sort of care that all human beings

Adapted from "On Removing Food and Water: Against the Stream," *Hastings Center Report* 14:11–13 (December 1984). Reprinted by permission.

owe each other. All living beings need food and water in order to live, but such nourishment does not itself heal or cure disease. When we stop feeding the permanently unconscious patient, we are not withdrawing from the battle against any illness or disease; we are withholding the nourishment that sustains all life.

The President's Commission does suggest that certain kinds of care remain mandatory for the permanently unconscious patient: "The awkward posture and lack of motion of unconscious patients often lead to pressure sores, and skin lesions are a major complication. Treatment and prevention of these problems is standard nursing care and should be provided." Yet it is hard to see why such services (turning the person regularly, giving alcohol rubs, and the like) are standard nursing care when feeding is not. Moreover, if feeding cannot benefit these patients, it is far from clear how they could experience bed sores as harm.

If this is true, we may have good reason to question whether the withdrawal of nutrition and hydration in such cases is properly characterized as stopping medical treatment in order to allow a patient to die. There are circumstances in which a plausible and helpful distinction can be made between killing and allowing to die, between an aim and a foreseen but unintended consequence. And sometimes it may make excellent moral sense to hold that we should cease to provide a now useless treatment, foreseeing but not intending that death will result. Such reasoning is also useful in the ethics of warfare, but there its use must be strictly controlled lest we simply unleash the bombs while "directing our intention" to a military target that could be attacked with far less firepower. Careful use of language is also necessary lest we talk about unconscious patients in ways that obscure our true aim.

Challenging those who have argued that it is no longer possible to distinguish between combatants and noncombatants in war, Michael Walzer has pointed out that "the relevant distinction is not between those who work for the war effort and those who do not, but between those who make what soldiers need to fight and those who make what they need to live, like the rest of us."[4]

Hence, farmers are not legitimate targets in war simply because they grow the food that soldiers need to live (and then to fight). The soldiers would need the food to live, even if there were no war. Thus, as Paul Ramsey has observed, though an army may march upon its belly, bellies are not the target. It is an abuse of double-effect reasoning to justify cutting off the food supply of a nation as a way of stopping its soldiers. We could not properly say that we were aiming at the soldiers while merely foreseeing the deaths of the civilian population.

Nor can we, when withdrawing food from the permanently unconscious person, properly claim that our intention is to cease useless treatment for a dying patient. These patients are not dying, and we cease no treatment aimed at disease; rather, we withdraw the nourishment that sustains all human beings whether healthy or ill, and we do so when the only result of our action can be death. At what, other than that death, could we be aiming?

One might argue that the same could be said of turning off a respirator, but the situations are somewhat different. Remove a person from a respirator and he may die—but, then, he may also surprise us and continue to breathe spontaneously. We test to see if the patient can breathe. If he does, it is not our task—unless we are aiming at his death—now to smother him (or to stop feeding him). But deprive a person of food and water and she will die as surely as if we had administered a lethal drug, and it is hard to claim that we did not aim at her death.

I am unable—and this is a lack of insight, not of space—to say more about the analogy between eating and breathing. Clearly, air is as essential to life as food. We might wonder, therefore, whether provision of air is not also more than medical treatment. What justification could there be, then, for turning off a respirator? If the person's death, due to the progress of a disease, is irreversibly and imminently at hand, then continued assistance with respiration may now be useless. But if the person is not going to die from any disease but, instead, simply needs assistance with breathing because of some injury, it is less clear to me why such assistance should not be given. More than this I am unable to say. I repeat, however, that to remove a respirator is not necessarily to aim at death; one will not go on to kill the patient who manages to breathe spontaneously. But it is difficult for me to construe removal of nutrition for permanently unconscious patients in any other way. Perhaps we only wish them dead or think they would be better off dead. There are circumstances in which such a thought is understandable. But it would still be wrong to enact that wish by aiming at their death.

SEPARATING PERSONHOOD AND BODY

Yet for many people the uselessness of feeding the permanently unconscious seems self-evident. Why? Probably because they suppose that the nourishment we provide is, in the words of the President's Commission, doing no more than "sustaining the body." But we should pause before separating personhood and body so decisively. When considering topics (care of the environment, for example) we are eager to criticize a dualism that divorces human reason and conciousness from the larger world of nature. Why not here? We can know people—of all ranges of cognitive capacity—only as they are embodied: there is no other "person" for whom we might care. Such care is not useless if it "only" preserves bodily life but does not restore cognitive capacities. Even if it is less than we wish could be accomplished, it remains care for the embodied person.

Some will object to characterizing as persons those who lack the capacity or, even, the potential for self-awareness, for envisioning a future for themselves, for relating to other selves. I am not fully persuaded that speaking of "persons" in such contexts is mistaken, but the point can be made without using that language. Human nature has a capacity to know, to be self-aware, and to relate to others. We can share in that human nature even though we may not yet or no longer exercise all the functions of which it is capable. We share in it simply by virtue of being born into the human species. We could describe as persons all individuals sharing our common nature, all members of the species. Or we could ascribe personhood only to those human beings presently capable of exercising the characteristic human functions.

I think it better—primarily because it is far less dualistic—to understand personhood as an endowment that comes with our nature, even if at some stages of life we are unable to exercise characteristic human capacities. But the point can be made, if anyone wishes, by talking of embodied human beings rather than embodied persons. To be a human being one need not presently be exercising or be capable of exercising the functions characteristic of consciousness. Those are capacities of human nature; they are not functions that all human beings exercise. It is human beings, not just persons in that more restricted sense, whose death should not be our aim. And if this view is characterized as an objectionable "speciesism," I can only reply that at least it is not one more way by which the strong and gifted in our world rid themselves of the weak, and it does not fall prey to that abstraction by which we reify consciousness and separate it from the body.

The permanently unconscious are not dying subjects who should simply be allowed to die. But they will, of course, die if we aim at their death by ceasing to feed them. If we are not going to feed them because that would be nothing more than sustaining a body, why not bury them at once? No one, I think, recommends that. But if, then, they are still living beings who ought not be buried, the nourishment that all human beings need to live ought not be denied them. When we permit ourselves to think that care is useless if it preserves the life of the embodied human being without restoring cognitive capacity, we fall victim to the old delusion that we have failed if we cannot *cure* and that there is, then, little point to continued *care*. David Smith, a professor of religious studies at Indiana University, has suggested that I might be mistaken in describing the comatose person as a "nondying" patient. At least in some cases, he believes lapsing into permanent coma might be a sign that a person is trying to die. Thus, though a comatose state would not itself be sufficient reason to characterize someone as dying, it might be one of several conditions which, taken together, would be sufficient. This is a reasonable suggestion, and it might enable us to distinguish different sorts of comatose patients—the dying, for whom feeding might be useless; the nondying, for whom it would not. Even then, however, I would still be troubled by the worry I raised earlier: whether food and drink are really medical treatment that should be withdrawn when it becomes useless.

Even when care is not useless it may be so burdensome that it should be dispensed with. When that is the case, we can honestly say—and it makes good moral sense to say—that our aim is to relieve the person of a burden, with the foreseen but unintended effect of a hastened death. We should note, however, that this line of argument *cannot* be applied to the cases of the permanently unconscious. Other patients—those, for example, with fairly severe dementia—may be made afraid and uncomfortable by artificial nutrition and

hydration. But this can hardly be true of the permanently unconscious. It seems unlikely that they experience the care involved in
feeding them as burdensome.

In short, if we focus our attention on irreversibly ill adults for
whom general nursing care but no more seems appropriate, we can
say the following: First, when the person is permanently unconscious, the care involved in feeding can hardly be experienced as
burdensome. Neither can such care be described as useless, since it
preserves the life of the embodied human being (who is not a dying
patient). Second, when the person is conscious but severely and irreversibly demented, the care involved in feeding, though not useless, *may* be so burdensome that it should cease. This requires
demonstration during a trial period, however, and the judgment is
quite different from concluding that the person's life has become
too burdensome to preserve. Third, for both sorts of patients the care
involved in feeding is not, in any strict sense, medical treatment,
even if provided in a hospital. It gives what all need to live; it is
treatment of no particular disease; and its cessation means certain
death, a death at which we can only be said to aim, whatever our
motive.

That we should continue to feed the permanently unconscious
still seems obvious to some people, even as it was to Karen Quinlan's
father at the time he sought removal of her respirator. It has not
always seemed so to me, but it does now. For the permanently unconscious person, feeding is neither useless nor excessively burdensome. It is ordinary human care and is not given as treatment for
any life-threatening disease. Since this is true, a decision not to offer
such care can enact only one intention: to take the life of the unconscious person.

I have offered no arguments here to prove that such a life-taking
intention and aim would be morally wrong, though I believe it is
and that to embrace such an aim would be corrupting. If we can face
the fact that withdrawing the nourishment of such persons is, indeed, aiming to kill, I am hopeful (though not altogether confident)
that the more fundamental principle will not need to be argued. Let
us hope that this is the case, since that more basic principle is not
one that can be argued *to*; rather, all useful moral argument must
proceed *from* the conviction that it is wrong to aim to kill the innocent.

NOTES

1. Sidney H. Wanzer et al., "The Physician's Responsibility Toward Hopelessly Ill Patients," *N. Engl. J. Med.* 310:958–96 (1984).
2. President's Commission for the Study of Ethical Problems in Medicine and Biomedical and Behavioral Research, *Deciding to Forego Life-Sustaining Treatment*, Washington, D.C.: U.S. Government Printing Office (1982).
3. Joanne Lynn and James Childress, "Must Patients Always Be Given Food and Water?" *Hastings Cent. Rep.* 13:17–21 (October 1983).
4. Michael Walzer, *Just and Unjust Wars*, New York: Basic Books (1977) (146).

Dan W. Brock, Ph.D., and Joanne Lynn, M.D.

20 The Competent Patient Who Decides Not to Take Nutrition and Hydration

Most patients for whom the best choice is to forgo food and water are unable to make their own choices due to incompetence. Furthermore, they are usually irreversibly ill and often near death, making the benefits of improved nutrition and hydration few and the burdens of the necessary procedures disproportionately large. The physician and family (or other surrogate) must decide on behalf of such a patient. Some patients, however, can personally make the choice as to whether or not treatment is desirable. The trend both in recent case law[1] and in bioethics discussions[2] has been to uphold, almost without exception,[3] the authority of a competent patient to refuse medical treatment. We support this trend and in this essay examine the considerations that come into play when a competent patient wishes to forgo food and water,[4] thereby hastening death.

COMPETENCE

What is meant when a patient is said to be "competent" to make medical treatment decisions? At its most elementary, such a determination requires that the patient be sufficiently mature to have fairly settled value commitments and priorities, have a normal capability to understand the situation and the likely effects of proposed interventions, have the ability to evaluate the desirability of various likely futures in relation to the pursuit of personal goals and value commitments, and be able to make and communicate a choice arising from these considerations.[5]

The competence determination establishes whether a patient will be permitted to decide about health care for himself or herself or whether a surrogate decision-maker will decide for the patient. To be competent does not mean that the patient must make decisions without errors. Society can and should tolerate some compromise of well-being in order to secure another important value—self-determination. Justice Brandeis said that the most fundamental free-dom is "the freedom to be left alone."[6] Protecting this authority to make choices about one's own life is important, so important that only when one's ability to consider the options is substantially im-paired and is likely to lead to serious harm should a person be pro-tected from his or her own choices.

Since the competence determination must balance patients' in-terests in avoiding the harmful consequences of their defective de-cisions against their interest in deciding for themselves, patients need not be completely free of indentifiable deficits in comprehen-sion and reasoning to be considered competent. Nor must patients measure up to some single predetermined standard of reasoning or understanding to have their choices be determinative. Rather, the determination as to competence must relate to the specific demands of the decision facing the patient at a particular time. As the con-sequences of the patient's choice entail more risks to the patient, an increasingly stringent standard of decision-making competence is naturally demanded.[7]

The most common origins of inadequate decision-making com-petence are immaturity, barriers to communication (e. g., language deficits or reduced consciousness), barriers to understanding (e.g., inadequate time in emergencies, information too complex or fright-ening for this patient to confront), barriers to reasoning (e.g., fixed erroneous beliefs as in psychotic or severe denial states), or inability to make and express a consistent[8] choice.

SITUATIONS WHERE COMPETENT PATIENTS MIGHT DECLINE FOOD AND WATER

Can there be competent patients who refuse the medical assistance necessary to provide nutrition and hydration (which will be assumed to be available and possibly successful)? This question reflects two different sorts of doubts about whether competent patients ever choose to forgo food and water. First, is it possible still to be com-petent while in such terrible medical condition that refusal of (usu-ally substantially intrusive) provision of nutrition and hydration is in one's best interests? Second, is it possible to make a competent decision to forgo nutrition and hydration (either by refusing to ingest food and water in the normal way although physically able or by refusing the medical procedures made necessary by physical disability) and therefore to die, even when such a decision does not seem to others to be in the patient's best interests?

The first case seems to be possible, though relatively rare, and not particularly controversial. For example, a patient could be dying of an illness that renders the gastrointestinal tract nonfunctional and also causes substantial anorexia (lack of appetite). Once having developed ketosis (a chemical change in the blood resulting from the breakdown of fats in the body), anorexia is even more complete. The patient might well find that he or she experiences no hunger or thirst and is quite comfortable without other efforts to improve intake, so long as ice chips or lubricant are applied to the patient's mouth. When approached about the possibility of total parenteral nutrition, requiring intravenous lines and involving various potential complications, the patient may well feel that this would be inappropriate to his or her condition, an inappropriate use of funds, overly burdensome to the patient or to his or her loved ones, or even a potential cause of relieving the patient's anorexia, which would incur more suffering.

Such a case must be quite rare, since most people so near to death have substantial clouding of the sensorium and diminished capacity for (and interest in) reasoning. However, such a case of refusal of food and water is both possible and, in our view, morally unproblematic. The patient's assessment of the merits of the alternatives should be binding. Indeed, it is hard to see how a case could be made that the patient's view should be overridden while leaving intact any significant loyalty to the value of self-determination which underlies the doctrine of informed consent.[9] Forcing treatment upon such a patient would be unacceptably inhumane, and all the more so if the patient were physically to resist. We believe that this reasoning holds in any case in which the patient remains competent while suffering from a mortal illness and judges that the life remaining is sufficiently short and distressing as to be worse than an early death, even allowing for whatever suffering may be unavoidable when death will result from forgoing nutrition and hydration.

The problem as presented by the second potential group of patients mentioned above, however, is more difficult, though even more rare. How should one view a person's willful refusal to sustain his or her life when that could readily be done and would be expected to succeed for a long time? Many scholars, courts,[10] and legislatures[11] have tried to restrict the authority to decline life-sustaining treatment to those who are "terminally ill," often with the additional requirement that they be "imminently dying." Left out are those who could yet live for a substantial period but who do not choose to do so. How should we respond to these cases? Such cases are very rare, since competent patients will less often choose to forgo life-support when a substantial period of life is possible, and they can and usually will choose a faster and more comfortable means of death, including direct suicide. When other means are not possible, as in the *Bouvia* case,[12] a competent person facing a long but personally unacceptable life might decide to refuse food and water.

It might be thought that this problem does not arise, because such a person could not be competent and therefore someone else can be authorized to override the patient's choice. This view, however, requires an arbitrary and indefensible extension of the concept of incompetence so as to include those who choose to curtail their lives, irrespective of whether they have settled values and goals, can understand the choice before them, and can reason and decide.

Certainly, patients can and do have settled values according to which longer life will only be of value if the quality of that life is adequate. Various states of existence may well be deemed worse than being dead, and the patient may be facing such an existence if life is sustained.

A person's decision to die is often evaluated differently by others depending upon what state of existence is being avoided or what is to be achieved through the death. If the purpose were to avoid betraying one's loved ones or community or to be loyal to a religious tenet, the action might well be praised (as with a religious or political martyr, for example). However, if it were only to avoid an impoverished life or having to grow older, the choice of a person to starve to death would be widely considered to be unjustified. Thus, public endorsement often relies not only upon the presence or absence of settled goals and values, but also upon a view of their merit. Perhaps the pursuit of some goals should not be tolerated in a society; but, if so, it would seem better to state and defend this position explicitly, rather than to hide such an assessment under the guise of an assessment of decision-making capacity, or competence. Whether society should forbid or respect a choice by a competent person to forgo food and water is the subject of the following section. But it does no violence to the everyday or legal notion of competence to claim that a person could competently make such a choice, reasoning from that person's settled and coherent values.

A person could quite competently come to understand his or her current situation and likely future and decide that the better course would be to refuse to eat or drink. Such a decision involves the conclusion that death is better than some kinds of life, that eating and drinking would only support a kind of life that is worse than being dead, and that dying from dehydration and malnourishment would not directly cause enough suffering to make early death a worse option after all. Such a situation is mercifully rare.[13] However, if such a patient is to be prevented from acting upon this conclusion, the nature of his or her choice itself provides no basis for justifying doing so by a finding of limited capacity to be self-determining, that is to say, a finding of incompetence. Honesty requires some other justification for preventing the patient from acting upon his or her competently chosen option. Three such justifications are commonly offered: that the patient is acting upon values that should not be tolerated by his or her society; that the patient's choice can be constrained because of the interests of others; or that the mode of death by refusal of food and water is unacceptable to others who are affected. These considerations are the subject of the ensuing sections of this chapter, which will start from the premise that some persons are competent even though they choose not to take nourishment or hydration, either in the normal way or through medical interventions.

BEING DEAD AS PREFERABLE TO BEING ALIVE

The competent person who claims that it would be better to refuse to eat and drink (or to refuse medical interventions to substitute for eating and drinking) has concluded that living out some kinds of life would be worse than having died. This is generally true of all choices to foreshorten life substantially—from disconnecting a respirator for a patient who might live for years to declining transfusions for an accident victim with religious objections to the necessary remedies. However, the imagery may well be starker when the patient's choice involves deliberate starvation.

What sorts of counterarguments can be given to this sort of patient? First, one can seek to convince the patient that he or she is in error in the assessment of the merits of living, either because one believes that to be true and wishes to convince the patient or because one wants to be sure that a patient choosing this course has considered the matter with great care. One way to ensure that all relevant considerations have been duly weighed is to advocate vigorously for life to be maintained.

However, what arguments remain if one believes that, from the perspective of the one intending to forgo food and water, to do so would actually further that person's own goals and values best? First, one can claim that it is psychiatrically abnormal to choose to cut short one's own life and that it is irrelevant that such a person is deemed to be competent. Second, one can claim that it would be incompatible with many prevalent conceptions of the nature of life, and of the good life, for a competent person whose life could be sustained for a substantial period without greatly burdensome interventions to choose to forgo that life. And third, one can claim that each person's life is so fundamentally intertwined with the lives of others that the interests of those others preclude allowing any one person to decide unilaterally to die. These arguments raise large and difficult issues that cannot be adequately explored here, but we will respond briefly to each.

THE PSYCHOLOGY OF SUICIDE

Suicidologists commonly claim that nearly every person who chooses to die is afflicted with a mental illness that warrants intervention to prevent loss of life.[14] Such persons are said to feel worthless to themselves and others and to consider their situations hopeless.[15] Then persons who choose to deny themselves basic sustenance are interpreted as doing so to validate feelings that their lives are doomed to be without value or to escape great but possibly remediable emotional pain, rather than as a result of a reasonable and thoughtful application of personal values to the situation. Moreover, the act itself of refusing basic sustenance, like other suicide attempts, often is not an expression of an intent to die, but instead is intended to be a dramatic, last-resort plea to others for help.

This interpretation may well be true for a large number of people who attempt to take their own lives. In fact, the difficulty that arises in both respecting autonomy and intervening to stop suicide illuminates a basic problem with the current theory of medical decision-making and with the informed consent doctrine in particular: medical decision-making, when based on an overly rational and emotionless perspective, often focuses upon the content of communication while ignoring the manipulative effects of communication and relationships. If a person claims to want to forgo a life-sustaining treatment, this may reflect a clear-eyed examination of the alternatives in light of the person's own values. However, it might instead be a test of the responses of others. Do they care enough to resist or even question the choice? Obviously, if others were thoughtlessly to take all communications at face value and respond only in a cool and rational manner with unquestioning deference to the person's expressed wishes, they may well inadvertently affirm the patient's feelings that others no longer care about him or her. On the other hand, if it is always assumed that patients are only testing the environment, their expressed choices would therefore be discounted and patient autonomy would be overwhelmed, thus authorizing widespread and unjustified paternalistic interventions. Nevertheless, people who express a wish to forgo food and water may be doing so in order to assess how others regard them or to garner support for a fragile sense of self-worth. It would certainly be unfortunate if their claim to autonomy were met with detachment and misunderstanding and their claim to want no food or water thereby inadvertently and inappropriately supported.

The view that feelings of hopelessness and worthlessness are signs of emotional ill-health assumes that persons normally feel that their lives are of value. Tragically, however, there are many people within this society whose lives are not much valued by others, and the views of others about us can importantly shape our own views of ourselves. While most decent persons bristle at discrimination against any unfortunate group, it is difficult to arouse the same level of concern for the foreshortening of the life of an old person as for a youth, for a multiply handicapped and dependent person as for an able-bodied person, or for a social misfit or troublemaker as for an upright and productive citizen. When such sources of devaluation are present, it may well be a very realistic assessment of the situation for the afflicted person to feel that he or she is not valued by others. This can lead to feelings that the world would be better off if one were to die, feelings that are often met with acceptance or even stronger affirmation.

In such cases, it may well be true that poor mental health is in evidence, but it also may well be that the locus of the malfunction is in the social assessment of worth rather than in the person feeling worthless.[16] This leaves a very difficult question: How should the society react to those whose quite reasonable response to societal attitudes toward them is to be self-destructive, responding correctly to expressions of societal values that often only pay lip service to life's high value? Certainly, the society might respond by redoubling efforts to cherish even the unlovable and unproductive. But, for the person for whom this does not happen or does not suffice, it would be difficult to defend empowering the society that helped originate and sustain the self-destructiveness to force the afflicted person to receive the treatments necessary to continue a life now felt to be intolerable or no longer of value.

Thus, the empirical claim that most people who intend to foreshorten life do so out of an abnormal feeling of self-hate or worthlessness does not warrant barring the choice. Some patients are not acting from this motive.[17] Furthermore, even those who are choosing to die because their lives now seem to be of so little value may be making a reasonable assessment of their situations, not mentally ill with a misperception of reality. As with other suicides, the most that is justified is temporary intervention to permit responses that improve the person's situation and to ensure that the person's choice is competently made and reflects a realistic understanding of his or her situation. Food and water seem to present no special problems for this line of argument, except perhaps that forgoing them is so dramatic as to ensure that others will respond if ever they can be brought to do so.

THE NATURE OR VALUE OF LIFE

Many people have either a conception of human good or an understanding of the nature of life that is incompatible with deliberately choosing to end one's life by refusing food and water. In some cases these beliefs are religious and founded in a belief in God: for example, that life is a gift from God and that each person is obliged to be a responsible steward of that gift, or that life is a period to endure and make the best of, but of no substantial importance compared to the eternal reward possible after death. In other cases, the beliefs are secular: for example, that life has value when it provides a balance of happiness or of pleasure over pain, or has value in itself independent of what the experience in that life is like. Many such beliefs are incompatible with choosing to end a life that could readily be sustained, even when a person competently chooses to do so.

However, we believe that public policies should not depend upon any single understanding of the nature of life or of the good life. Instead, autonomous persons must be free to affirm some such conception for themselves. These are ultimately and properly matters of personal choice, all the more so in a society that values religious freedom and is pluralistic in the classical liberal sense of not enforcing one single conception of the good life, but of ensuring conditions in which persons can pursue their differing and sometimes conflicting views of the good life. Thus, even if the deliberate choice to forgo food and water may be seen as an affront by holders of some particular conception of the nature or meaning of life or of the good life, public policy should not prohibit that choice to persons who do not share that conception of life.

COMMUNITY CONCERNS IN DECISIONS TO DIE

Another group of responses to the person who wishes to die by refusing to take food and water is that deciding for oneself to do so assumes an unrealistic view of persons as autonomous individuals, entitled to decide for themselves what weight, if any, effects on others should have in their decisions. In this line of argument, people are instead viewed as more fundamentally interrelated, existing by necessity in communities, families, and societies. We believe that the fact that people live in interrelated groups with effects upon one another justifies the society preventing individuals from acting in ways that cause significant harm to others. A decision to forgo food and water that will result in death does not generally cause significant harms to others of the sort that should properly be prevented by law. Although any death of this sort might be seen as a harm to the community, it would be such only in a symbolic and metaphorical sense inadequate to justify foreclosing the choice by law. Those who view any such death as a harm to the community should certainly undertake concerted action to ensure that few persons are ever so bereft of better options that death by starvation or dehydration is appealing.

In health care cases, courts have held that there are "state interests" in the preservation of human life, the prevention of suicide, the protection of dependent third parties, and the protection of the ethical integrity of the medical profession.[18] The strength of these interests when arrayed against so important a choice of a competent patient as to forgo food and water seems to be quite limited. The state interest in the preservation of human life, for example, seems clear and substantial in the prevention or punishment of ordinary homicide, where the victim has not freely chosen to die. However, we believe there is no significant state interest in forcing the continued existence against that person's will of someone who has freely and competently decided that life is no longer tolerable.

If there were good evidence that a person's death was likely to lead inexorably to a substantial and widespread devaluation of human life, a state interest could be sustained. However, only in extraordinary circumstances would there be sound reason to believe that a person who chooses to die by refusing to eat would have any such effect. And even if there were, the state interest would have to be sufficiently strong to justify using the person in this way against his or her will. The state interest in preserving human life has not been held in actual court cases to be sufficiently strong or direct as to overrule a competent person's choice. In medical contexts, the state interest in preventing suicide has been seen as a special case of the interest in preserving life[19] and has been similarly ineffectual in justifying preventing persons from choosing to end life by forgoing life-sustaining medical treatments. The relation of forgoing life-sustaining treatment to suicide is complex, but courts have commonly held that forgoing treatment is not suicide, because it merely allows the disease to take its natural course, death does not result from a self-inflicted injury, and death need not be intended. In this analysis, any state interest in preventing suicide does not arise when a life-sustaining medical treatment is forgone.

If there are persons, especially minor children, who are dependent upon the patient for their well-being, the state might claim an interest in the well-being of these persons to bar the patient from removing himself or herself from the supporting role. This would protect the community by preventing dependents from seeking support from it instead of from the patient who had the responsibility by virtue of some established relationship. However, we believe that it is problematic whether a community's interest in avoiding burdens of support is ever substantial enough to justify forcing continued life on a competent person who finds that life intolerable. Only a few court cases have seen a person forced to stay alive largely because the welfare of dependents was at stake.[20] Perhaps there are few persons who are so bereft of hope as to wish to die while still having meaningful relationships and persons dependent upon them. Moreover, continued life forced under these circumstances will often be of doubtful benefit to dependents.

The proffered state interest in the ethical integrity of the medical profession has at least two facets: protection of the rights of individual health care professionals, just as patients' rights are protected, and special protections for health care providers as necessary to enable the health care system to continue to benefit the community. These issues are taken up at greater length in chapter 21 concerning the responses of caregivers to the forgoing of food and water. Here it is only important to state that the rights of caregivers to refuse to be involved in activities that they find to be morally offensive ordinarily requires only that patients be offered the opportunities of transfer or discharge. In some very rare cases, these options might be insufficient, in which case a serious and difficult conflict between the patient's right of self-determination and a professional's right of conscience would exist. We believe that which right or interest should prevail can then only be determined in the particular case. Fortunately, in nearly all cases it is possible to arrange alternatives such as transfer or discharge that avoid having to choose between these rights of patient and professional.

Some court cases[21] mention a concern for the ethical integrity of the medical profession, but no treatment (or nontreatment) options have been found by a court to be permissible for persons to choose but impermissible for physicians and other health care professionals to be involved in. Thus, the state interests as developed in case law to date do not serve to bar the forgoing of food and water by a competent person. Nor do there seem to be sound moral grounds for extending arguments of state interests or the interests of others so as to create such a constraint upon choice.

RELEVANCE OF THE MODE OF DYING

The objection to a person choosing to die by refusing nutrition could be not only that it would be wrong to choose to be dead, as could be claimed whenever one chooses to forgo an opportunity to sustain life, but also that it would be wrong to choose to die in this particular way. Insofar as this consideration relates to the suffering induced by malnutrition or dehydration, it raises no distinctive considerations, since other modes of dying may have similarly uncomfortable dying processes. However, there are two additional considerations that might make it unacceptable to allow persons to choose to die in this way, though they might be allowed to choose other courses that lead to death.

First, to refuse nutrition and die will usually require the cooperation of others. To be called upon to assist in such an endeavor may be profoundly unsettling. Acquiescing in a death that is expected to be so distressing to the person dying[22] is understandably difficult for health care professionals. Assisting in making the dying more tolerable by providing sedation or tranquilizers could raise serious questions as to the appropriateness of using medical skills to help people to tolerate deliberately self-induced suffering, an image that might be disruptive to patient trust and a coherent professional self-image. Furthermore, the medications themselves are likely to hasten death, which might be seen by some as implicating the health care professional in the death. Making this death easier might also have the effect of encouraging the choice of forgoing food and water. Such a role could lead to physicians being seen as providers of easy deaths, which might (though it need not) lead to a diminution in the trust of patients that physicians will expend every effort in their behalf.

Nevertheless, it is important to see that all of the preceding considerations arise in forgoings of other kinds of life-support in which physicians' participation is already widely acknowledged and accepted. Physicians commonly give medications to ease suffering in the final stages of life when other forms of life-support are withdrawn, those medications often hasten death, and giving them could likewise encourage forgoing those other forms of life-support by making death easier. While such considerations might justify a particular health care professional refusing to assist a person forgoing food and water who is not otherwise dying, they do not in our view warrant barring all professionals from lending assistance in these cases.

Second, giving and receiving food and water is an exchange that is central to the human community. The symbolism is pervasive and powerful, and refusal of this gift may seem to be a profound repudiation of the human concerns of those who would give. To give food is in many ways to give of oneself, and to be refused may seem to be a personal repudiation. For loved ones and for health care providers, this refusal may well be distressing. To some extent, the same could be said of the central and symbolic importance of health care generally in providing care and comfort to the sick. This consideration cannot justify forcing health care generally, or food and water in particular, upon a competent patient who has concluded that it is no longer of benefit to him or her. To do so would demean the gift, transforming it into a torment and a means of using a person for the benefit of others.

CONCLUSION

There certainly can be dying persons for whom the choice to forgo food and water seems not to be unreasonable because to maintain nutrition and hydration would have little effect on the length of life and would probably make the remaining life more uncomfortable. When the patient is competent, his or her own assessment of the relative merits of taking or forgoing nourishment should be binding.

There probably also can be persons who are far from dying but who find the potential futures they face so unrewarding that it would be better to die soon, even if dying requires voluntarily forgoing food and water. There is no justification for a social policy that attempts to thwart such persons. Health care providers would ordinarily find it very difficult to collaborate in deliberate starvation, but that does not justify force-feeding. Certainly, all concerned can and probably should redouble efforts to improve the life prospects of a person who is not otherwise near death but who concludes that deliberate starvation is his or her best choice. However, if that is not sufficient and the person is competent and informed, then he or she has the authority to take this course and curtail life.

NOTES

1. See, e.g., *In re* Plaza Health and Rehabilitation Center, Sup. Ct., On-andaga County, Syracuse, N.Y. (February 2, 1984); *In re* Quackenbush, 156 N.J. Super. 282, 383 A.2d 785 (1978); *In re* Conroy, 98 N.J. 321, 353, 486 A.2d 1209, 1225 (1985).

2. See, e.g., Richard W. Besdine, "Decisions to Withhold Treatment from Nursing Home Residents," *J. Am. Geriatr. Soc.* 31:602–606 (1983); Albert

R. Jonsen, Mark Siegler, and William J. Winslade, *Clinical Ethics*, New York: Macmillan Publishing Co., Inc. (1982).

3. Bouvia v. County of Riverside, Sup. Ct. Cal. Civ. No. 159780 (County of Riverside, 1984); Application of President and Directors of Georgetown College, Inc., 331 F.2d 100, 1008 (D.C. Cir.), *cert. denied*, 377 U.S. 978 (1964).

4. The same considerations are to be applied to the forgoing of food alone. It is probably not a practical possibility to forgo water alone, as any reasonably normal amount of food brings with it generally adequate quantities of water.

5. President's Commission for the Study of Ethical Problems in Medicine and Biomedical and Behavioral Research, *Making Health Care Decisions*, Washington, D.C.: U.S. Government Printing Office (1982).

6. Olmstead v. United States, 277 U.S. 438, 471 (1928).

7. James F. Drane, "Competency to Give an Informed Consent," *J.A.M.A.* 252:925–927 (1984).

8. Vacillation alone has been specifically rejected as a reason to consider a patient incompetent. Lane v. Candura, 376 N.E.2d 1232, 1236 (Mass. App. 1978); *In re* Bartling, 209 Cal. Rptr. 220 (1984).

9. See, e.g., Cobbs v. Grant, 8 Cal.3d 229, 242; Barber v. Superior Court, 147 Cal. App. 3d 1006, 1015; Satz v. Perlmutter, 362 So.2d 160, 163, *aff'd.* 379 So.2d 359 (Fla. 1980).

10. See also *In re* Conroy, 98 N.J. 321, 486 A.2d 1209 (1985).

11. See, e.g., legislation establishing "living wills" in The President's Commission for the Study of Ethical Problems in Medicine and Biomedical and Behavioral Research, *Deciding to Forego Life-Sustaining Treatment*, Washington, D.C.: U. S. Government Printing Office (1983), 310–387.

12. Bouvia v. County of Riverside, No. 159780 (Sup. Ct. Cal., 1984).

13. The court in Bouvia v. County of Riverside, *supra*, held that Elizabeth Bouvia's is such a case.

14. See, e.g., Harvey M. Schein and Alan A. Stone, "Psychotherapy Designed to Detect and Treat Suicidal Potential," *Am. J. Psychiatry* 125:1247–1251 (1969); but see Thomas Szasz, "The Ethics of Suicide," *Antioch Rev.* 31:7–17 (1971).

15. Bernard Sochet, "Recognizing the Suicidal Patient," *Modern Med.* 38:114–123 (1970).

16. Bouvia v. County of Riverside, No. 159780 (Sup. Ct. Cal., 1984).

17. E.g., Elizabeth Bouvia; see Declarations of Robert B. Summerour, M.D., and of Thomas M. Heric, M.D., in Bouvia v. County of Riverside, *supra*.

18. *In re* Conroy, 98 N.J. 321, 348, 486 A.2d 1209, 1223 (1985).

19. *Id.* at 25–26.

20. Application of President and Directors of Georgetown College, Inc., 331 F.2d 1000, 1008 (D.C. Cir.), *cert denied*, 377 U.S. 978 (1964).

21. See *In re* Conroy, 98 N.J. 321, 353, 486 A.2d 1209, 1225 (1985).

22. Starvation and dehydration cause suffering for a relatively healthy person who chooses this as a means to end life. It seems to be much more comfortable for seriously ill and dying patients. See chapter 3.

Joanne Lynn, M.D.

21 Those Who Provide Medical Care

While it seems true that life-sustaining mechanical feedings can justifiably be stopped for some patients, it is also true that some persons will have to disconnect the apparatus and care for the person as he or she dies. The professionals who provide medical care have their own rights, concerns, and consciences, which shape the alternatives that they are willing to provide to patients, perhaps especially those choices about forgoing life-sustaining nutrition and hydration.[1]

Law construes the physician-patient relationship as a fiduciary contract involving occasional services rendered over an indefinite time period. While either party is free to withdraw from the relationship, a physician who wishes to withdraw is obliged to provide sufficient notice to allow the patient to secure other medical treatment.[2] Morally, other health care providers and hospitals are in much the same position as are physicians—having interests and scruples but being obliged to continue to provide services to patients. Perhaps nurses, who attend to the patient continuously, have an especially strong claim to be allowed the opportunity to be comfortable with the care plan or to be able to withdraw from involvement.[3]

Providing care in these situations poses some troubling and, in health care at least, uncommon issues. Are there some choices which are justifiable for the patient but which no health care provider should provide? If a particular practitioner is unwilling to cooperate in providing an option chosen by or on behalf of a patient, how should the practitioner respond? What aspects of the decision-making process should be the responsibilities of the professionals involved? What should be the impact of financial considerations upon the choices made and the services rendered? What responses to these questions should be made by health care systems and institutions? These questions arise in other situations where a life-sustaining treatment is at issue. How, if at all, are these questions answered differently when the treatment concerns life-sustaining nutrition and hydration?

CHOICES INAPPROPRIATE FOR
HEALTH CARE PROVIDERS

Are there any choices which are legally acceptable and morally justifiable but which should not be available if they require the involvement of a health care provider—in other words, a choice in which all health care providers should decline to be involved?

How could such an alternative arise? It would have to be that those who provide health care have special characteristics which would make it wrong, or at least imprudent, to have them involved. The strong claim that it would be wrong for them (but not for others) to be involved in a particular action, irrespective of the outcomes of that action, relies upon there being some distinction between the moral commitments of health care providers and others.

Some have argued that this is so, especially that health care providers must always advocate for continued life. However, this is clearly not the case: good health care can certainly lead to an earlier death,[4] e.g., the forgoing of resuscitation in persons dying of cancer or the discontinuation of respirator support. However, allowing health care providers to be involved in effectuating a choice to die for lack of nutrition and hydration might nevertheless be imprudent because doing so would lead to undesirable outcomes for other patients. Providers may well be trusted in large part because they are presumed to act in defense of their patients' lives. For providers to condone a dying that can seem so avoidable and so distressing as many people assume is the case with malnutrition and dehydration might lead to a distrust of health care professionals generally and thereby to other harms, though estimating the likelihood of this transpiring would be quite speculative.

PROTECTIONS FOR THE CONSCIENCES OF PROVIDERS

Individual providers may well be unwilling to effectuate certain choices, whether made by patients, their surrogates, or the courts. Elizabeth Bouvia's[5] psychiatrists, for example, were unwilling to attend to her other needs while she starved to death under their care.[6] Although some caregivers were willing to carry out the court order to force-feed her, it should be possible also to refuse involvement in that activity as well.

How should such a clash be resolved? Certainly, if there can be found an acceptable transfer or other accommodation that allows all concerned to exercise their options without compromise, that should be pursued. If, however, there is no availing compromise, what should be done? George Annas has said that the disadvantaged position of patients justifies requiring physicians to accommodate the preferences of patients.[7] But that would be unacceptable, for it would require treating physicians as mere automatons, having no legitimate moral agency or conscience that deserves protection. For the same reasons this society respects the choices of competent patients—respecting the authority of each person to shape his or her own preferences and to live in accord with them—it must respect the choices of physicians and other health care providers.

If both the patient's legitimate choice and the provider's conscience are to be respected, how should a situation be resolved in which a treatment choice is unacceptable to the provider and no transfer or accommodation is possible? I cannot find any uniform resolution that is satisfactory. Instead, in the rare case when unresolvable conflict is unavoidable, it should be addressed with full recognition of the seriousness of the conflict and the legitimacy of the claims on each side. No presumption or rule will be adequate. Instead, the search must be for a creative compromise, or at least for minimizing the abrogations of rights and for minimizing other harms to all concerned.

Should the considerations be different when the issue is food and water instead of another life-sustaining intervention? Although it is a difference in degree and not in kind, forgoing nutrition and hydration may well be more difficult for a health care practitioner to tolerate or assist. The rich symbolism of feeding mixes nursing, comforting, supporting, sharing, and other laudable elements of caregiving. To be barred from doing those things and required to watch death occur thereby might be incompatible with the self-image and self-esteem of many in health care, even if a particular caregiver is not afflicted with the common, though unrealistic and undesirable, denial of death. Of course, if it were only the medical procedures that were foreclosed by the patient's choice, and oral feedings could continue (although expected to be inadequate), most of the unpleasant symbolism would be erased. Also, if the patient is so near death that feedings are irrelevant or contraindicated, or if feedings would cause substantial suffering, lack of eating may pose no problem for caregivers.

Some of the resistance of providers to accommodate to patients forgoing nutrition or hydration stems from fear of legal action. *Conroy* should do much to reduce such fears. However, civil and criminal penalties are still possible and perhaps are most likely in situations where emotions run high, as is often the case in a decision against life-sustaining fluids and nutrition. Self-protection of this sort is sometimes justifiable, but it does have three unfortunate effects: it can deny a patient a legitimate option; it can induce deception of self and of patients because honest explanations are so difficult; and, if widespread, it eventually establishes noninvolvement of caregivers as a standard of care. If this last effect is achieved, even in this thoughtless way, it may become harder for other providers to comply with justifiable forgoings of this form of treatment.

PROVIDERS' ASSISTANCE IN DECISION-MAKING

What roles should providers play in making choices about nutrition and hydration? Simply, the roles should be the same as for any other choice about treatment. Caregivers routinely consider discontinuing a respirator for a patient who is suffering greatly while dying and who has no hope of recovery. The thought of abandoning nutritional support does not surface as often. If forgoing procedures to supply nutrition and hydration to patients is not considered by providers, it usually cannot become an option for the patients (or their surrogates). Thus, caregivers must be open to the possibility that their methods to normalize nutrition and hydration may not be beneficial to the patient.

Caregivers probably know less about the effects of dying with dehydration or malnutrition than they know about other ways of dying. Only if this ignorance is corrected can relevant information be conveyed to patients and better empirical data be generated. The limitations and side effects of the interventions now available also need to be more adequately researched and more widely known. People often ask searching questions about other technologies, but it is all too easy to create the expectation that no additional information would be relevant to a decision to ensure adequate nutrition and hydration by using medical procedures.

Caregivers also have the responsibility to effectuate further review or intervention if the decision-making process seems to have gone awry. Some prominent cases have arisen because of such action,[8] though unduly aggressive pursuit of the caregiver's perspective may lead to sanctions.[9] Both caregiving individuals and institutions have the responsibility to institute procedures that serve to ensure good decision-making.

EFFECTS OF FINANCING

Whether or not a patient is using a medical means of supporting nutrition or hydration often has dramatic, and sometimes perverse, effects upon financing the patient's medical care, including the nutrition and hydration itself as well as other forms of care, and upon financing basic supportive care. For example, intravenous alimentation for a baby would probably justify paying for continued hospitalization, while feeding through a gastrostomy would not, perhaps not even qualifying for funds for dressings and food preparation. Switching an elderly nursing home resident from a nasogastric feeding tube to the more comfortable and safe gastrostomy tube often causes a reduction in the "level of care" determination, which may not only reduce the nursing home's reimbursement but may also require transfer of the patient to a facility certified to provide a lower level of care.

Should these considerations have any effect upon the choices to be made? Pretending that such effects could be avoided would be foolish. Surely the decision-makers must be informed that a patient will have to leave the hospital if he or she does not undertake a medical procedure to provide adequate nutrition, or that the patient's estate will be bankrupted by the costs of long-term support made possible by tube feedings. These facts can be considered only to the extent that the patient wants (or would want, if the patient is incompetent).

But what of the patient who has never been competent or for whom there is no reliable evidence of his or her preferences in this regard? To refuse to consider finances would absolutely prevent costs from becoming an overwhelming consideration but would also create an artificially "cost-free" arena that would encourage overuse of the technology. On the other hand, to consider financial aspects might well dictate nontreatment too often. In the frequent ambiguous situations, even a "tie-breaker" in the decision could determine the outcome. Perhaps the best resolution is to refuse to consider costs in any one case, but to create policy that is sensitive to costs and that publicly bans certain options when the yields are small and the costs great or when the benefits to the patients are routinely uncertain.

CONSIDERATIONS FOR INSTITUTIONS AND SYSTEMS

Institutions and health care systems have a responsibility to consider the issues raised herein and to generate thoughtful policy responses. Just as individuals can refuse to provide certain options which are legal, so could institutions, though the likelihood of this arising may well be less. An institution which defines its mission in terms of advancing self-determination could refuse to comply with a court order to force-feed a patient, as could one with a strongly life-supporting mission refuse to support a patient who chooses to die by starvation. The hospital involved in the recent *Bartling* case, in which a competent, respirator-dependent man sought to have the respirator disconnected, made such a contention: ". . . Glendale Adventist is a Christian hospital devoted to the preservation of life, and it would be unethical for Glendale Adventist's physicians to disconnect life-support systems from patients whom they viewed as having the potential for cognitive, sapient life."[10] Although this case did not finally force the issue, as the patient died during the court proceedings, it should be possible for an institution to refuse to comply with a patient's request, even if some staff members might be willing to comply and the request is legal.

Institutions sometimes balk at accepting unusual or emotion-laden clinical situations, out of fear of unknown problems ahead or just because doing otherwise disrupts routines. After what is taken to be a landmark case affirming the authority of her father to decide her treatment, Karen Quinlan was maintained on a respirator against her parents' wishes until she was gradually weaned from it. Then, no long-term care facility was willing to take her as a patient until finally one accepted her on a number of conditions, including that her parents agree to "the continuance of maintenance and sustenance therapy."[11]

Institutions also have a responsibility to try to ensure that the incentives that they work within are those most conducive to good decisions being made. In this respect, they bear a responsibility to secure adequate surrogates, to make available adequate information, and to ensure honesty in presenting information to the decision-makers. Probably most important, institutions have a responsibility to be aware of the multiple allegiances that affect the institution's behaviors and those of the staff and to act responsibly to mitigate any untoward impact of these upon patients.

CONCLUSIONS

The ethical concerns of caregiving professionals and health care institutions must be considered in decisions to forgo life-sustaining nutrition and hydration. No one should be required to assist in another's dying or being kept alive by means that the caregiver finds reprehensible. This will occasionally lead to clashes of rights between caregivers and patients which, made more important by the symbolic meaning of food and water, will test the wisdom of societal practices and institutions.

Caregivers and health care institutions should redouble efforts to enhance the quality of decision-making, which will require better objective information, more introspection, and improved communication with patients.

NOTES

1. The author gratefully acknowledges the contributions of a discussion at the symposium involving Joseph L. Mintzer, A.C.S.W.; Eleanor M. Toohey, R.N., M.S.N.; Joan Monaghan, R.N., M.S., C.S.; and Chaplain Dan D'Arment.
2. To fail to do so incurs the civil charge of abandonment.
3. Jonathan Kirsch, "A Death at Kaiser Hospital," *Calif. Mag.* 79–81, 164–175 (November 1982).
4. Darrel W. Amundsen, "The Physician's Obligation to Prolong Life: A Medical Duty without Classical Roots," *Hastings Cent. Rep.* 8:23–30 (1978).
5. Bouvia v. County of Riverside, No. 159780 (Super. Ct. Cal., 1984)
6. See Deposition of Donald E. Fisher, M.D., in Bouvia v. County of Riverside.

7. George J. Annas, "When Suicide Prevention Becomes Brutality: The Case of Elizabeth Bouvia," *Hastings Cent. Rep.* 14:20–21 (1984).

8. Barber v. Superior Court, 147 Cal. App. 3d 1006, 195 Cal. Rptr. 484 (1983).

9. The nurses in the *Spring* case were sued successfully for invasion of privacy after divulging confidential facts about the patient to the news media. (See "Home Loses 'Right to Die' Case," *Am. Med. News* (Dec. 10, 1982) at 20.

10. *In re* Bartling, 209 Cal. Rptr. 220 (1984).

11. Harold L. Hirsch and Richard E. Donovan, "The Right to Die: Medico-Legal Implications of *In re* Quinlan," *Rutgers L. Rev.* 30:267–303, at 289 (1977).

Part V *In Re* Claire C. Conroy: A Case Study

22 *In re* Conroy:
History and Setting of the Case

Famous legal cases have often snatched from obscurity people whose lives were otherwise ordinary. Their names are splashed across newspaper headlines, eventually to become enshrined in cases familiar to judges, lawyers, and generations of law students who cut their teeth on the style cases collected in textbooks. In the annals of medical law, Brother Fox,[1] Joseph Saikewicz,[2] Abraham Perlmutter,[3] and, of course, Karen Ann Quinlan[4] have all become familiar names.

While Claire Conroy's name may not be a household word, her situation resulted in a case perhaps as important as Karen Quinlan's. What follows is a descriptive account of how Claire Conroy's case arose and how it was presented in court. Ensuing chapters will analyze the legal principles developed in the context of three levels of court review.

Claire Conroy's case garnered little media attention, especially in comparison to Karen Quinlan's, the only other such case to wind its way up to the New Jersey Supreme Court. Miss Conroy was elderly. She was virtually friendless, with few family members. At life's end she was minimally responsive and suffering from an array of physical ailments, including gangrene. There was no poignant high school yearbook picture to rivet the public's attention as there had been with Karen Quinlan, and her drama was cut short when she died while the court's resolution was still awaited. Nevertheless, the New Jersey Supreme Court recognized the dimensions of the problem before it when it noted that:

> decisions like these are an awesome responsibility that can be undertaken only with a profound sense of humility and reserve. The case of Claire Conroy raises moral, social, technological, philosophical, and legal questions involving the interplay of many disciplines. No one person or profession has all the answers.[5]

The court record is rather barren as to what kind of person Claire

Conroy was. By all accounts she led a simple, even cloistered, life. She was born in 1900 and lived in the same home in Belleville, New Jersey, from childhood until she was placed in a nursing home in 1979. She was employed by the same cosmetics company from her teenage years until she retired at age 62 or 63. Although she had few friends, she had been devoted to her three sisters, with whom she had shared a house. All her sisters died before Claire was admitted to the Bloomfield, New Jersey, nursing home. According to her only surviving blood relative, Thomas C. Whittemore (her nephew), all that Miss Conroy and her sisters "wanted was to . . . have their bills paid and die in their own house."[6]

Thomas Whittemore was appointed Claire Conroy's guardian in 1979, primarily for the purpose of having her admitted to Parklane Nursing Home, a thirty-bed institution. According to Mr. Whittemore, Conroy had never before visited a doctor, indeed she had "scorned medicine" all her life. Her only brushes with organized medicine in any sense came when Whittemore's wife, a registered nurse, "would try and get her through whatever she had," including pneumonia.[7]

When admitted to the nursing home, Miss Conroy was suffering from an organic brain syndrome occasioning intermittent periods of confusion. According to Dr. Ahmed Kazemi (a family practitioner) and Catherine Rittel (a registered nurse and nursing home administrator), Miss Conroy was in relatively good physical condition upon admission, sufficiently aware to converse and follow directions and able to walk on her own. Thereafter, her condition deteriorated and she could no longer communicate, becoming increasingly disoriented and physically dependent.

On two occasions, Miss Conroy's condition became serious enough to warrant transfer to Clara Maas Hospital. She was admitted for the first time on July 23, 1979, for a urinary tract infection and dehydration, was treated, and was released on August 8, 1979. She was again transferred from the nursing home to the hospital on July 21, 1982, this time for an elevated temperature and dehydration. A physical examination revealed necrotic gangrenous ulcers on her left foot. Orthopedic surgeons warned that these were life-threatening; they predicted she would die soon unless an amputation were performed. Mr. Whittemore, believing Miss Conroy would not have wanted to undergo an amputation, refused to consent to the procedure. Despite their dire, albeit mistaken, prognosis, the doctors involved acquiesced in Whittemore's refusal, in stark contrast to their reaction when it was later proposed that tube feeding be discontinued. They did not press for amputation in the discussions with Mr. Whittemore, which involved only a few brief phone conversations. Claire Conroy lived on despite gangrene and a host of other serious but not life-threatening illnesses. She was discharged from her second stay in the hospital on November 17, 1982.

During this second hospitalization, she was for the first time fed by a nasogastric tube. The tube, which was also used to provide antibiotics to forestall further infection, was removed for a two-week trial period in October. It was replaced on November 3, when it became apparent that she could not take sufficient quantities of food by mouth to survive. Thus, when she was discharged to the nursing home for the second time, on November 17, it was with a feeding tube. Yet another trial removal of the tube in January of 1983 proved futile. According to Dr. Kazemi, "even a person with great time and patience could probably not have coaxed her into absorbing enough fluids and solid foods by mouth to sustain herself."[8]

This was the situation when Thomas Whittemore beseeched Dr. Kazemi to remove the feeding tube. Mr. Whittemore had known his aunt for over fifty years. He or his wife had visited her every week for the four or five years before her admission to the nursing home and continued to visit her regularly there, although less frequently when it became apparent that she didn't know they were there.

All of the parties to the court case which eventually resulted from the nephew's request agreed that Whittemore was possessed of unalloyed good intentions, harboring no conflicts of interest. In a footnote, the appeals court observed that not only was Whittemore acting in "good faith" with "utmost sincerity," he was not "mistaken in concluding that Conroy would have asked to terminate treatment if she were able."[9]

Dr. Kazemi refused to accede to Thomas Whittemore's request to remove the feeding tube to allow Claire Conroy to die. Nursing home administrators and staff followed the physician's orders, remaining "essentially neutral on the issue of the removal of the tube" and stating that they would not oppose any court order to that effect. Transfer to another facility was not readily available, due to a moderate bed shortage and her dwindling financial reserves. Nephew

Whittemore, as guardian, brought an action to obtain a court order allowing removal of the tube.

The case came before Judge Reginald Stanton of the Chancery Division of Essex County's\Superior Court. Judge Stanton appointed a guardian *ad litem*, attorney John J. Delaney, Jr. Judge Stanton issued an opinion after hearing two days of testimony and making a visit to the bedside of Miss Conroy. Judge Stanton heard from Mr. Whittemore, Dr. Kazemi, and Catherine Rittel, the nursing home administrator and a registered nurse, as well as from Dr. Bernard Davidoff, an internist retained by the court-appointed guardian, and Rev. Joseph Kukura, a Roman Catholic priest and ethics committee member.

Judge Stanton's response to Claire Conroy was moving and eloquent:

> I think it fair to say that everyone involved in this case wishes that this poor woman would die. This wish does not flow from any lack of concern for Claire Conroy. On the contrary, it flows from a very deep sympathy for her sad plight. The disagreement among the participants involves differences in perception about what helping the patient means under the circumstances of this case.[10]

The medical testimony which brought Judge Stanton to this conclusion was supplied by Drs. Davidoff and Kamezi. Clearly Miss Conroy was not "brain dead"; nor was she in a persistent vegetative state or permanently unconscious. Thus, she did not fit within the ambit of the *Quinlan* decision. She was described as suffering from "organic brain syndrome," which the appellate court later defined as "[a] syndrome resulting from diffuse or local impairment of brain tissue function, manifested by alteration of orientation, memory, comprehension and judgment."[11] None of the tests needed to confirm the diagnosis were mentioned in the transcript, nor was the diagnosis rendered with any greater precision.

Her many physical ailments were described in this way: She was bed-bound and in a semi-fetal position, suffering from hypertension, diabetes, and arteriosclerotic heart disease. She had extensive bedsores (decubitus ulcers) on her left foot, leg, and hip, and her left leg was gangrenous to the knee. She had no bowel or bladder control, and had a urinary catheter.[12]

A subject of less agreement was the extent of Claire Conroy's mental life and her ability to think and respond to her environment, to feel pain, or to suffer. Her behavior was subject to differing interpretations.

> [S]he interacted with her environment in some limited ways: she could move her head, neck, hands and arms to a minor extent; she was able to scratch herself, and had pulled at her bandages, tube and catheter; she moaned occasionally when moved or fed through the tube or when her bandages were changed; her eyes sometimes followed individuals in the room; her facial expressions were different when she was awake from when she was asleep; and she smiled on occasion when her hair was combed, or when she received a comforting rub.[13]

Miss Conroy's behavior was interpreted differently by the two physicians who testified. Dr. Davidoff found her unable to respond to verbal stimuli, severely demented without higher functioning or consciousness. Dr. Kamezi thought her to be somewhat more responsive, testifying that, although unaware and confused, she was able to respond.

Testimony was similarly equivocal on the critical question of Miss Conroy's ability to experience pain. Were the skin sores or the feeding tube a source of pain or discomfort? Were her severely contracted legs a source of or a reaction to pain? Dr. Davidoff thought these were open questions and testified that she might be in a great deal of pain, since she apparently responded to noxious or painful stimuli by withdrawing and/or moaning. Judge Stanton did not wait for the testimony of a neurologist, which the plaintiff had offered to provide.

The judge also queried the caregivers as to the ethics of continued treatment, in what seemed at one point to be almost a straw poll with a need for a tie-breaker. Dr. Davidoff characterized the tube feeding as extraordinary and optional and Dr. Kazemi thought the removal of the feeding tube would violate professional canons and Claire Conroy's right to life.[14]

A witness called to testify further as to the ethics of continued feeding was Reverend Joseph Kukura, a Roman Catholic priest. Although the record is nearly silent on the depth and nature of Miss Conroy's religious beliefs, she was a Roman Catholic. Reverend Kukura described for the court the distinctions between ordinary and extraordinary care in Catholic moral theology and described the test laid out in the Vatican Declaration on Euthanasia to balance benefits and burdens of treatments. Reverend Kukura testified that, in Miss Conroy's case, the feeding tube was extraordinary and therefore

could be withdrawn—even if the death which would inevitably ensue would be painful.[15]

Although not without "some misgivings," Judge Stanton issued
an order allowing removal of the feeding tube on February 2, 1983.
The order was stayed, and while an appeal was pending Claire Conroy died on February 15, the feeding tube still in place. An autopsy
disclosed no definite cause of death and noted her height to be 4
feet, 11 inches and her weight to be 116 pounds.

Reviewing the case despite her death, a three-judge appellate panel
overruled Judge Stanton. On January 17, 1985, the New Jersey Supreme Court reversed the appeals court in a six-to-one decision, with
Justice Handler concurring in part and dissenting in part.[16]

This sort of litigation carries costs that warrant consideration.
This case cost tens of thousands of dollars, including a substantial
amount of public money expended upon salaries of those in the
Public Advocate's Office and in the judiciary who were involved in
the case. More than a score of expert witnesses, attorneys, and judges
were involved. Eight organizations filed *amicus curiae* briefs when
the case was before the state Supreme Court.

The Conroy case is also interesting for what it says about "medical
ethics" and how personal and professional moral and religious views
should determine medical outcomes. One of the commonly cited
state interests in requiring medical treatments is that of upholding
the ethics of the medical profession.[17] "Dr. Kazemi thinks it would
be a violation of medical ethics to remove the tube. Dr. Davidoff
believes that . . . the tube should be removed. Nurse Rittel would
be reluctant to see the tube removed. The guardian thinks it is wrong
to keep his aunt alive through the use of the tube."[18] This apparent
deadlock may have troubled the court and been the source of some
of the judge's "misgivings." This avenue of inquiry may be misguided, according to the New Jersey Supreme Court.

> If the patient rejected the doctor's advice, the onus of the decision would
> rest on the patient, not the doctor. Indeed, if the patient's right to in-
> formed consent is to have any meaning at all, it must be accorded respect
> even when it conflicts with the advice of the doctor or the values of
> the medical profession as a whole.[19]

Claire Conroy's case is illustrative of the many challenges and
tensions involved when medical decision-making is brought into

the courtroom. A number of commentators have been skeptical of the courts as a forum for resolving such dilemmas, citing inherent differences in the medical and legal processes.[20] Such criticisms center upon the public and adversarial process of law being antithetical to the private and collaborative process of health care.[21] A "lightning" fast decision concerning medical treatment brings to mind a resuscitation order and a "crash cart" careening down a hospital corridor. In legal proceedings, the same term might be applied to a case argued and decided in hours or days. Sometimes court orders are issued at the bedside within hours of the judge's first knowledge of the case, with an opinion written after the fact. However, very few cases move so quickly. (One rare example was the New York case of Baby Jane Doe, in which hearings by all three levels of state courts and a ruling by the state's highest court occurred within a week.)[22]

In Claire Conroy's case, Mr. Whittemore filed his petition on January 24. A guardian was appointed on January 26 and oral arguments were heard before Judge Stanton on January 31 and February 1. The judge decided the case on February 2. Judge Stanton's order to remove the nasogastric feeding tube was stayed pending further review by a three-judge intermediate court of appeals. Although the courts had moved as quickly as possible, while the appeal was being pursued, Claire Conroy died on February 15, 1984, nasogastric tube still in place.

Despite substantial efforts by each of the parties involved with the initial proceedings, the records from the trial court are as revealing for what they failed to explore as for what they do tell us about Claire Conroy as a person and as a patient. The New Jersey Supreme Court was aware of the failure to explore Claire Conroy's personal values sufficiently when it declined to say how she would have fared under its substantive guidelines and elaborate procedural roadmap:

> More information should, if possible, have been obtained by the guardian with respect to Ms. Conroy's intent. What were her religious beliefs? She did try to refuse initial hospitalization, and indeed had "scorned medicine." However, she allowed her nephew's wife, a registered nurse, to care for her during several illnesses. It was not clear whether Ms. Conroy permitted the niece to administer any drugs or other forms of medical treatment to her during these illnesses. Although it may often

prove difficult, and at times impossible, to ascertain a person's wishes, the Conroy case illustrates the sources to which the guardian might turn. For example, in more than eight decades of life in the same house, it is possible that she revealed to persons other than her nephew her feelings regarding medical treatments, other values, and her goals in life. Some promising avenues for such an inquiry about her personal values included her response to the illnesses and deaths of her sisters and others, and her statements with respect to not wanting to be in a nursing home.[23]

Courts and decision-makers face a difficult task in trying to divine the wishes of incompetent people who have failed to leave explicit instructions. On this score the Conroy court explicitly overruled itself in Quinlan. In the Quinlan case the court had heard testimony about Karen Ann's views on life-sustaining medical technologies and medical care at the end of life in the context of cases of family friends who had died. The Quinlan court found this evidence to be too "remote" to be "probative."[24] Subsequent court cases and discussions have sometimes turned on what a particular person would want if in Karen Quinlan's situation (e.g., Brother Fox).[25] The Conroy court ruled that such statements ought to be explored, while recognizing the "remoteness, consistency, and thoughtfulness of the prior statements or actions and the maturity of the person at the time of the statements or acts."[26]

The New Jersey Supreme Court limited its ruling to those persons who are elderly, incompetent residents of nursing homes, who have severe and permanent mental and physical impairments indicating a life expectancy of less than a year, and who were once competent. While the New Jersey Supreme Court ruling applies directly only to such persons residing in New Jersey, there is every reason to believe that the substantive standards will be more broadly construed.

NOTES

1. Eichner v. Dillon, 52 N.Y. 2d 363, 420 N.E. 2d 64 (1981).
2. Superintendent of Belchertown State School v. Saikewicz, 373 Mass. 728, 370 N.E. 2d 417 (1977).

3. Satz v. Perlmutter, 363 So. 2d 160, *aff'd* 379 So. 359 (Fla 1978).

4. *In re* Quinlan, 70 N.J. 10, 355 A.2d 647 *cert. denied*, 429 U.S. 922 (1976).

5. *In re* Conroy, 98 N.J. 321, 343–44, 486 A.2d 1209, 1220 (1985).

6. *Id.* at 1218.

7. *Id.*

8. *Id.* at 1217.

9. *In re* Conroy, 190 N.J. Super. 453, 464 A.2d 303, 306 n. 4 (App. Div. 1983).

10. *In re* Conroy, 188 N.J. Super. 523, 526, 457 A.2d 1232, (Chancery Div. 1983).

11. *In re* Conroy, 190 N.J. Super 453, 464 A.2d 303, 304 n. 1 (App. Div. 1983).

12. *In re* Conroy, 98 N.J. 321, 337, 486 A.2d 1209, 1217 (1985).

13. *Id.* at 1217.

14. *Id.*

15. *Id.* at 1218.

16. *In re* Conroy, 98 N.J. 321, 486 A.2d 1209 (1985).

17. *Id.* at 1224–25.

18. *In re* Conroy, 188 N.J. Super. 523, 526, 457 A.2d 1232 (Chancery Div. 1983).

19. *In re* Conroy, 98 N.J. 321, 352–3, 486 A.2d 1209, 1225 (1985).

20. Arnold Relman, "The Saikewicz Decision: A Medical Viewpoint," *Am. J. Law & Med.* 4:233– (1978); Allen Buchanan, "Medical Paternalism or Legal Imperialism: Not the Only Alternatives for Handling the Saikewicz-type Cases," *Am. J. Law & Med.* 5:97–117 (1979).

21. But see Charles H. Baron, "Medical Paternalism and the Rule of Law: A Reply to Dr. Relman," *Am. J. Law & Med.* 4:337–365 (1978).

22. Weber v. Stony Brook Hospital, 60 N.Y. 2d 208, 469 N.Y.S.2d. 63, 456 N.E.2d 1186, *cert. denied*, 104 S. Ct. 560 (1983).

23. *In re* Conroy, 98 N.J. 321, 385-86, 486 A.2d 1209, 1243 (1985) (citation omitted).

24. *In re* Quinlan, 70 N.J. 10, 21, 355 A.2d 647, *cert. denied*, 429 U.S. 922 (1976).

25. Eichner v. Dillon, 52 N.Y.2d 363, 420 N.E.2d 64 (1981).

26. *In re* Conroy, 98 N.J. 321, 362, 486 A.2d 1209, 1230 (1985).

Robert C. Cassidy, Ph.D.

23 *Conroy* on Appeal: Two Contrasting Perspectives by the Appellate Court and the State Supreme Court

REGULATORS AND THE APPELLATE COURT

If courts were divided into two kinds, one could distinguish between Regulators and Liberators. A commitment to defining and enforcing limits on the individual's judgment and actions marks the regulatory court. Its primary motif is a perceived duty to protect "society," "community values," "the tradition," and "others" from unbalanced subjectivity and unchecked autonomy. Its heroes are Plato and Hobbes. Its decisions are laced with talk of precedent, slippery slopes, and camels' noses.

Such a regulatory disposition was manifest in the 1983 decision by the Appellate Division of the Superior Court of New Jersey in the matter of Claire C. Conroy. The court held that discretion could be permitted only in the treatment of "incurable, and terminally ill patients who are brain dead, irreversibly comatose or vegetative, and who would gain no medical benefit from continued treatment."[1] All others must be given all medically indicated treatment, regardless of their so-called quality of life.

In this view, distinctions must be defended; regulations must be enforced. Otherwise, the subjective judgments of self-approving and self-serving individuals could be used to justify putting others out of our misery. Ultimately, the appellate court feared that this could well set us on the slippery slope toward the benevolent extermination of large groups of the disabled, the impaired, and all those judged as having a life not worth living, and so not worth serving.

The *Conroy* court at the appellate level affirmed a number of categories used to demarcate right from wrong actions: ordinary/extraordinary; unconscious/severely limited awareness; valuing life/assessing quality of life; terminal/chronic illnesses; and passive/active means. While the merit of some of these distinctions is quite uncertain in this setting, the court seemed bent upon shoring up defenses against possible abuse.

LIBERATORS AND THE SUPREME COURT

Liberators, by contrast, feel the weight of their responsibility on the other side of that delicate balance between protecting the rights of the individual and preserving the security of society. Such courts tend to espouse the essential libertarian belief in the endemic goodness and reasonableness of persons. With Mill (and, possibly, Jefferson), they share the egalitarian dogma that each person is the best judge of his or her own best interests. They defend individuals' rights to shape their own lives and deaths by the constructive application of their own principles, not by restrictive submission to paternalistic regulations. They tend to champion the personal perspective, which sees fit to judge and reject any established order, tradition, or law which does not meet the test of practical personal utility. The decisions of such courts resonate with invocations of integrity, liberty, privacy, and "self," as in self-determination, self-fulfilling, and self-satisfying.

It is just such a strikingly strong sense of the reality and significance of the individual self which initially marks the New Jersey Supreme Court's reversal of the appellate court's restrictive decision. The keynote of the opening movement of this landmark decision is an apparently bold championing of the rights of patients or their surrogate decision-makers to control their own medical care. Beginning with an extended analysis of the constitutional, common law, and ethical bases for the competent patient to consent to or dissent from recommended treatment, the court systematically eliminates or radically diminishes the restraints previously set on patients' self-determination by the competing claims of state interests, caregivers' professional integrity, tradition-fixed rules of treatment, and paternalistic interventions. Going far beyond the case at hand, the court virtually liberates the patient from compulsory medical service when it recognizes that

> a competent adult patient generally has the right to decline to have *any* medical treatment initiated or continued.[2]

The basic concern determining care should not be what sort of treatment this is, or what classification of patient this is. Rather, the court proposes, so clearly and simply, two determinative questions: the autonomy question—Is this what this patient, this person, wants—and the therapeutic question—Will this treatment on balance produce net benefit or net harm?

The individual's rights and best interests are to be of primary concern in the care of the incompetent patient. We must not deny respect and relief to clearly suffering patients because they can no longer speak for themselves. Neither can forgoing burdensome care be restricted only to the comatose. Clinical, legal, and semantic rubrics must not be allowed "to foreclose the possibility of humane actions."[3]

In this spirit of rational and humane and courageous dedication to doing whatever on balance is best for each patient, the New Jersey Supreme Court overrules the appellate court's traditional, inflexible, and cautious distinctions between obligatory and optional life-sustaining treatment. The court seems to have gone beyond every other major decision in the extent to which it promises to refocus attention on the needs of this suffering person and to restore authority for deciding about this person's care to those most personally invested.

And yet, when the court turns directly to Miss Conroy's case, it produces a surprisingly conservative judgment. When the court works through its own new guidelines and procedures, it ends up deciding that Miss Conroy did not qualify for relief. Despite being unable to communicate and having multiple afflictions, had Miss Conroy lived, she would still have had to be kept hooked up to that artificial life-support equipment. After all the bold defense of surrogate decision-making for the incompetent, the court cautiously decides not to allow Miss Conroy's lifelong friend and attentive legal guardian to decide how best to serve her best interests.

Is this an anomaly? Perhaps it is only the incidental elements of this particular situation which prevented the personal perspective from working through the innovative decision-making process to reach an autonomous and therapeutic conclusion. Or, perhaps, when it finally came down to the real practice of euthanasia, to the reality of killing an old woman, the court's sense of regulatory responsibility overruled its own theoretical liberation.

PERSONAL RIGHTS AND STATE INTERESTS

The appellate court had viewed the ultimate question to be whether Claire Conroy's right of privacy outweighed the state's interest in preserving life.[4] In doing so, they fixed on what we have called "the *Quinlan* formula," set in the New Jersey Supreme Court's 1976 decision.

> We think that the State's interest . . . weakens and the individual's right to privacy grows as the degree of bodily invasions increases and the prognosis dims. Ultimately there comes a point at which the individual's rights overcome the State's interest.[5]

According to this formula, the presumptive determinant is not the individual's right to choose how to live or die, but the state's interest in preserving life. The state will only be forced by an overwhelming imbalance in the costs and benefits of the treatment to give up its paternalistic overriding of the individual's self-determination. Paradoxically, almost the only patients allowed to control their lives (and deaths) will be those with almost no life left.

The contrast with the 1985 New Jersey Supreme Court decision in *Conroy* is striking. Here the starting point is a determination of "what rights a competent patient has to accept or reject medical care."[6] This court begins not by focusing on a severely debilitated Karen Quinlan or Claire Conroy, but by taking the strong, alert, articulate, and competent patient as the model of the self-determining person to be served by the court. Building on the competent person's right to "control his own body,"[7] the "common-law right to self-determination,"[8] and, to a lesser degree, the right to privacy, the court comes down forcefully and almost categorically on the side of liberating patient autonomy.

Indeed, the court explicitly declares that if Miss Conroy were competent, her interest in "freedom from nonconsensual invasion of her bodily integrity" would overrule any state interest.

SURROGATE JUDGMENT: THREE TESTS

In the case before the court the patient was clearly not competent. The aim of the court, therefore, is to delineate the rights of the *incompetent* patient, and also to specify the guidelines and procedures by which those rights may be made realities.

This leads the court to specify three tests, at least one of which must be met before life-support may be withheld or withdrawn.[9]

The first test to determine if life-sustaining therapy may be withheld or withdrawn is called the "subjective" test: "when it is *clear* that the particular patients would have refused the treatment under the circumstances involved."[10] And here, with the stress on "clear," regulatory caution begins to circumscribe the surrogates' freedom. The court describes numerous ways in which the no-longer-competent patient's wishes could be made "clear," with the prescriptive stress strongly on a living will or some other verifiable form of "evidence" which will have "probative value," which will be "clear proof."[11] Evidence should be tested as to its remoteness, consistency, thoughtfulness, maturity, and specificity.[12] In addition to this evidence, the surrogate must also have full and accurate information about the patient's current physical, sensory, emotional, and cognitive functioning; degree of pain with and without treatment; life expectancy, treatment options, and so on.[13]

The second and third tests are called "limited-objective" and "pure-objective," and one will be required when the person's wishes cannot be clearly established. Briefly, the limited-objective test requires "*some* trustworthy evidence" that the patient would have refused treatment, as well as evidence that the "net burdens" of his prolonged life (i.e., pain with treatment minus pain of withdrawing treatment) "markedly outweigh" any possible "physical pleasure, emotional enjoyment, or intellectual satisfaction."[14] In sum, the test is whether it is clear that the burdens of this life outweigh the benefits.

Absent any trustworthy evidence at all of this patient's wishes, the "pure-objective" test must be satisfied. For this, in addition to the proof that the burdens "clearly and markedly" outweigh the benefits, the "recurring, unavoidable and severe pain of the patient's life with the treatment should be such that the effect of administering life-sustaining treatment would be inhumane."[15] The court concludes this section with the injunction that whenever the person's wishes or physical or mental condition is equivocal, "it is best to err, if at all, in favor of preserving life."[16]

How cautious and demanding the court's standards are to be in practice becomes clear when the court examines Mr. Whittemore's evidence regarding his aunt's wishes and condition. After four detailed and penetrating pages of challenges, the court orders her lifelong friend, only living relative, and legal guardian to go back to produce more compelling evidence to support his judgment of her wishes, as well as more incontrovertible expert testimony as to the balance of pain and pleasure in this "mentally and physically severely impaired" woman.

Perhaps ambivalence is the true keynote of this decision. For, having almost baldly asserted its support of the rule of patient self-determination and patient's best interests as determinative in the care of the incompetent, the court then sets the regulatory standards so high as to reimpose in practice the restrictions it removed in principle. Unless convincing proof is given, caregivers and guardians are bound to continue giving the patient the treatment.

THE SEMANTICAL MILIEU—TERMINATING THE DISTINCTIONS

The focus of the appellate court's decision was an insistence upon setting fixed limits to discretion by means of fixed terminological distinctions. In a remarkably liberating series of broad strokes, the New Jersey Supreme Court proceeds to erase these traditional distinctions one by one, drawing heavily upon the recommendations of the President's Commission for the Study of Ethical Problems in Medicine and Biomedical and Behavioral Research.[17]

On the grounds that these terms are too ambiguous, elusive, nebulous, and variable to be of use in real clinical decision-making, the court systematically releases guardians and caregivers from the constraints of the distinctions between active and passive euthanasia,[18] between withholding or withdrawing treatment,[19] between extraordinary and ordinary treatment,[20] and, finally, between artificial care and natural care, such as feeding.

The basic message is that caregivers need to be liberated from the "semantical milieu" in which caring about distinctions takes precedence over caring for patients. The legal perspective and, indeed, the medical perspective itself may have become bewitched by these linguistic landmarks. However, the court insists, it is not the type of the procedure that matters; it is the purpose. Nothing should be

categorically excluded as the means to achieve the goal of the pre-
eminent therapeutic responsibility of doing whatever serves the patient's best interests, and no more.

DUE PROCESS IN THE NURSING HOME

Throughout this long substantive decision, the court continually
reminds us that it is only determining how to make life-support
decisions for severely impaired patients in nursing homes. The special environmental characteristics of the nursing home shape the
last section of the supreme court's decision.

The nursing home, in the somewhat Dickensian view of the court,
lacks the involved, caring family members and the enforced guild
standards of humane care necessary to guarantee that closed-door
decision-making will truly protect severely debilitated patients from
abuse.

Since New Jersey had already established by statute the Office of
the Ombudsman for the Institutionalized Elderly, vested with the
responsibility and powers to guard against the "abuse" of such patients,[21] the regulatory vehicle for reviewing and controlling life-
support decisions about nursing home patients was available. Again,
the regulatory side of the court's balanced concern (or frustrating
ambivalence) comes forth to constrain the decision-making authority of the most immediately involved family and caregivers.

In brief, the process requires that there must first be a judicial
determination of the patient's incompetency and an assignment of
a "general guardian." A further court determination must be made
as to whether, despite general incompetency, the patient may still
be competent to make this particular medical decision and, if not,
whether that "general" guardian is competent to make this particular surrogate decision.

When the guardian or "another interested party" believes that life-
sustaining treatment should be withheld or withdrawn, that person
must notify the Office of the Ombudsman, who "should treat every
notification . . . as a possible 'abuse.' " The ombudsman must in-
vestigate and report to the Commissioner of Human Services within
24 hours. All relevant "evidence" from the attending physician and
nurses is collected, and the ombudsman appoints two unaffiliated
physicians to "confirm the patient's medical condition and prognosis."[22] All these persons must concur if the subjective test is being

used. In addition, if the limited-objective or pure-objective is the basis for nontreatment, then all the patient's family must also concur. This section concludes with a final acute note of regulatory anxiety and admonition: "The ombudsman can refer cases of questionable criminal abuse to the county prosecutor."[23]

CONCLUSIONS

The New Jersey Supreme Court's *Conroy* decision impacts upon our most basic personal and family values, rights, and fears. Further, it proposes substantive modifications of the established guidelines and procedures by which professional caregivers and institutions have struggled to manage this most ancient and yet most modern human dilemma. Why and how we decide to preserve a human life, or not to, is paradoxically both the most intensely personal experience and also the most socially resonant event.

The ambivalence of the court is understandable, if not inevitable. With one eye it sees and responds to the anguish of Claire Conroy and Thomas Whittemore. Mirroring his benevolent concern and personal perspective, the court courageously asserts the rights of individuals to be truly individual, truly free both to find our own way and to do whatever is most humane and rational for those in our care.

But the other eye is more wary, more judicious. Fearing the potential for the fatal abuse of our most vulnerable citizens, the court turns back to set new limits on the new freedom. Virtually the court's last word is: "Guardians—and courts, if they are involved—should act cautiously and deliberately in deciding these cases."[24] And so the superior court's regulating distinctions are removed, but the Mr. Whittemores are sent back to gather more complete, clear evidence. Patient self-determination will be honored, but only after we have conclusively proven that this is the informed wish of the authentic self. Finally, even the feeding—and the lives—of those in our care can be stopped. But let us take on this awesome responsibility only after our most rational and humane judgments have been tried by our most rigorous and regulated procedures.

Unfortunately, the complexity of the regulatory process and the stringency of the evidentiary requirements raise the real possibility that this decision will further inhibit the person-centered decision-making the court clearly intended to increase. Finally, the court's fear of abuse may have placed greater restrictions on the use of rational and humane judgment in the care of severely impaired nursing home patients. As philosopher George Santayana wrote: "We compose our public figures timidly, in fear and trembling, and more to escape damnation than to achieve salvation."[25]

NOTES

1. *In re* Conroy, 190 N.J. Super 453, 464 A.2d. 303, 310 (App. Div. 1983).
2. *In re* Conroy, 98 N.J. 321, 486 A.2d 1209, 1222 (1985).
3. *Id.* at 1231.
4. *In re* Conroy, 190 N.J. Super. 453, 464 A.2d 303, 306 (App. Div. 1983).
5. *In re* Quinlan 70 N.J. 10, 355 A.2d. 647 *cert. denied* 429 U.S. 922 (1976).
6. *In re* Conroy, 98 N.J. 321, 346, 486 A.2d 1209, 1221 (1985).
7. *Id.*
8. *Id.* at 1223.
9. It should be noted that although the question of *withholding* treatment did not arise in the Conroy case, the court consistently speaks of deciding to "withhold or withdraw," and requires its guidelines and procedures to be followed for either decision.
10. *In re* Conroy, 98 N.J. 321, 486 A.2d 1209, 1232 (1985).
11. *Id.* at 1230.
12. *Id.*
13. *Id.* at 1231.
14. *Id.* at 1232.
15. *Id.* at 1233.
16. *Id.*
17. President's Commission for the Study of Ethical Problems in Medicine and Biomedical and Behavioral Research, *Deciding to Forego Life-Sustaining Treatment,* U.S. Government Printing Office: Washington, D.C. (1983).
18 *In re* Conroy, 98 N.J. 321, 369, 486 A.2d 1209, 1234 (1985).
19. *Id.*
20. *Id.* at 1234–35.
21. *N.J.S.A.* 30:13–1 to –11, and *N.J.S.A.* 52:27 G-1, G-2a.
22. *In re* Conroy, 98 N.J. 321, 384, 486 A.2d 1209, 1242 (1985).
23. *Id.*
24. *Id.* at 1243–44.
25. George Santayana, *The Last Puritan: A Memoir in the Form of a Novel,* New York: Scribners (1936).

William Strasser, J.D.

24 The *Conroy* Case: An Overview

The New Jersey Supreme Court in *Quinlan*[1] held that, if physicians attending a patient whose vital processes were being sustained by a mechanical respirator conclude that there is no reasonable probability of the patient emerging from her comatose condition to a cognitive, sapient state, then the life-support apparatus could be discontinued. In the *Conroy*[2] case, I asserted on behalf of Mr. Thomas Whittemore, nephew and guardian of Claire Conroy, that the right to refuse medical treatment for a terminally ill person is the same as that established by *Quinlan*.

Immediately after Mr. Whittemore's withholding of consent for amputation of Claire Conroy's gangrenous leg, Mr. Whittemore requested the treating physician, Dr. Kazemi, to remove her nasogastric tube, since he felt that his aunt would not have wanted her life prolonged under the circumstances. Dr. Kazemi refused to remove the nasogastric tube, except for a two-week trial period in October 1982.

Representing Thomas Whittemore, I demanded of Dr. Kazemi on November 4, 1982, that the nasogastric tube be removed. Dr. Kazemi agreed that Claire Conroy's prognosis was "zero" and that there was no hope of recovery; however, he advised that Miss Conroy should be transferred to her nursing home, where the nasogastric tube could be removed.

On November 17, 1982, Claire Conroy was discharged from Clara Maas Hospital and readmitted to Parklane Nursing Home, Bloomfield, New Jersey. Although requests that the nasogastric tube be removed were made to the institution's administrative officials by Mr. Whittemore, the nursing home refused to do so without Dr. Kazemi's authorization, which he would not give. Dr. Kazemi and all other medical personnel involved agreed that Claire C. Conroy was terminally ill and that death was imminent. However, Conroy continued to defy all medical predictions regarding the time of her death.

On January 24, 1983, I filed on Thomas Whittemore's behalf a Complaint and Order to Show Cause, seeking a judicial declaration that the guardian, Thomas C. Whittemore, had the right to effect the discontinuance of the nasogastric tube which was inserted in the person of Claire C. Conroy. After three days of testimony, the trial court on February 2, 1983, so declared.

On February 3, 1983, the guardian *ad litem* filed an appeal and obtained a stay blocking implementation of the trial court judgment. On February 15, 1983, thirteen days after the decision of the trial court, Claire Conroy died. On that day, the New Jersey Public Advocate intervened in the appeal. The decision of the Appellate Division reversed the decision of the trial court and severely limited the right of a conscious individual to refuse medical treatment and limited the forgoing of nutrition to those who are permanently unconscious.[3]

BASIS OF THE NEW JERSEY SUPREME COURT APPEAL

Mr. Whittemore and I believed that the decision of the Appellate Division was an incorrect application of the law, and Mr. Whittemore wanted the situation improved so that others might have less difficulty than he had experienced in caring for his aunt. The appeal of the Appellate Division decision filed on behalf of Mr. Whittemore was based on facts which I believe to have been sufficiently established in the lower court record and by legal premise.

The record clearly established that Claire Conroy was neither brain dead, comatose, nor described as being in a persistent vegetative state. The focus of the appeal in *Conroy* was that an individual who is terminally ill and facing imminent death is entitled to the same right of privacy as an individual who is comatose, such as Quinlan. As in *Quinlan*, the state's interest weakens as the prognosis dims; and, with Miss Conroy, her right of privacy surpassed the state's interest in preserving life.

The appeal contended that the nasogastric tube is medical treatment which, under the constitutional right to privacy, an individual has the right to refuse. Furthermore, to do so is in accordance with accepted moral and ethical standards. Therefore, a nasogastric tube may be refused or removed under the individual's right to privacy whenever the tube is imposing a great burden on the patient and offering no hope of benefit or cure to the ailment that the individual is suffering.

THE DECISION OF THE NEW JERSEY SUPREME COURT

On January 17, 1985, the New Jersey Supreme Court rendered its decision, setting the benchmark in this area of the law, not only for the State of New Jersey, but also for the country and the world.[4] The court agreed that medical provision of nutrition and hydration was medical treatment and set forth procedures to guide future cases of this sort.

The *Conroy* ruling also encourages the New Jersey legislature to develop and frame a comprehensive plan for resolving the life-and-death decision-making problems in a variety of other situations that were not before the court in *Conroy*. The court restricted its holding to elderly nursing home patients like Claire Conroy who were suffering from serious and permanent mental and physical impairments, who will probably die within one year even with treatment, and who, though formerly competent, are now incompetent to make decisions about their life-sustaining treatment and are unlikely to regain such competence.[5] An important side effect of *Conroy* is the underscoring of the importance of living-will legislation, which has been turned back many times by the state legislature. Although the court in its *Conroy* decision has set down the basic legal tenet to answer any and all questions relating to medical treatment decisions, the procedures for termination of medical treatment for patients in hospitals, nursing homes (patients under 60), hospices, and state institutions for the handicapped remain unresolved. The procedure set down by the court in clarifying the role of the state ombudsman in the decision-making process for termination of medical treatment for nursing home patients resolves the serious question with regard to nursing home patients, who, as studies have shown, are in many cases left without family and/or friends to act as decision-making individuals in their personal cases of medical treatment termination.

The New Jersey Supreme Court's decision in *Conroy* certainly will have many ramifications, not only in the State of New Jersey but also across this country. Mr. Whittemore and I are pleased with the outcome and have every expectation that others in the position of he and his aunt will benefit.

NOTES

1. *In re* Quinlan, 70 N.J. 10, 355 A.2d 647, *cert. denied*, 377 U.S. 978 (1976).
2. *In re* Conroy, 188 N.J. Sup. 523, 457 A.2d 1232 (Chancery Div., 1983).
3. *In re* Conroy, 190 N.J. Sup. 453, 464 A.2d 303 (App. Div. 1983).
4. *In re* Conroy, 98 N.J. 321, 486 A.2d 1209 (1985).
5. *Id.* at 1231.

John J. DeLaney, Jr. J.D.

25   The Role of the Guardian *Ad Litem*

The New Jersey Supreme Court's decision in *In re* Quinlan[1] created a whole new awareness of modern technology's ability to prolong the dying process. However, few persons ever fully examine its ramifications and the myriad surrounding issues until thrust into the controversial decision-making process regarding a similar case. My opportunity to do so arose on January 26, 1983, when Judge Reginald Stanton made a telephone request that I serve as the guardian *ad litem* (court-appointed attorney) for Claire C. Conroy.[2] The facts of the case and its progress through the courts are recounted in the preceeding chapters. I did not realize that courts had never been asked to grant a request for discontinuing feeding a patient and that doing so would force a reexamination of the limits of medical choices, especially as developed in *Quinlan.*

ROLE OF THE GUARDIAN *AD LITEM*

The guardian *ad litem* serves a very important safeguard function.[3] In New Jersey, the function of a guardian *ad litem* is to ensure the protection of the rights and interests of a litigant who is apparently incompetent to prosecute or defend the lawsuit.[4] The New Jersey Supreme Court in *Quinlan* entrusted the decision of whether to continue artificial life-support to the person's guardian, family, attending doctors, and hospital "ethics committees,"[5] but case law does not specify the role of the guardian *ad litem* in medical treatment cases underlying withdrawal of life-support from incompetent patients.

Other jurisdictions have recognized the importance of the guardian *ad litem* in these kinds of cases, and generally two views on the role and function of a guardian *ad litem* have developed. Under the first view, the guardian *ad litem* should be an advocate and play a true adversarial role.[6] Under the other view, the guardian *ad litem* should be an investigator and a reporter of the relevant facts to the court.[7]

The adversarial role of the guardian *ad litem* has been adopted in Massachusetts.[8] Such a view stems from that jurisdiction's philosophy of mandating judicial resolution on whether potentially life-prolonging treatment should be withheld from a person incapable of making his or her own decision.[9] This philosophy contrasts with that developed by the New Jersey Supreme Court in *Quinlan*, which encouraged the directly affected parties to resolve most such questions. The guardian *ad litem* is responsible in Massachusetts for presenting to the trial court, after as thorough an investigation as time will permit, all reasonable arguments in favor of administering treatment to prolong the life of the individual involved. A report should also be prepared and made available to the trial judge prior to the hearing on the ultimate issue of treatment. This procedure will ensure that all viewpoints and alternatives will be aggressively pursued and examined at the subsequent hearing where it will be determined whether treatment should or should not be allowed.[10]

In contrast, Washington has adopted an alternative view. There, the guardian *ad litem*'s role is to discover all the facts relevant to the decision to withdraw life-sustaining treatment and to present them to the court.[11] Such facts would include, but are not necessarily limited to (a) facts about the incompetent, i.e., age, cause of incompetency, relationship with family members and other close friends, attitude and previous statements concerning life-sustaining treatment; (b) medical facts, i.e., prognosis for recovery, intrusiveness of treatment, medical history; (c) facts concerning the state's interest in preserving life, i.e., the existence of dependents, other third-party interests; and (d) facts about the guardian, the family, other people close to the incompetent, and the petitioner, i.e., their familiarity with the incompetent, their perceptions of the incompetent's wishes, any potential for ill motives. Under this view, the guardian *ad litem* would not necessarily play a true adversarial role, but would serve as an investigator and a reporter of relevant facts to the court.[12]

In undertaking my responsibility as the guardian *ad litem* for Miss Conroy, I initially chose to act as the investigator and reporter of relevant facts to the court. However, after I had completed my investigation and had analyzed the law in New Jersey and the nation, I realized that the state of the law required that I advocate for Miss

Conroy's interests in continuing to live and oppose removal of the feeding tube.

THE TRIAL COURT HEARING

Investigation for the hearing was accomplished within five days, as the plaintiff had claimed that treatment was causing the patient pain and distress. In light of the facts learned during the investigation and the absence of legal precedent, I decided to argue strongly against removal of the feeding tube, even though this meant opposing the conclusion of my expert physician.

Only seven days passed from the appointment of the guardian *ad litem* to the entry of the judgment by the trial court. While Judge Stanton is to be commended for his prompt and well-reasoned, though incorrect, decision, the guardian *ad litem* made a critical error in not requesting leave of court to fully brief the issues, as well as to require the testimony of the neurologist that plaintiff's counsel had consulted. Time should have been taken to memorialize both the results of the investigation and analysis of the law.

THE APPEAL

Immediately after Judge Stanton delivered his opinion, I moved for and was granted a stay for forty-eight hours pending the filing of a Notice of Appeal and Notice of Motion for a Stay Pending Appeal. The Appellate Division ordered an accelerated appeal and continued the stay pending appeal.

Numerous legal arguments were presented to the Appellate Division by the guardian *ad litem*. First, as previously discussed and argued to the trial court, the decision appeared to violate the *Quinlan* principles and guidelines. Second, the uniqueness of Judge Stanton's order (at the time) was undisputed. There was not one reported decision in any jurisdiction which authorized the removal of feeding tubes, let alone removal of a feeding tube from a person who was not brain dead, comatose, or in a chronic vegetative state. Never before had a court taken the extraordinary and immutable step of direct deprivation of food, water, and medicine to a patient.[13]

Third, Judge Stanton's opinion was written in language so broad as to create a framework and basis for legitimizing conduct inimical to the fundamental rights and liberties of all persons as guaranteed by the federal and state constitutions. The broad language of the opinion creates a standard of choice—life or death—based on the subjective determination as to whether the life in issue is still "meaningful." No court has ever, or, for that matter, should ever cross such a threshold.

Judge Stanton stated that he did not believe that senile persons or retarded persons of all ages should have basic feeding and care wrongfully withheld from them; however, he used the "quality of life" test, that such persons be able to give and accept love, and have cognitive ability to merit continued care and feeding.[14] Therefore, the trial court's opinion left open the door to cases which would terminate basic care for these groups as well. By saying, "we have to be very careful about premature and wrongful withdrawal of treatment,"[15] Judge Stanton intimated that there are times and tests to permit such withdrawal and in fact require us to make these choices.[16]

A reading of the language of the trial court decision leaves one with the fearful and frightening conclusion that the trial court made the decision to actively terminate life based on its "meaningful level" and on whether the life is worth preserving. Such a decision is fatally flawed. Such a decision violates all legal and moral principles, which serve as the foundation of our society, our ethics, and various religious beliefs. A state's interest in the protection of human life attaches by virtue of the existence of that life, not by virtue of its subjective quality.

Fourth, the trial court's decision appeared inconsistent not only with *Quinlan*, but with other areas of the law as well. Courts and legislatures are having great difficulty in imposing the death penalty, even for those who have committed the most heinous of crimes.[17] Further, our courts have ruled that prisoners are not permitted to starve themselves to death.[18] It would be ironic and confusing to see our courts refuse to permit a convicted and incarcerated felon to starve himself to death and at the same time *order* an elderly woman to be deprived of food and water in her final period of life.

Fifth, the trial court's decision is euthanasia in that it authorizes a direct and intentional positive act that would ultimately cause death. If Judge Stanton's decision stood, it might be applied excessively, as it was in the Nazi regime in Germany.[19]

The impact of the trial court's decision and the broad language of the opinion would extend far beyond the case. There are thousands, if not millions, of handicapped veterans, quadriplegics, mental incompetents, severely retarded children, and elderly who may not attain the "meaningful level of intellectual functioning" or the intangible standards required by the trial court's decision. Despite the admonitions contained in the trial court's opinion, and the admirable and compassionate motives of Judge Stanton, the trial court's decision provides a rationale to condemn the weaker members of our society to death by starvation or by denial of basic ordinary care.

Sixth, as Judge Stanton noted, "life is our most basic possession."[20] Indeed, one of our most deeply held beliefs is that life is more precious than nonlife.[21] The Declaration of Independence states as a self-evident truth that all men "are endowed by their Creator with certain unalienable Rights, that among these are *Life,* Liberty and the pursuit of Happiness." The trial court, in ordering Miss Conroy to a painful death by starvation and/or dehydration, sanctioned a denial of this fundamental right.

Finally, although not argued at the trial level, removal of the feeding tube could have subjected Mr. Whittemore and the health care professionals to criminal liability. The issue was raised in *Quinlan,* wherein the court stated:

> We conclude that there would be no criminal homicide *in the circumstances of this case.* We believe, first, that the ensuing death would not be homicide but rather *expiration from existing natural causes.* Secondly, even if it were to be regarded as homicide, it would not be unlawful. (emphasis added)[22]

The *Conroy* case was different. Miss Conroy was simply being fed. She would not die "from existing natural causes" but from an intentional act, the intentional deprivation of food and water.

THE APPELLATE DIVISION DECISION

The New Jersey Superior Court, Appellate Division, reversed Judge Stanton's decision, declaring that his order amounted to "the authorization of euthanasia,"[23] although the court rejected the guardian *ad litem's* contention of possible criminal exposure.[24] The appeals court issued the decision despite the mootness of the case, because of the public importance of the issues.[25]

THE NEW JERSEY SUPREME COURT

The final determination of the *Conroy* case was in the hands of the New Jersey Supreme Court, which once again took the opportunity to fully discuss and clarify the principles outlined in *Quinlan*. The New Jersey Supreme Court is to be commended for its in-depth and courageous ruling.

The supreme court reaffirmed and expanded upon the *Quinlan* principles and reversed the Appellate Division by holding that life-sustaining treatment may be withheld or withdrawn from an incompetent patient when it is clear that the particular patient would have refused the treatment under the circumstances ("subjective test"). The court also held that life-sustaining treatment may also be withheld or withdrawn from such a patient if either of two "best interest" tests—a "limited objective" test or "pure objective" test—is satisfied. The court found, as advocated by the guardian *ad litem* and ruled upon by the Appellate Division, that the record in the case did not satisfy any of those standards and, thus, that authorization for removal of the feeding tube should not have been given. Additionally, the court specifically rejected any decision-making process based on assessments of personal worth or social utility of another's life.[26]

In making its decision, the court recognized its own limitations and noted that the legislature is better equipped to handle all of the relevant contingencies in resolving requests to terminate life-sustaining treatment for incompetent patients.[27]

NOTES

1. *In re* Quinlan 70 N.J. 10, 355 A.2d 647 *cert. denied* 429 U.S. 922 (1976).

2. *In re* Conroy, 188 N.J. Super. 523, 457 A.2d 1232 (Chancery Div.), *rev'd* 190 N.J. Super. 453, 464 A.2d 303 (App. Div. 1983).

3. E.g., *In re* Grady, 85 N.J. 235, 264, 426 A.2d 467, 482 (1981), where the Supreme Court of New Jersey ruled that when application is made for authorization to sterilize an allegedly incompetent person, the court should appoint an independent guardian *ad litem* as soon as possible. The guardian must have the full opportunity to meet with the incompetent person, to

present proofs, to cross-examine witnesses at the hearing, and to represent zealously the interests of his or her ward in other appropriate ways.

4. *In re* Commitment of S.W., 158 N.J. Super. 22, 26, 385 A.2d 315 (App. Div. 1978).

5. *In re* Quinlan 70 N.J. 19, 55, 355 A.2d 647, 666.

6. Superintendant of Belchertown State School v. Saikewicz, 370 N.E.2d 417, 433–434 (Mass. 1977). See also Charles Baron, "Assuring Detached But Passionate Investigation and Decision; The Role of Guardians *Ad Litem* in Saikewicz-type Cases," *Am. J. Law & Med.* 4:111 (1978).

7. *In re* Welfare of Colyer, 99 Wash.2d 114, 660 P.2d 738, 748–749 (1983).

8. Superintendent of Belchertown State School v. Saikewicz, *supra* n. 6.

9. *Id.*

10. *Id.* at 433–434.

11. Matter of Welfare of Colyer, supra n. 7.

12. *Id.*

13. *See* Power of Court to Order or Authorize Discontinuation of Extraordinary Means of Sustaining Human Life, 79 A.L.R.3d, 237 (1977).

14. *In re* Conroy, 188 N.J. Super. 523, 530–531, 457 A.2d 1232, 1236 (Chancery Div. 1983).

15. *Id.* at 531.

16. *Id.* at 529.

17. Berman v. Allen, 80 N.J. 421, 429–430, 404 A.2d 8, 13 (1979).

18. Von Holden v. Chapman, 37 A.D.2d 66, 450 N.Y.S.2d 623, 626 (4th Dept. 1982).

19. See Yale Kamisar, "Some Non-Religious Views Against Proposed 'Mercy-Killing' Legislation," *Minn. L. Rev.* 42:969–1042 (1958).

20. *In re* Conroy, 188 N.J. Super. 523, 527, 457 A.2d 1232, 1234 (Chancery Div. 1983).

21. Berman v. Allen, 80 N.J. 421, 429–430, 404 A.2d 12 (1980).

22. *In re* Quinlan, 70 N.J. 18, 51, 355 A.2d 647, 669–670 *cert. denied* 429 U.S. 922 (1976).

23. *In re* Conroy, 190 N.J. Super. 453, 461, 464 A.2d 303, 307 (App. Div. 1983).

24. *Id.* at 460 n. 4.

25. *Id.* at 459.

26. *In re* Conroy 98 N.J. 321, 367, 486 A.2d 1209, 1222–23 (1985).

27. *Id.* at 1220, 1244.

Joseph H. Rodriguez, Jr., J.D.

26 Role of the Public Advocate

New Jersey was the first state to implement a federally aided program of advocacy for the developmentally disabled. One of five major advocacy divisions, it provides a variety of services for thousands of victims of mental retardation and lifelong disabilities and is empowered to litigate in the public interest on behalf of its clients.

In *Conroy*, a superior court judge had ruled that an eighty-four-year-old semicomatose woman residing in a nursing home could be disconnected from the nasogastric tube which had been sustaining her life for about six months. The Office of Public Advocate moved to intervene in the case at the appellate level because of our strong view that the court should establish guidelines governing termination of life and the right of a patient to receive basic nourishment.

Furthermore, I and my associates were concerned as advocates with how a decision which would allow a patient to die of dehydration or starvation would affect severely disabled persons, handicapped infants, and the mentally ill.

During oral argument before the Supreme Court, I contended that there is a substantial difference, a humanitarian difference, between comforting the dying and treating the sick.

In my opinion, the state has valid interests in preserving life, in protecting the helpless, in preventing suicide, and in maintaining the integrity of the medical profession. In most instances, these interests yield to the privacy rights of a competent individual, particularly when that person is fully aware of the disease or illness process that he or she is confronting and decides to surrender to that process. But there are limits. Even competent persons cannot legally commit suicide.

In my view, a humane society must recognize and preserve the basic care which comforts the dying. An ill person is not denied hygienic care. I would include food and fluids in this category of care.

Some would say that food and fluids may be discontinued when the patient's condition is terminal. However, a key question arises out of the *Conroy* case: How do we define the "terminal" condition of a person? Lou Gehrig's disease is terminal because it involves an inexorable process, but death might not occur for five years or more. As Public Advocate, I asked the New Jersey Supreme Court to establish guidelines for future decisions. I asked that the court tell us what a terminal condition is and what its legal significance is in the area of life-sustaining treatment.

I believe that food and fluids can be permanently withdrawn only when these two conditions are met: death is imminent and any other course of action would induce additional suffering. If the the kidneys are not functioning, for instance, food and fluids should be discontinued so that we do not drown the patient. Medical procedures for nutrition and hydration may have a destructive impact on the body and make the overall effect of continued feeding harmful to the patient and therefore be contraindicated.

The trial court judge recognized that Claire Conroy might live for a year or more. (As it turned out, she died shortly after the decision was handed down, but no one could know that this would happen at the time.) Should a court rule that basic nourishment and fluids can be withdrawn because the patient's life is not worth living? If such an action is legally permissible, why not simply end it all with a lethal injection? The interests of nursing home patients, the severely handicapped, and all of the other people in our society that I represent as Public Advocate dictate that we not permit such termination of life.

Despite the court decision that allowed for discontinuation of a respirator, Karen Ann Quinlan remained alive for ten years, sustained by the same type of feeding tube system that sustained Claire Conroy. And yet Karen Ann Quinlan was in a much less sentient state than was Claire Conroy when the trial court ordered that feeding could be suspended. Claire Conroy nodded, smiled, and scratched herself. There was no neurological testimony in *Conroy* that even suggested that mere reflex responses were mimicking intellectual power.

We should recognize that we are dealing with an emotional subject. The first response of a newborn infant is to feeding. Society has traditionally used food as a method of friendship. If the court is to make judgments on whether or not a person should be fed, it should make the decisions only under clear guidelines and with a full record before it.

The New Jersey Supreme Court stated with clarity what forms of life-sustaining care or treatment can be denied. Under appropriate circumstances, any form of care or treatment—including tube feeding—can be denied or rejected. Although it went further than I had advocated—to permit the termination of feeding not only when it might cause the patient new harm but also when it would be contrary to the prior wishes of an incompetent patient—it did so in a way that was both compassionate and which fully protected the interests of persons with disabilities.

Conroy is not a right-to-die decision. The court held that, as a general rule, patients have a right to determine the course of their treatment and, in so doing, can refuse or discontinue treatment if they wish. More properly, *Conroy* involves the right of patients to make treatment decisions and control what will be done to their bodies.

Perhaps the most significant aspect of *Conroy* is the rejection of such treatment labels as "ordinary" versus "extraordinary" or "artificial" versus "natural." The court noted that such terms confuse the issue and stand in the way of clear analysis.

The New Jersey Supreme Court in *Conroy* extended the right of self-determination in a carefully limited way to incompetent patients. Surrogate decision-makers may refuse treatment for the patient when the wishes of the patient are known, and life expectancy is short, and appropriate procedures have been followed. Where the wishes are not known with precision, several rigorous tests must be met which involve the patient's medical condition. These tests and standards mirror what I asked the court to adopt. In fashioning them, the court followed the analysis used in its 1981 *Grady* decision, involving the sterilization of the retarded—a case in which the court adopted in their entirety the standards advocated by my department.

In applying these tests to Claire Conroy, the New Jersey Supreme Court concluded that the record developed before the trial court was insufficient to establish whether a feeding tube should have been removed from Claire Conroy and the court vacated the trial court judgment.

Other portions of my argument also were consonant with *Conroy*. The court encouraged the use of written directives prepared by patients while competent and expressly invited the legislature to adopt living will or other suitable legislation that would help patients record their views on the subject. The *Conroy* court established an innovative procedure for surrogate decision-making on behalf of elderly nursing home residents that involves family, health care providers, the courts, and the Ombudsman for the Institutionalized Elderly. But because the ombudsman's jurisdiction is restricted to nursing home residents age 60 or older, the *Conroy* court necessarily limited the procedure to that population. Again, the court explicitly invited the legislature to develop procedures governing other situations such as those involving younger nursing home residents, patients in hospices, institutions for the developmentally disabled, and hospitals that lack ethics committees.

One last aspect of *Conroy* must be mentioned. I am comforted that the court embraced the Public Advocate's request to clearly distinguish severely handicapped persons from the dying. The court expressly declined to authorize decision-making based on assessments of quality of life or social utility. To do so would, according to the court, "create an intolerable risk for socially isolated and defenseless people suffering from physical or mental handicaps."

New Jersey now has a workable framework in which to analyze treatment decisions, and a rudimentary procedure to permit decision-making on behalf of elderly incompetent persons has been established. What we need now is comprehensive legislation that brings all of these pieces together and establishes the procedures necessary to implement them. Beyond this, I personally think we must begin to help people with terminal illnesses spend their final days at home or in a hospice or other comforting place instead of in the sterile and laboratory-like world of hospitals.

Russell L. McIntyre, Th.D.

27 The *Conroy* Decision: A "Not-So-Good" Death

The New Jersey Supreme Court's recent decision in the case of Claire C. Conroy[1] significantly broadens its famous *Quinlan*[2] decision and represents bold advances in the development of legal medicine and health law. But the procedural requirements in arriving at a decision to terminate or withhold medical treatment from a dying patient are confusing, unnecessarily burdensome, and represent such an unwarranted intrusion into the physician-family relationship that the actual impact of the patient's death on the family may be more traumatic.

In *Quinlan*, the court said, first, that the *focus* of the decision ought to be on prognosis—on whether the patient is "beyond being restored to a cognitive, sapient state." Second, the *locus* of decision-making resides with the family. If the family requests that life-sustaining equipment be removed, an "ethics" committee at the hospital should meet to confirm the prognosis.

Since 1976, major questions have arisen regarding some of the details of how "termination of medical treatment" decisions are to be made. The *Conroy* decision attempts to address many of these questions but incurs four shortcomings.

ETHICS COMMITTEES OR " 'GRANDPA DOE' SQUADS"?

The *Quinlan* decision required review of decisions by a hospital "ethics" committee. In 1977, the Attorney General and Commissioner of Health for New Jersey published "Guidelines for Health Care Facilities to Implement Procedures Concerning the Care of Comatose Non-Cognitive Patients." The guidelines were optional and no institution—hospital or nursing home—was required to form such a committee.[3]

The *Conroy* decision, however, assigns no role whatsoever to such an institutional ethics committee. What it does instead is to create a "geriatric" version of the "Baby Doe" squads by assigning an investigatory role to the State Office of the Ombudsman whenever a family or physician wants to withhold or withdraw life-sustaining medical therapy from an elderly nursing home patient who is expected to die within a year. With full subpoena powers, a team of investigators from Trenton must conduct an official investigation with, according to the court decision, the presumption that "abuse" of the patient is possibly being committed. "The Ombudsman should treat every notification that life-sustaining treatment will be withheld or withdrawn from an institutionalized, elderly patient as a possible 'abuse'."[4]

Why the court ignored the role of the ethics committee is not clear from the decision itself. The court did recognize that nursing homes are quite different from hospitals. Very few nursing homes have established ethics committees, but neither the court nor the state has created any incentive for nursing homes to form such committees.

Possibly the court did not realize how well the ethics committee model was working in hospitals. Instead of assigning the role of reviewing difficult or worrisome patient care decisions to an ethics committee, it has forced a very unwelcome official state investigation upon the dying patient and the grieving family. With the presumption of "abuse," the investigation itself becomes abusive.

THE ISSUE OF NUTRITION AND HYDRATION

A second major criticism of the *Conroy* decision involves the issue of whether the continued feeding of a dying patient is always required or may be optional. A national debate has been developing since the 1983 indictment of two California physicians who removed a nasogastric feeding tube from a patient with severe brain damage.[5] The physicians were charged with manslaughter for "starving" their patient to death. The charges were brought and dismissed, then reinstated and finally dismissed on appeal, but the indictments themselves touched a very sensitive public nerve regarding what is minimally required of us as human beings when we are caring for others.

The *Conroy* decision states that in the care of the clearly dying patient (i.e., one who is expected to die within one year even with treatment), feeding either by tube or vein is an artificial means of prolonging life and, as such, is equivalent to a respirator or dialysis and, therefore, can be removed or withheld. The court used an "ends versus means" analysis and argued that if the ends were the same, i.e., the artificial prolongation of life or delay of death, then any of these treatments could be unnecessary and not required.

Any individual may not be disturbed by the decision to remove nutrition from a patient who is irretrievably comatose and dying, because removing nutrition at this stage does not seem to cause the patient to experience increased pain or suffering. However, the *Conroy* decision rather glibly dismisses some rather strong and powerful public sentiments about feeding as part of what is minimally required of us as human beings. Hans Jonas once said that "the patient must never feel that his physician might become his executioner." This sentiment is also held by many physicians and was the cornerstone of the appeals court decision in *Conroy* which stated that feeding was never optional.[6]

Law must reflect accepted standards of knowledge as well as social attitudes, as long as these attitudes are not unjust. The *Conroy* decision dismissed—or, rather, trivialized—this rather profound public sentiment concerning feeding when, in fact, it might have had another choice, although there is no evidence in the decision that the court even considered this possibility. Claire Conroy was being kept alive by feeding and by medications for heart disease, diabetes, and hypertension. The nasogastric tube which passed through her nose and into her stomach carried nutrition and hydration but was also the conduit for her medications. Under *Quinlan* principles, the court could have permitted the removal of the medications—which might have permitted her to die from her underlying diseases—yet still have required nutrition and hydration for the strong symbolic meaning they have to others, most notably, in this case, the physician and the nursing staff.

IN THE PATIENT'S "BEST INTEREST"

The third major criticism of the *Conroy* decision concerns the way in which the court expanded the inquiry as to what was in the patient's best interest. The court redefined standard legal categories and came up with a new form of the "substitute judgment test" which it called the "subjective test" and two forms of the "best interest test" which it termed the "limited objective test" and the "pure objective test."

A. The Subjective Test

The validity of this test arises from some form of personal declaration, either expressed or implied, that can be attributed to the patient. The most well-known form is the "living will," in which the patient states that if he or she becomes terminally ill, can no longer participate in decision-making, and has lost the ability to benefit from continued medical treatment, then this patient elects "not to be subjected to resuscitation, surgery, or receive strong antibiotics or other medications" for the sole purpose of postponing death. The patient requests instead to receive only pain medication that would make dying more comfortable.

Many states have already passed legislation making a "living will" legally binding, if properly executed. New Jersey does not have such a statute, but the *Conroy* court stated clearly that this was an acceptable form of decision-making. The court also expanded the concept beyond a "living will" to include an "oral directive" conveying the patient's wishes, or the appointment of a proxy through a "durable power of attorney."

In addition to a direct written or oral statement, the *Conroy* court declared that the patient's authentic wishes could also be deduced from such situations as (1) the known reaction of the patient to other situations in which a patient was in similar circumstances; (2) the patient's own religious beliefs; and (3) the patient's consistent pattern of conduct and prior decisions about his or her own medical care.[7]

The court, however, was concerned about the appropriateness of each of these categories and, therefore, required that *all* of the above criteria for the subjective test (including the "living will") be judged by qualifying standards of "remoteness," "consistency," "thoughtfulness," "maturity" of the patient at the time the declaration was made, and "specificity." One notes that the "subjective test," then, is to be judged by other criteria which are more objective and measurable. Therefore, even a signed "living will" could be disqualified if it failed the court's measure for being not recent enough, not logically consistent, or not specific enough. The court did not address how one would judge the patient's "thoughtfulness" or level

of "maturity" when the document was issued. The "subjective test,"
then, is to be evaluated by rather precise external criteria.

B. The "Limited Objective Test"

When there is no specific declaration by the patient as to what he
or she would want when unable to participate in his or her own
medical decisions, then either the "limited objective test" or the
"pure objective test" applies.

The "limited objective test" may be used, according to the court,
when there is "some trustworthy evidence" that the patient would
have refused the medical treatment. Although this sounds similar
to the "subjective test," in this case the "evidence" is too vague to
be considered "absolute proof."[8] This test would allow evaluation
of casual statements or informally expressed statements.

In addition, "the decision-maker" (actually, the ombudsman; see
above) must be satisfied that "the burdens of a patient's continued
life with the treatment outweigh the benefits of that life for him."[9]

C. The "Pure Objective Test"

The court stated that when there is "no trustworthy evidence as to
what the patient would have wanted," then the decision-maker (the
ombudsman) must be satisfied that "the net burdens of the patient's
life with the treatment should *clearly* and *markedly* outweigh the
benefits that the patient derives from life" (emphasis added).[10] And,
in addition, the recurring, unavoidable pain of the patient's life with
the treatment should be such that the effect of administering life-
sustaining treatment would be inhumane.

Note the terribly subjective nature of the "objective" tests. For
example:

   a. "Some trustworthy evidence. . . ." Who determines and by
      what criteria?
   b. "The burdens of a patient's life with treatment. . . ." How do
      we judge "burdens"?
   c. ". . . outweigh the benefits of life. . . ." How do we evaluate
      "benefits"? Perhaps we can do this for ourselves, but can we
      really do it for others?
   d. ". . . clearly and markedly outweigh. . ."
   e. ". . . humane."

The "subjective test" is to be constrained strictly by objective
criteria. And, now, the so-called "objective tests" become entirely

the subjective determination of the State Ombudsman or someone in his or her office. All of this acts to preempt the decision-making of the family and physician, possibly working with an "ethics committee," who would clearly know the patient much more thoroughly and be in a better position to act in his or her best interest.

LEGISLATIVE INITIATIVES

My last criticism of the *Conroy* decision is that the court abdicated its responsibility for establishing the procedures through which these principles can be implemented. Instead of designing adequate procedures, the court stated that the primary responsibility for this rests not with the court but with the legislature. As prone as the legislative process is to the political ambitions of the members, it is very doubtful that the kind of legislation that is needed could be established without constant redefinition from the courts.

In fact, legislation in this field has been needlessly bottled up in both houses of the New Jersey Legislature for the last five years, primarily because many politicians perceive it to be an unpopular cause and most misunderstand it. The *Conroy* decision, in itself, will do little to change this perception and may even make it more difficult to get appropriate legislation.

CONCLUSIONS AND RECOMMENDATIONS

The *Conroy* decision is a major precedent in determining medical and social responses to patients whose lives are being prolonged artificially by advances in medical technology. However, further refinements are needed to assure that neither patients nor families become victimized by the prolonged use of technology when all meaningful life is over, or by a bureaucratic system that is insensitive to the tragedies of these families in crisis. A much more rational and effective approach is needed.

First, institutional ethics committees ought to be required to review all life-threatening nontreatment decisions for patients in all health care facilities, including hospitals and nursing homes. This would ensure that the people who are most affected by the decision can share perspectives and insights and come to what they believe is the most ethically appropriate solution. Second, the decision-making process must be kept at the local level. This would be much less intimidating to a grieving family and caring physicians than an official state investigation, especially one which presumes "abuse" by family and caregivers who are considered guilty until proven innocent. Third, the "geriatric 'Baby Doe' squad" mentality must be removed, otherwise doctors and institutions, for fear of liability, will force increased use of life-sustaining measures because they do not want to be involved in a state investigation.

Since the *Conroy* decision was handed down, in January 1985, several key individuals in New Jersey have called upon Governor Kean and the legislature to establish a "blue ribbon panel" to evaluate the needs of dying patients and their families and to make recommendations on a series of legislative initiatives which would protect the rights of all persons while preserving the state's interests in protecting and preserving life. This would be a beneficial development.

Until this is accomplished, despite the *Quinlan* and *Conroy* decisions, the rights of patients and the responsibilities of physicians and health care institutions will remain in confusion and disarray.

N O T E S

1. *In re* Conroy, 98 N.J. 321, 486 A.2d 1209 (1985).
2. *In re* Quinlan, 70 N.J. 10, 355 A.2d 647 *cert. denied*, 429 U.S. 922 (1976).
3. New Jersey State Department of Health, "Guildelines for Health Care Facilities to Implement Procedures Concerning the Care of Comatose Non-Cognitive Patients," available in Ronald E. Cranford and Edward A. Doudera (eds.), *Institutional Ethics Committees and Health Care Decision Making* (Ann Arbor, Mich.: Health Administration Press, 1984), 388–391.
4. *In re* Conroy, 98 N.J. 321, 383, 486 A.2d 1209, 1242 (1985).
5. Barber v. Superior Court, 195 Cal. Rptr. 484 (Cal. App. 1983).
6. *In re* Conroy, 190 N.J. Super. 453, 464 A.2d 303, 312 (App. Div. 1983).
7. For example, in the trial proceedings, Claire Conroy was reported never to have sought medical care during her entire life. This, presumably, could qualify as acceptable evidence for rejecting care when she was comatose, if so determined by the ombudsman. The court did say that the evidence presented during the trial was insufficient; the court would not have authorized the removal of Miss Conroy's nasogastric tube but would have remanded the case back to the trial court for additional evidence.
8. *Id.* at 1232. Of course, one must wonder if some of these "subjective test" categories really constitute "absolute proof,"
9. *Id.*
10. *Id.*

Jacqueline J. Glover, Ph.D., and Joanne Lynn, M.D.

Afterword
Update since *Conroy*: 1985–1988

In the three short years since this collection was first published, the issues surrounding artificial nutrition and hydration have passed from being ignored to being widely discussed. These few years have seen dozens of court cases and professional articles on the subject. Thus far, the cases brought to public attention have been resolved in favor of letting nutrition and hydration be forgone whenever the patient's present or past views indicate a preference that such be done or whenever the patient would be more burdened than bene-fited by artificial nutrition and hydration.

On the whole, this seems to have been salutary for patient care. Discussions of forgoing artificial nutrition seem often to be done carefully and dying is undoubtedly more comfortable for many pa-tients because this option is made available.

However, the dark side of allowing death to occur by forgoing artificial nutrition and hydration now looms as a larger risk. As the issue is decided more often, it must not be decided perfunctorily or injudiciously. Nor should this be a choice made to spare others the burden of caring for disabled people. Callahan, in this volume, warns against allowing the forgoing of nutrition and hydration to become the "forgoing of choice" for the "biologically tenacious." And, in this regard he is right.

Always making the right choice for the right reasons is a difficult goal, though one that we must pursue. Now that it is often possible to choose to forgo life-sustaining nutrition and hydration, the chal-lenge is to do so whenever that is what ethically should be done, and only then.

SINCE *CONROY*

Since the landmark case of Claire Conroy in 1985,[1] at least 45 cases in 21 states have dealt with the issue of the withdrawal of artificial hydration and nutrition (see table 3). Of the 39 states that have living

Table 3

Case	Patient Condition	Initial Ruling	Final Ruling	Other Notes
1. Alderson (Kimbrough) *In re Application of Alderson* (Kimbrough), No. 90193/86 (N.Y. Sup. Ct. N.Y. County Aug. 3, 1988) (Ciparick, J.); N.Y.L.J. Aug. 9, 1988 at 18, col. 2.	Vegetative	Against withdrawal		No clear and convincing evidence of condition or wishes
2. Barber *Barber v. Superior Court*, 147 Cal. App. 3d 1006 195 Cal. Rptr. 484 (Ct. App. 1983)	Coma	Physicians had to answer to charges of murder and breach of legal duty, but charges dismissed	No breach of legal duty; no further action against physicians	
3. Bayer *In re Bayer*, No. 4131 (N.D. Burleigh County Ct. Feb.5 and Dec. 11, 1987) (Riskedahl, J.)	PVS (persistent vegetative state)	In favor of withdrawal		Physician removed nasogastric tube and then instituted oral feedings with "cuffed tracheostomy tube"; family returned to court to discontinue tracheostomy tube; hospital served complaint for unpaid balance; Bayer responded with complaint for medical and legal fees and emotional distress
4. Bouvia *Bouvia v. Superior Court* (Glenchur), 179 Cal. App. 3d 1127, 225 Cal. Rptr. 297 (Ct. App. 1986), *review denied* (Cal. June 5, 1986)	Competent; disabled with cerebral palsy	Against withdrawal	In favor of withdrawal	Refusal isn't suicide

Case	Patient	Decision	Notes
5. Brooks (Leguerrier) *In re Application of Brooks* (Leguerrier) (N.Y. Sup. Ct. Albany County June 10, 1987) (Conway, J.)	Competent nursing home resident; no serious illness	Against order to force-feed	Refused force-feeding; not suicide
6. Brophy *Brophy v. New England Sinai Hospital, Inc.*, 398 Mass. 417, 497 N.E.2d 626 (1986)	PVS	Against withdrawal	Hospital cannot be forced to comply
7. Cantor *Cantor v. Weiss*, No. 626 163 (Cal. Super. Ct. Los Angeles County Dec. 30, 1986) (Newman, J.)	Incompetent	In favor of withdrawal	Court ordered institution to comply with living will
8. Clark *In re Clark*, 210 N.J. Super. 548, 510 A.2d 136 (Super. Ct. Ch. Div. 1986); 212 N.J. Super. 408, 515 A.2d 276 (Super. Ct. Ch. Div. 1986), *aff'd*, 216 N.J. Super. 497, 524 A.2d 448 (Super. Ct. App. Div. 1987)	Incompetent; partial paralysis, brain damage	Enterostomy in patient's best interests	No trustworthy evidence of patient's wishes; no concurrence of family/physician/hospital optimal care committee
9. Conroy *In re Conroy*, 98 N.J. 321, 486 A.2d 1209 (1985)	Incompetent; elderly, demented	Against withdrawal	In favor of withdrawal in general although Clair Conroy would not meet established standards	Established procedures for withdrawal

Table 3—*continued*

Case	Patient Condition	Initial Ruling	Final Ruling	Other Notes
10. Corbett *Corbett v. D'Alessandro*, 487 So. 2d 368 (Fla. Dist. Ct. App.), *review denied*, 492 So. 2d 1331 (Fla. 1986)	PVS	Against withdrawal	In favor of withdrawal	Right to refuse artificial feeding not limited by state living will statute
11. Cruzan *Cruzan v. Harmon*, 70813 (Mo. Supp. Ct. Nov. 16, 1988)	PVS	In favor of withdrawal	Against withdrawal	State's interest in preserving life takes precedence in a case where patient not being burdened by treatment and not terminally ill
12. Culham *In re Culham*, No. 87–340537-AZ (Mich. Cir. Ct. Oakland County Dec. 15, 1987) (Breck, J.)	Competent; ALS	In favor of withdrawal		
13. Delio *Delio v. Westchester County Medical Center*, 129 A.D.2d 1, 516 N.Y.S.2d 677 (2d Dep't 1987)	PVS	Against withdrawal	In favor of withdrawal	Court initially distinguished feeding and ventilator; ruling reversed
14. Drabick *In re Conservatorship of Drabick*, 200 Cal. App. 3d 185, 245 Cal. Rptr. 840 (Cal. Ct. App. 1988), *review denied* (Cal. July 28, 1988), *application for stay of remittitur filed* (Cal. Ct. App. July 28, 1988)	PVS	Against withdrawal	In favor of withdrawal	Review denied by court of appeals but application for stay of remittitur filed

Case	Condition			Comments
15. Jane Doe (PA) *In re Jane Doe*, 16 Phila. 229 (Pa. Ct. Com. Pl. 1987)	Competent; ALS	In favor of withdrawal	In favor of withdrawal	Patient did not request termination of artificial feeding, but court mentioned it in ruling
16. Jane Doe (GA) *In re Jane Doe*, No. D 56730 (Ga. Super. Ct. Fulton County July 13, 1988) (Williams, J.)	PVS	In favor of withdrawal	In favor of withdrawal	Court ruled in favor of withdrawal in spite of state living will statute
17. Fuhrman *Fuhrman v. Kean*, No. 86–1951 (D.N.J. July 13, 1987) (Cowen, J.)	Incompetent; elderly, demented	Removed Mr. Fuhrman as his mother's guardian		
18. Gardner *In re Gardner*, 534 A.2d 947 (Me. 1987)	PVS	In favor of withdrawal	In favor of withdrawal	Clear and convincing evidence of patient's wishes
19. Gary *Gary v. California* (Hirth), No. 576 123 (Cal. Super. Ct. San Diego County March 5, 23), *modified in part* (April 15, 1987) (Milkes, J.)	Comatose	In favor of withdrawal	In favor of withdrawal	Physician first ordered to comply and then original order amended so physician was no longer compelled
20. Grant *In re Guardianship of Grant*, 109 Wash. 2d 545, 747 P.2d 445 (1987)	Incompetent; Batten's disease	Against withdrawal	In favor of withdrawal	No provider required to participate but cannot interfere with transfer
21. Gray *Gray v. Romeo*, Civ. 82–0573B-F. Supp.-(D. RI 1988)	PVS	In favor of withdrawal	In favor of withdrawal	Defends U.S. constitutional right of privacy

Table 3—*continued*

Case	Patient Condition	Initial Ruling	Final Ruling	Other Notes
22. Hazelton *Hazelton [sic] v. Powhatan Nursing Home, Inc.,* No. CH 98287 (Va. Cir. Ct. Fairfax County Aug. 29, 1986), *order signed* (Sept. 2, 1986) (Fortkort, J.) *appeal denied,* Record No. 860814 (Va. Sept. 2, 1986), 6 Va. Cir. Ct. Op. 414 (Aspen 1987)	Coma; inoperable brain tumor	In favor of withdrawal		Only court interpretation of language in state natural death act
23. Helstrom *Helstrom v. Florida Life Care,* No. 88–1870-CA-01 (Fla. Cir. Ct. Sarasota County May 10, 1988) (Boylston, J.)	PVS	In favor of withdrawal		Right to refuse artificial feeding not limited by state living will statute; patient has right not to be moved or discharged against his will
24. Hier *In re Hier,* 18 Mass. App. 200, 464 N.E.2d 959 (Ct. App.), *review denied,* 392 Mass. 1102, 465 N.E.2d 261 (1984)	Incompetent; long history of mental illness	In favor of withdrawal		Guardian appointed to authorize antipsychotic drugs but not gastrostomy; considered patient's expression of discomfort and attempts to remove nasogastric tube
25. Hoffmeister *Hoffmeister v. Satz,* No. 87–28451 CR (Fla. Cir. Ct. 17th Dist. Broward County Feb. 22, 1988)	Incompetent; Alzheimer's disease	In favor of withdrawal		Right to refuse artificial feeding not limited by state nursing home regulation
26. Jobes *In re Jobes,* 108 N.J. 394, 529 A.2d 434 (1987)	PVS	In favor of withdrawal	In favor of withdrawal	First ruling, nursing home entitled to refuse to comply; decision reversed

Case	Condition	Court decision	Status	Notes
27. Kerr (O'Brien) *In re Application of Kerr* (O'Brien), 135 Misc. 2d 1076, 517 N.Y.S. 2d 346 (N.Y. Sup. Ct. N.Y. County 1986)	Incompetent	Against withdrawal		Court unwilling to consider patient's gestures of irritation and annoyance with nasogastric tube
28. Chetta (LaSala) [LaSala] *In re Chetta* [Wickel], No. 1086/87 (N.Y. Sup. Ct. Nassau County May 1, 1987, Feb. 16, 1988) (Becker, J.); N.Y.L.J. March 9, 1988, at 15, notice of appeal filed (N.Y. App. Div. 2d Dep't March 17, 1988)	PVS	*Against withdrawal*	*Pending*	*First ruled clear and convincing evidence of wishes but could not withdraw based on Delio; after Delio reversed ruling, evidence of wishes did not meet higher standard*
29. Laws *In re Laws*, No. 226215 (Mass. Probate Ct. May 4, 1987) (Buczko, J.)	Incompetent; moderately to severely retarded since birth	In favor of withdrawal		Court considered patient's resistance to nasogastric tube as sign of preference to forgo treatment
30. Licopoli (Akullian) *In re Application of Licopoli* (Akullian), No. 1172–88 (N.Y. Sup. Ct. Albany County March 10, 1988) (Prior, J.)	PVS	In favor of withdrawal		Clear and convincing evidence of patient's wishes
31. McConnell *McConnell v. Beverly Enterprises*, No. 0293888 (Conn. Super. Ct. Danbury Jud. Dist. July 8, 1988) (Dranginis, J.), *on appeal.* Nos. SC 13477, 13478 and 13479 (Conn.)	PVS	In favor of withdrawal	Pending	Right to refuse artificial feeding not limited by state living will statute

Table 3—*continued*

Case	Patient Condition	Initial Ruling	Final Ruling	Other Notes
32. Newman *Newman v. William Beaumont Army Medical Center*, No. EP-86-CA-276 (W.D. Tex. Oct. 30, 1986) (Hudspeth, J.)	PVS	Against withdrawal		Federal law applied to patient in military hospital; one isolated conversation not sufficient evidence of patient's wishes
33. Peter *In re Peter*, 108 N.J. 365, 529 A.2d 419 (1987)	PVS	Against withdrawal	In favor of withdrawal	Clear and convincing evidence of patient's wishes
34. Plaza Health and Rehabilitation Center *In re Application of Plaza Health and Rehabilitation Center* (N.Y. Sup. Ct. Onondaga County Feb. 2, 1984) (Miller, J.)	Competent	Against order to force-feed		Health care facility ordered not to attempt to force-feed
35. Prange *In re Estate of Prange*, 166 Ill. App. 3d 1091, 520 N.E. 2d 946 (Ill. Ct. App.), *vacated*, 121 Ill. 2d 570 (Ill. 1988)	PVS	Patient died; case dismissed as moot	In favor of withdrawal (vacated)	Clear and convincing evidence of patient's wishes; ruling vacated without explanation; petition for reconsideration filed
36. Putzer *In re Putzer*, No. P21–87E (N.J. Super. Ct. Ch. Div. Essex County July 9, 1987) (Margolis, J.)	Competent; "locked in" syndrome	In favor of withdrawal		

Case	Condition	Ruling		Notes
37. Rasmussen *Rasmussen v. Fleming*, 154 Ariz. 207, 741 P.2d 674 (1987)	Comatose	In favor of withdrawal	In favor of withdrawal	Initial ruling, priority list of surrogates, later eliminated
38. Rekstad *Rekstad v. Florida Life Care, Inc.*, No. 87–4285-CA-01 (Fla. Cir. Ct. Sarasota County Sept. 18, 1987) (Walker, J.)	Incompetent; elderly	In favor of withdrawal		Right to refuse artificial feeding not limited by state nursing home regulation
39. Requena *In re Requena*, 213 N.J. Super. 475, 517 A.2d 886 (Super. Ct. Ch. Div.), *aff'd*, 213 N.J. Super. 443, 517 A. 2d 869 (Super. Ct. App. Div. 1986) (per curiam)	Competent; ALS	In favor of withdrawal and against hospital compelling patient to leave	Against compelling patient to leave	Offending sensibilities of hospital personnel subordinate to harm to patient
40. Rodas *In re Rodas*, No. 86PR139 (Colo. Dist. Ct. Mesa County Jan. 22, 1987, as modified, April 3, 1987) (Buss, J.)	Competent; "locked in" syndrome	In favor of withdrawal		Right to refuse artificial feeding not limited by state living will statute
41. Sanchez *Sanchez v. Fairview Developmental Center*, No. CV 88–0129 FFF (Tx) (C.D. Cal. March 30, 1988) (Fernandez, J.), *notice of motion for preliminary injunction filed*, No. 563–313 (Cal. Super. Ct. Orange County July 27, 1988) (McDonald, J.)	Incompetent; profoundly mentally retarded, semicomatose	Against withdrawal		Federal court denied relief for violation of constitutional rights; case refiled in state court

Table 3—*continued*

Case	Patient Condition	Initial Ruling	Final Ruling	Other Notes
42. Strauss *In re Strauss*, No. 8378/87 (N.Y. Sup. Ct. Bronx County July 1, 1987) (Tompkins, J.)	Incompetent; Alzheimer's disease	In favor of withdrawal		Clear and convincing evidence of patient's preference; ruling advocated more formal written documents
43. Sullivan (Stoppe) *Sullivan v. St. John's Mercy Medical Center* (Stoppe), No. 561631 (Mo. Cir. Ct. St. Louis County June 8, 1987) (Weinstock, J.)	Comatose	Against withdrawal		Credible evidence of patient's wishes but cannot withdraw artificial feeding because of state living will statute (although could withdraw ventilator)
44. Visbeck *In re Visbeck*, 210 N.J. Super. 527, 510 A.2d 125 (Super. Ct. Ch. Div. 1986)	Incompetent	Against withdrawal		Quality of patient's life sufficiently high to make withholding tube feeding unacceptable; son named as surrogate but directed to authorize feeding tube
45. Vogel *In re Vogel*, 134 Misc. 2d 395, 512 N.Y.S.2d 622 (Sup. Ct. Nassau County 1986), *declined to follow in Delio v. Westchester County Medical Center*, 129 A.D.2d 1, 516 N.Y.S.2d 677 (2d Dep't 1987)	Comatose	Against withdrawal		Would not remove nasogastric feeding tube because patient not terminally ill or brain dead

Case	Condition	In favor of withdrawal	Against withdrawal	Notes
46. Westchester County Medical Center (O'Connor) / *In the Matter of Mary O'Connor, Westchester County Medical Center v. Helen Hall,* 312 (N.Y. Ct. App. Oct. 14, 1988)	Incompetent		Against withdrawal	Establishes standard for clear and convincing evidence in New York State
47. Wilcox / *Wilcox v. Hawaii,* Civ. No. 860116 (Hawaii Cir. Ct. 5th Cir. June 16, 1986) (Hirano, J.)	Competent; terminally ill	Dismissed		Hospital willing to concede to patient's wishes; court dismissed because no case or controversy
48. Workmen's Circle Home (O'Conner) / *Workmen's Circle Home and Infirmary for the Aged v. Fink,* 135 Misc. 2d 270, 514 N.Y.S.2d 893 (Sup. Ct. Bronx County 1987), *declined to follow in Delio v. Westchester County Medical Center,* 129 A.D.2d 1, 516, N.Y.S.2d 677 (2d Dep't 1987)	Incompetent; semi-comatose; inoperable tumor		Against withdrawal	Granted authority to refuse to connect gastrostomy tube but not to remove IV feeding tube
49. Zahn / *In re Zahn,* No. 85–3723 (Fla. Cir. Ct. Broward County Nov. 20, 1986) (Hare, J.)	PVS	In favor of withdrawal		Right to refuse artificial feeding not limited by state living will statute

Table 4

State Living Will Statutes and Artificial Nutrition

Clearly states that artificial feeding can be withdrawn	Language of Uniform Rights of Terminally Ill Act may be interpreted to authorize withdrawal of artificial feeding	Artificial feeding linked with comfort care, may be interpreted to prohibit withdrawal of artificial feeding	Artificial feeding not a procedure that may be rejected in living will	Enacted special statute to prohibit withdrawal of artificial feeding, not linked to state living will statute
Alaska Idaho Illinois Tennessee	Arkansas Montana Oregon	Arizona* Florida* Hawaii* Indiana Iowa Maryland New Hampshire Oklahoma South Carolina Utah West Virginia Wyoming	Colorado* Connecticut* Georgia* Maine* Missouri Wisconsin	Oklahoma

*Court cases have allowed refusal of artificial feedings, in spite of state statute.

will statutes, 25 make some mention of artificial feeding (see table 4). Many articles and professional organization pronouncements have also been published. Several themes are increasingly evident regarding decisions to forgo life-sustaining therapy, including artificial feeding.

The first theme is the nature of artificial feeding as a medical intervention. A consensus is emerging that artificial hydration and nutrition are forms of medical treatment that can be withheld or withdrawn following the guidelines that govern the use of life-sustaining therapy generally.

A second theme is the role that patient prognosis should play in decisions regarding life-sustaining therapy. Patients and their families, health care professionals, courts, and legislatures struggle to balance the benefits and burdens of therapy in determining patients' best interests. Prognosis often serves as a measure of the formality of decision-making procedures required, as for example in *Conroy*.[2] Additionally, prognosis is central in balancing the patient's interests and preferences against state interests in preserving life.

The issue of prognosis and best interests is particularly troublesome when incompetent patients are involved, making a third theme of surrogate decision-making. Who should speak for incompetent persons, and what standards should be used? A consensus is emerging that the patient's own views should take precedence when possible, but practical implementation faces problems of reliable evidence and may not be possible for the majority of patients who do not prepare advance directives. Consensus has not developed as to how to determine the best interests of an incompetent patient who has not made preferences known.

A fourth theme involved in decisions to forgo life-sustaining therapies is the balance between state interests and the rights or interests of patients. Four major state interests have been identified, the most pertinent being the states' interest in preserving life.

A fifth theme is defining the role of the courts in decision-making. Should we look to the courts to make actual decisions, for the development of guidelines, or for resolution of only the most intractable problems?

The sixth and final theme deals with disagreement among caregivers. When health care providers disagree with a decision to withdraw artificial feeding, their rights must be balanced against the rights of patients.

Various parties are beginning to take an active part in the discussion. Professional organizations have produced guidelines and regulatory and financing bureaucracies are beginning to address the issue. Although the majority of professional organizations support the withdrawal of artificial feeding, disagreement remains. The discussion that follows is a summary of the major themes related to decisions to forgo nutrition and hydration as they are reflected in developments since the Conroy case.

ARTIFICIAL HYDRATION AND NUTRITION AS MEDICAL TREATMENT

The final appellate court in every case but one since *Conroy* has decided there is no distinction between the forgoing of artificial hydration and nutrition and the forgoing of other life-sustaining medical treatments.[3] Most courts have adopted the reasoning of the *Conroy* court that artificial feedings are medical procedures which have inherent risks and possible side effects and which are instituted by skilled health care providers to compensate for impaired physical functioning. Some state statutes and professional organization pronouncements also follow this reasoning.

Since artificial hydration and nutrition have uniformly been considered medical treatments, patients can decline their use as they could any other treatment. This right to refuse treatment is usually based on a constitutional (state or federal) right of privacy and/or a common law right of self-determination or informed consent or a state regulation.[4] Cases regarding hydration and nutrition rely upon and confirm the emerging legal consensus that the right to refuse treatment is not lost with incompetency.

Part of the debate surrounding artificial feeding has involved the patient's response when feeding is forgone. Evidence presented to courts supports the claim that patients with malnutrition and dehydration do not seem to suffer hunger or thirst, and the forgoing of artificial feeding may lessen, rather than increase, uncomfortable symptoms in the dying patient.[5] The American Academy of Neurology has also issued a statement that affirms that patients in a persistent vegetative state (PVS) do not have the capacity to experience pain or suffering.[6]

THE ROLE OF PATIENT PROGNOSIS

The patient's prognosis, with or without artificial nutrition or hydration, is the cornerstone of good decision-making. Although every patient has the right to reject medical intervention, the prognosis would ordinarily be what determines whether the patient does (or probably would) want artificial feedings. This is true for competent patients deciding for themselves or for those who need others to make decisions for them.

The clearest cases involve competent patients. Every case involving a competent terminally ill patient has been decided in favor of withdrawal.[7] Even cases where a competent patient was not terminally ill have been decided in favor of not force-feeding. These cases include those in which the patient was severely disabled, such as *Putzer* and *Rodas* (who were in a "locked-in" condition, unable to move, talk, or eat, but able to think and, with difficulty, to communicate), and *Bouvia* (who is incapacitated with cerebral palsy).[8]

But not all cases involve disabled patients. A court decided in *Brooks*[9] that a competent 80-year-old nursing home resident who was not suffering from any serious illness did not have to be force-fed, even though she began to refuse to eat or drink. A similar decision was made in *In re Application of Plaza Health and Rehabilitation Center.*[10] The consensus is that competent adults have a right to refuse life-sustaining treatment, regardless of age, medical condition, or prognosis.

Cases that involve incompetent patients are more difficult, but those in which patient preferences to withdraw treatment are sufficiently clear have all been decided in favor of withdrawing artificial hydration and nutrition.[11]

The most difficult cases involve patients who are incompetent, do not have clear advance directives, and also are not terminally ill, including patients who are permanently unconscious or severely mentally and physically disabled.[12] In light of the possibility of miscommunication and error, surrogates and caregivers are understandably more cautious about withdrawing treatment on behalf of a patient who is not soon dying and who has not given sufficient evidence of his or her preferences.

Calling persons who are permanently unconscious "terminally ill" sometimes appears to make the decision-making easier, particularly in a state with a living will statute applying to the terminally ill. Some confusion on this point has arisen. The court in *Corbett* actually called Mrs. Corbett's persistently vegetative condition "terminal" without any discussion,[13] even though they did include the AMA's statement on the withdrawal of hydration and nutrition that mentions that withdrawal is permissible even when death is not imminent if the coma is irreversible.[14]

In the *McConnell* case a physician testified that the coma would cause Mrs. McConnell's death,[15] that all of her organ systems were in jeopardy as a result of the coma, and that she was in a terminal condition, even though she was not presently in the final stages of dying. The court decided, however, upon further examination, that the physician's position was actually consistent with the position of the American Academy of Neurology that PVS patients are not terminally ill.[16] All other cases dealing with permanently unconscious patients agree that they are not terminally ill.[17] All also require evidence, sometimes clear and convincing, that the condition is irreversible and that there is no reasonable possibility that the patient will return to cognitive and sapient life.[18]

While many are concerned about permanently unconscious patients because they are not terminally ill, and not suffering, and preserving life might therefore seem appropriate (the exact argument of the *Cruzan* court), the court in *Delio* makes an interesting argument.[19] The court claims that the absence of terminal illness may serve to reinforce the decision to withdraw artificial feeding because of the potentially long and indefinite period that the patient may continue to live in a vegetative condition in which there is no benefit beyond mere existence, while the patient continues to suffer the indignities and dehumanization created by helplessness.

In each of the cases involving permanently unconscious patients where no controversy arose as to the patient's wishes (except *Cruzan*), the withdrawal of artificial feeding was permitted.[20]

A final category of patients, and perhaps the most difficult, includes those incompetent patients who are neither terminally ill nor permanently unconscious but who are irreversibly physically and mentally disabled.[21] These cases are most like *Conroy* and wrestle with the same issues of evidence of patient preference and the determination of best interests. In general, where patient preferences were known, authority was given to withdraw artificial hydration and nutrition.[22] In cases where preferences are not considered clear, there is considerable disagreement about how the patient's prognosis and condition are to be translated into a measure of the patient's best interests.

In *Kerr* (O'Brien), for example, the court was unwilling to make any judgment about best interests in the absence of clear patient preference. "When a person is not competent to make such a life or death decision, the court must intervene in favor of life prolonging treatment despite the feelings and desires of those closest to the patient."[23] In *Clark*,[24] where there was disagreement among family members and guardians, the court ruled that an enterostomy was in the best interests of a patient with partial paralysis and organic brain damage. The court pointed out that there was no evidence the patient was presently suffering recurring, unavoidable, or severe pain, and that he would continue to derive some benefits from prolonging his life, as the enterostomy was not likely to cause other than normal postoperative pain. In *Visbeck*,[25] the court would not allow the patient's son to refuse a gastrostomy tube on her behalf, because the proposed surgical procedure was simple and would not result in significant pain, and the patient demonstrated some awareness, responsiveness, and minimal comfort. The court claimed that Mrs. Visbeck's quality of life was sufficiently high to make withholding of tube feeding unacceptable to many responsible and caring people. This is considerably different from the decision in *Hier*, [26] which allowed the refusal of a gastrostomy tube for a 92-year-old incompetent woman with a long history of mental illness whose other chronic illnesses were truly minor (a hiatal hernia and a large cervical diverticulum).

DECISION-MAKING PROCESS FOR INCOMPETENT PERSONS

As is apparent from the above discussion of the role of prognosis, the central question before the courts has most often concerned how to make appropriate decisions for incompetent patients. Who is an appropriate surrogate, and what standards should be used? What constitutes sufficient evidence of a patient's preference?

WHO CAN DECIDE

In most of the decisions concerning incompetent patients, legal guardians or family members who were named legal guardians were empowered to make surrogate decisions. However, there is no explicit instruction that a surrogate must be named a legal guardian. In fact, several cases specifically say that prior court approval of decisions is not appropriate and decisions are best left to patients, families, and physicians.[27]

One exception of a sort is the *Peter* case,[28] where the court ruled that if the patient did not clearly designate a surrogate, then a family member could act as surrogate. If there is no family, then a guardian must be appointed by the court. If the patient's surrogate should be a friend, the physician cannot designate that person; instead, a court must appoint a guardian. This is also the ruling in *Jobes*.[29] Since *Conroy*,[30] the *Peter* case and all others in New Jersey must involve the Ombudsman in seeking the forgoing of life-sustaining treatment for nursing home patients over 60 who are expected to live less than a year. A recent advisory letter published by the New Jersey Office of the Ombudsman for the Institutionalized Elderly would require that *every* proposal to forgo life-sustaining medical diagnosis or treatment for any psychiatric hospital or nursing home patient age 60 and over who has not been currently and *legally* determined to be competent be reported to the Ombudsman's office as a possible case of patient abuse. This ruling would apply regardless of who proposes that treatment be discontinued and regardless of whether the patient has a living will or other written or oral instructions or indications.[31]

In the *Kerr* (O'Brien) case,[32] the court made a clear distinction between family members who could be surrogates without court approval, and friends, who could not. In *Visbeck*[33] the court acknowledged the surrogate role of Mrs. Visbeck's son, but then directed him to authorize the implantation of the feeding tube against his initial wishes.

The *Rasmussen* case[34] initially included a priority list governing surrogate decisions, including first a judicially appointed guardian of the patient, then a person designated in writing by the patient, then (in order) the patient's spouse, adult children, parents, nearest living relative, and finally (if none of the above) someone at the discretion of the attending physician. The Supreme Court of Arizona in reviewing the case, however, removed the priority list.

Decision Standards

The central question regarding decision-making for incompetent persons is what standard should be used. Following *Conroy*, the two extremes proposed are a subjective standard, which applies the preferences of the specific patient, and a best-interests standard, which employs the general preferences of the so-called "reasonable person." In *Conroy* three possibilities were articulated. The preferred test is called "subjective" and seeks to ascertain whether the patient's own known views would have clearly decided the issue. When this is not possible, one is to use the "limited objective" test, which combines some trustworthy evidence of patient preferences with an analysis of the net burdens and benefits. Net burdens must outweigh benefits from what can be known of the patient's perspective in order for life-sustaining treatment to be forgone. The "pure objective" test is reserved for use when patient preferences cannot be known. Burdens of sustaining life through treatment must clearly and markedly outweigh benefits and the effect of administering life-sustaining treatment must be inhumane.[35]

Most cases since *Conroy* have adopted this framework, looking first toward the subjective standard and moving to a best-interests standard only when preferences cannot be known.

One exception is *Drabick* in California,[36] which is somewhat unusual in its emphasis on the primacy of the surrogate decision and in its rejection of the subjective standard. According to *Drabick*, it is the surrogate's responsibility to consider the patient's known preferences together with other information bearing on the patient's best interests. If there is no information about patient preferences, it is still the surrogate's right and duty to make treatment decisions. The court writes, "The statutory delegation of power to the conservator should not be confused with the different idea—which we do not accept—that an incompetent person's own prior informal statements *compel* either the continuance or cessation of treatment in a particular case."[37]

The *Drabick* court pointed out several problems with a subjective standard approach. First, they found no authority—other than cases on the subject of life-sustaining treatment—to support the idea that a person can exercise (or waive) a fundamental constitutional and common law right (to refuse treatment) unintentionally through informal statements years in advance. The court calls this "a dangerously unpredictable precedent."[38] Second, if one relies on the theory that an evidentiary hearing can reveal the patient's own hypothetical choice, one is left with no consistent basis for a decision when a patient has been silent. Third, the approach is contrary to the apparent intention of California Probate section 2355, which is to give the conservator "exclusive" authority for medical treatment decisions.[39]

Most other cases accept the validity of the subjective standard and struggle with the difficult problem of whether there is sufficient evidence of patient preference.

The clearest evidence of patient preference is some type of advance directive, such as a living will or a durable power of attorney. In only two cases, *Culham* and *Peter*,[40] were there durable powers of attorney in effect. The power of attorney was not influential in the first case since Culham was still competent, and in the second it was used as evidence for the subjective standard. In only one other case, *Prange*,[41] was there a living will. Although technically invalid since it lacked the required number of witnesses, the living will was still used as evidence.

The majority of cases relied upon the testimony of family and friends to establish the patient's preference, and also found such testimony to be sufficient.[42] Following *Conroy*,[43] the courts looked to such evidence as oral directives to family, friends, or health care providers, reactions that the patient voiced regarding medical treatment administered to others, religious beliefs and tenets of that religion, or the patient's consistent pattern of conduct with respect to previous decisions about his or her own medical care.

Most debate centers around previous statements and whether they are sufficiently specific. In *Brophy*,[44] for example, the court relied on Mr. Brophy's discussions with family and friends of the quality of life of Karen Quinlan, of a fire victim Mr. Brophy had rescued (he was an EMT), and of a local teenager put on a life support system. Mr. Brophy had also stated to one of his daughters within twelve hours after transport to the hospital, "If I can't sit up to kiss one of my beautiful daughters, I may as well be six feet under."[45] Although the evidence was regarded as sufficient, none of the statements specifically referred to feeding methods.

In the case of *Delio*,[46] the court also relied upon the testimony of family and friends about Mr. Delio's discussion of the Quinlan case. But here Mr. Delio specifically talked about artificial hydration and nutrition and his belief that the destruction of the cortex was equivalent to the cessation of life. Mr. Delio also talked about his wishes in connection with the death of his father.

The struggle to establish a standard of evidence for patient preferences is more apparent in other cases. In *Gardner*,[47] for example, the court found the evidence of Mr. Gardner's preferences provided by the testimony of family and friends to be clear and convincing. But in a dissenting opinion, Justice Clifford (with Justices Roberts and Wathen joining) disagreed, pointing out that the evidence was not written and even the conversations were casual and of a general nature. This is particularly relevant in *Gardner* since it was based entirely on the common law right of informed consent, and the dissenting judge argued that Mr. Gardner's refusal was not truly informed. This dissenting opinion, like the *Drabick* case,[48] raises some important issues about prior consent.

In the *Strauss* case as well,[49] the court found the testimony of family to be clear and convincing. But the opinion also included some interesting warnings about such testimony and the court advocated more formal written documents like living wills or special institutional admission forms in appropriate circumstances.

Expressing concern about the general nature of conversations used as evidence, the court in *Newman v. William Beaumont Army Medical Center* ruled that one isolated conversation was not sufficient evidence of Mrs. Newman's wishes.[50]

In an interesting reversal of opinion that may speak to the court's unease with evidence of patient preference, the *LaSala*[51] court initially ruled that evidence that the patient would not want artificial feeding was clear and convincing, but that tube feeding could not be withdrawn because of the precedent of the *Delio*[52] case (which at that time was on appeal from a decision against removal of artifical feeding). When *Delio* was reversed and the *LaSala* case reheard, however, the judge then decided that the standard of clear and convincing evidence put forth in *Delio* was higher than had been achieved in *LaSala*. According to the court, there was "no proof of an expressed intent to have a particular method of life prolongation terminated."[53] And unlike *Delio*, no witness testified that Mrs. LaSala made any specific statement relating to the termination of life.

Using similar reasoning, another New York court ruled that general attitudes did not constitute sufficient evidence. In *Alderson*[54] the court ruled that the family's testimony that Mr. Kimbrough was intolerant of people who are less than perfect and expressed the view that physically or mentally handicapped people should not live was not sufficient evidence that he would want to have his own life-sustaining treatment withheld.

A case recently decided by the New York Court of Appeals has helped clarify the standard of clear and convincing evidence, at least in that state. In *O'Connor*[55] the trial court and the first appellate court ruled that the testimony of family and friends was clear and convincing evidence, even though it did not specifically mention artificial feeding. The court ruled that the testimony showed that

Mrs. O'Connor demonstrated through discussions that she would want *any* life-sustaining treatment withheld in her current unresponsive state.

However, the highest New York appeals court ruled that the evidence was *not* clear and convincing. By a close margin the court decided that the evidence did not show that the patient held a firm and settled commitment concerning the termination of life under circumstances like those presented. The court said that the clear and convincing standard of evidence should be applied and would require that the strength and durability of belief be such that it makes a change of heart unlikely. Persistence, seriousness, and inferences from the surrounding circumstances are factors which should be considered. The court said written directives are best, but oral directives are also acceptable. Both need not include information about the precise condition or particular treatment. But both must discuss illnesses and procedures that are qualitatively similar to the ones at issue in the decision. In a dissenting opinion, Judge Hancock argued that this "specific-subjective-intent rule" is fundamentally flawed because it requires patients to anticipate their illnesses and because courts cannot adequately discover, as a factual matter, the exact intent of the incompetent patient.

The reaction of the patient to the proposed feeding is another type of evidence of patient preference that is considered in some cases. In the controversial *Hier*[56] case, which preceeded *Conroy*, the court allowed as evidence Mrs. Hier's repeated struggles against the feeding tube. Such expressions of opposition by an incompetent person do not amount to an exercise of the right to refuse treatment; nevertheless, the court directed that they be considered in applying the substituted judgment test on the grounds that they were indicative of the burden the patient felt. *Laws*, another Massachusetts case, followed this precedent.[57] In *Kerr*,[58] however, a New York case, the court said it was not prepared to order the discontinuance of life support based upon gestures of irritation or annoyance.

In the *Jobes*[59] case there is an analysis of the evidence of patient preference using the standards established in *Conroy*. The court found the evidence not clear and convincing since the statements attributed to Mrs. Jobes were remote, general, spontaneous, and made in casual circumstances. In fact, they were described as close to the types of statements mentioned in *Conroy* as specifically unreliable, namely, "an off-hand remark about not wanting to live under certain circumstances made by a person when young and in the peak of health" and "informally expressed reactions to other people's medical condition and treatment."[60]

While *LaSala* and *Newman*[61] denied the withdrawal of artificial feeding on the basis of lack of evidence of the patient's wishes, *Jobes* went on, following *Conroy*, to discuss the patient's best interests. But *Jobes* also stresses the importance of keeping the patient's preferences central, insofar as that is possible. Within this context, the court makes several important points about the role of family as surrogate decision-makers. Using family as surrogates "effectuates as much as possible the decision that the incompetent patient would make if he or she were competent" and "Our common human experience informs us that family members are generally most concerned with the welfare of a patient. It is they who provide for the patient's comfort, care, and best interests, and they who treat the patient as a person, rather than a symbol of a cause."[62]

Other cases rely explicitly on a best interests standard. *Grant*,[63] for example, involves a terminally ill 22-year-old who had been progressively incompetent since age 14. In determining Ms. Grant's best interests, the court used criteria established in *Conroy*, including

> Evidence about the patient's present level of physical, sensory, emotional, and cognitive functioning; the degree of physical pain resulting from the medical condition, treatment, and termination of treatment, respectively; the degree of humiliation, dependence, and loss of dignity probably resulting from the condition and treatment; the life expectancy and prognosis for recovery with and without treatment; the various treatment options; and the risks, side effects, and benefits of each of those options.[64]

In *Visbeck*[65] and *Clark*,[66] two New Jersey cases, the courts also relied on *Conroy*. In *Visbeck* the judge was also the trial judge in *Conroy*. The opinion represents an interesting comparison of the condition and prognosis of the two women, Mrs. Conroy and Mrs. Visbeck, and the way it influenced the determination of best interests. Mrs. Visbeck's son was named the surrogate and also ordered to authorize the feeding tube. As the court explained, the procedure was simple and not accompanied by significant pain, and the patient demonstrated awareness, responsiveness, and minimal comfort. In

Clark as well, the feeding tube was regarded as in the patient's best interests because there was no evidence Mr. Clark was presently suffering pain that was recurring, unavoidable, and severe.

STATE INTERESTS

A right to refuse medical treatment is not absolute. Many cases examine whether they should constrain this right in order to defend legitimate state interests. These interests include the preservation of life, the prevention of suicide, the protection of innocent third parties, and the safeguarding of the integrity of the medical profession.[67] In only one case since *Conroy*—*Cruzan*[68]—has a patient's right to self-determination or best interests actually been limited by state interests.

The courts are very clear in cases dealing with competent patients or incompetent patients whose wishes are known. In *Culham*[69] the court ruled that when a competent adult patient refuses treatment, that decision generally outweighs any state interest. The same is true for incompetent patients whose wishes are known. The *Peter* court,[70] for example, found it difficult to conceive of a case in which the state would have a strong enough interest to subordinate a patient's right to choose not to be sustained in a persistent vegetative state. In *Delio*[71] the court mentioned that since the patient was not terminally ill, the state's interest in preserving life might be expected to prevail, but that interest was outweighed by the individual's right to avoid being preserved in a condition which he considered degrading and without human dignity. In *Bayer*[72] the court said that Mrs. Bayer's own expressed wishes together with the invasive nature of the treatment and her irreversible condition outweighed the state's interest in preserving life. It is of interest that "invasive" was understood to refer not to the passing of instruments into her body or to the discomfort caused, but to the violation of the patient's expressed wishes.

Other cases follow *Quinlan*[73] in balancing the state's interest in the preservation of life and the patient's right to self-determination. In *McConnell*[74] the court said that societal interest in preserving life could take precedence if the prognosis for recovery was good and benefits to the patient outweighed burdens, even though this was not the case for Mrs. McConnell. In *Grant*[75] the court said the state's interest in preserving life may require life-saving treatment, but this interest weakens if the treatment merely postpones death for a person with a terminal illness or if the treatment will be highly invasive and intrusive. In *Brophy*[76] the court said the state's interest in preserving life is waived when the underlying affliction is incurable. Additionally, the state's interest in life encompasses a broader interest than mere corporeal existence. The burden of maintaining such an existence degrades the very humanity it is meant to serve.

Taking direct issue with this line of reasoning, the Supreme Court of Missouri ruled in the *Cruzan* case[77] that the state's interest in preserving life is unqualified and pertains both to the length of life and to life's sanctity, meaning its worth regardless of its quality. Because Nancy Cruzan is in a persistent vegetative state, the continuation of feeding is not heroically invasive, and she is clearly not terminally ill, the state has an overriding interest in preserving her life. The state supreme court disagreed with the trial court about the reliability of evidence concerning Nancy Cruzan's preferences. The court also denied a state or federal constitutional right of privacy permitting the refusal of therapy by a guardian. The court overturned the initial rulings on the basis that they had erroneously declared the law.

As one dissenting judge pointed out, this does seem rather ironic in light of the fact that more than 50 appellate decisions from 16 jurisdictions (which the Missouri Supreme Court itself cites) support and validate the trial court's findings of fact, conclusions of law, and the judgment in this case, and the state supreme court fails to cite even one case that supports its declaration of the law.

Regarding the remaining three state interests, in no decision was the withdrawal of artificial hydration and nutrition considered suicide, nor were there overriding harms to third parties or to the medical profession. Now that many professional organization pronouncements have been in favor of allowing the forgoing of nutrition and hydration in certain circumstances,[78] it would be difficult to claim that the profession's integrity would be jeopardized by the court's decision to withdraw feeding.

ROLE OF THE COURTS AND OTHER INTERESTED THIRD PARTIES

Among the cases since *Conroy* there is little consensus about what constitutes clear and convincing evidence of the patient's preferences or what constitutes the patient's best interests. Some common descriptive language has emerged, but there remains wide variability in application. The very complex question arises about what the role of the courts should be. Should courts establish general guidelines for decision-making, or should they make decisions? What role do other parties, like professional and political organizations, have in the determination of standards?

PRIOR APPROVAL

For the most part, courts have been reluctant to become involved in the personal health care decisions of particular patients. No court has stated that patients or their surrogates must come to the court before having artificial hydration and nutrition withdrawn. In general, courts see themselves as dealing with cases where unresolved conflict exists among decision-makers. Most cases do not address the question of prior approval. But where it is mentioned, all courts agree that prior approval is not necessary unless there is some kind of dispute among decision-makers.[79] The *Grant* court,[80] for example, states that prior authorization is not needed and that decisions are best left to the patient's guardian, immediate family, and physician. Most courts seem to agree that medical decisions are private and the court's role should be minimal.

There is even question about how involved courts should become in the development of specific guidelines. Although guidelines would be useful in avoiding litigation, some would argue that the role of developing guidelines more appropriately belongs to state legislatures and falls to courts only by default. Courts are more likely to see their role in limited terms.

The *Cruzan* court,[81] for example, argued extensively for a limited role of the court, stressing that issues of treatment termination are more properly addressed by representative assemblies. The *Drabick* court,[82] with its emphasis on surrogacy, saw its role only as ensuring that the surrogate (conservator) made a good-faith decision. The *Culham* court,[83] which dealt with a competent patient, saw its role as making sure the patient was competent, properly informed, and uncoerced. But it did establish a standard for the determination of competence by requiring evidence from two non-attending psychologists. Even when a court does not regard itself as developing guidelines for decision-making, its interpretation of certain key terms, like competence, is influential. The whole concept of the role of the court is complicated in that anything a court decides may have influence on future decisions through our system of common law.

Some courts clearly describe their role as the development of guidelines for decision-making. Like the *Conroy* court in New Jersey, with its development of particular standards and procedures, the *Jobes* court (also in New Jersey) viewed its role as establishing criteria for decision-making. The recently published opinion of the New Jersey Ombudsman is consistent with this goal of developing decision-making criteria.[84] But perhaps the necessary involvement of an Ombudsman stretches the court's differentiation between developing criteria for decisions and actually making the decisions. The *Jobes* court stated it was not the role of the trial court to decide whether to withdraw treatment.

In *Brophy* as well, the Massachusetts court said that the state's role is limited to ensuring that treatment refusal does not violate legal norms.

> It is antithetical to our scheme of ordered liberty and to our respect for the autonomy of the individual for the State to make decisions regarding the individual's quality of life. It is for the patient to decide such issues. Our role is limited to ensuring that a refusal of treatment does not violate legal norms.[85]

THE ROLE OF THE GUARDIAN AD LITEM

The guardian ad litem in the *Conroy* case interpreted his function as ensuring the protection of the rights and interests of a litigant who was apparently incompetent to prosecute or defend the lawsuit.[86] Many have translated this into a claim that the guardian ad litem must always argue in favor of continued treatment. Since *Conroy*, several courts have explicitly stated this is not the case. In the *Jobes* case, for example, the attorneys for the nursing home sought the appointment of a "life advocate" who would fight for the continuation of all available means of medical treatment.[87] The request was denied. The *Drabick*[88] court said the guardian ad litem was not required to advocate continued medical treatment. The *Rasmussen*[89] court also said the guardian ad litem was not necessarily an advocate for continued treatment; rather, his or her role was to gather facts.

STATE STATUTES REQUIRING ARTIFICIAL HYDRATION AND NUTRITION

There are currently 39 living will statutes in existence; 25 of these make some mention of artificial hydration and nutrition (see table 4). Four states (Alaska, Idaho, Illinois, and Tennessee) clearly say artificial feeding not necessary for comfort may be withdrawn. Three states (Arkansas, Montana, and Oregon) can fairly be interpreted to authorize rejection of artificial feeding. They use the language of the Uniform Rights of the Terminally Ill Act, which was adopted by the National Conference of Commissioners of Uniform State Laws in 1985, and the commissioners have commented that artificial hydration and nutrition not necessary for comfort may be withdrawn.[90]

Twelve states (Arizona, Florida, Hawaii, Indiana, Iowa, Maryland, New Hampshire, Oklahoma, South Carolina, Utah, West Virginia, and Wyoming) associate artificial hydration and nutrition with comfort care and seem to prohibit their withdrawal. Some would argue that since these statutes are typically worded to exclude artificially administered sustenance or the administration of medication or the performance of any medical procedure necessary to provide comfort, artificial feeding (as a medical procedure) may be withdrawn if it is not necessary for comfort.[91]

Six states (Colorado, Connecticut, Georgia, Maine, Missouri, and Wisconsin) clearly state artificial hydration and nutrition are not procedures that may be rejected through a living will.[92] Oklahoma has gone further in enacting in 1987 the Nutrition and Hydration for Incompetent Patients Act, which states that artificial hydration and nutrition *must* be provided to all incompetent patients unless: 1) the physician knows by clear and convincing evidence that the patient, when competent and with a specific illness or injury, decided that artificial feeding should be withheld or withdrawn based on information sufficient to constitute informed consent; 2) in the reasonable medical judgment of the patient's attending physician and a second, consulting physician, either artificial feeding would cause severe, intractable, and long-lasting pain or such hydration or nutrition is not medically possible; or 3) in the reasonable medical judgment of the patient's attending physician and a second, consulting physician the patient is chronically and irreversibly incompetent, in the final stage of terminal illness or injury, and the death of the patient is imminent.[93]

In the six states that have statutes that prohibit the withdrawal of artificial feeding, court cases (except *Cruzan* in Missouri) have been decided in favor of the withdrawal of artificial feeding in spite of the statute.

In the first ruling by a state supreme court, in *Corbett*[94] the court ruled that the Florida constitutional right of privacy extends to incompetent persons unable to exercise that right on their own behalf and cannot be denied by the state living will statute. That statute was intended to provide a method for competent adults to provide advance directives and was not intended to encompass the entire spectrum of instances in which those rights might be exercised. The *Zahn*[95] case (also in Florida) followed the precedent of *Corbett*.

In the *Cruzan*[96] case in Missouri, the most recent state supreme court ruling, the court overturned the trial court's judgment that the state statute was unconstitutional. The supreme court said it intended no judgment as to whether a common law right to refuse medical treatment is broader than the living will statute, since it regarded the statute as not being at issue in the case.

The *McConnell*[97] court in Connecticut ruled that the constitutional right to privacy overrides any statutory consideration. According to the court, the statute was not enacted to encompass the entire spectrum of instances in which rights are exercised.

The *Gardner*[98] court in Maine addressed the issue only in a footnote, stating that the Living Will Act was not relevant to the question of withdrawing artificial hydration and nutrition in this case because the patient did not have a living will and the statute makes no presumption about the wishes of people who do not have living wills. Additionally, the court said that the Living Will Act did not limit the court's power to read more broadly under Maine common law the right of a patient to make decisions concerning life-sustaining care. According to the court, since the court was basing the decision on Maine's common law doctrine of informed consent, the Living Will Act did not speak to the question in this case.

A decision in Colorado also limited the application of that state's Medical Treatment Act. In the *Rodas*[99] case the court ruled that none of the Act's limitations regarding artificial feeding applied, since the Act only referred to incompetent patients and even then did not apply to living wills that specifically rejected nutrition and hydration.

Finally, a recent case in Georgia also permitted the withdrawal of artificial feeding in spite of that state's statute to the contrary.[100]

A Virginia case, *Hazelton v. Powhatan Nursing Home, Inc.*,[101] has been the first case to interpret the language of a state natural death statute that did not specifically mention artificial feeding. The court concluded that artificial feeding was a "life-prolonging procedure," within the meaning of the statutory phrase, and therefore could be forgone. The court also developed a definition for "imminent," another word appearing in the statute. The court ruled that Mrs. Hazelton's death was imminent because her condition had "in less than six months reduced her from a normally functioning person to a comatose state within a few months of death." To say her death was not imminent would be to reduce that definition to "immediate, at once, within a day," and this would destroy the intent of the statute. The court wrote, "It is precisely people like Harriet Hazelton who lie between life and death, enjoying nothing of the sweetness of life, while her body slowly gives up its remaining functioning to the advance of a brain tumor, whom the legislature seeks to protect from the indignity of the artificial prolongation of life."

Two additional cases challenged state statutes regulating nursing home care that require the provision of hydration and nutrition in nursing homes. In the *Drabick*[102] case in California the court ruled that the withdrawal of artificial feeding should not be considered a violation of the California Administrative Code for Long Term Care Facilities when a patient is reliably diagnosed and when the patient's record contains clear and written evidence of that prognosis, consultation between the physician and the surrogate, consideration of the patient's expressed desires or best interests, the surrogate's determination, and the physician's order.[103]

In the *Hoffmeister v. Satz*[104] case in Florida the nursing home sought injunctive relief from a state regulation which required that nursing homes always provide sustenance to residents. The Secretary of State of Florida promulgated a proposed rule allowing the withdrawal of artificial feeding that was accepted in this case. This proposed rule was adopted on July 1, 1988.[105] An earlier case in Florida, *Rekstad*,[106] had also ruled that the nursing home could withdraw artificial feeding in spite of the Florida statute.

STATEMENTS BY PROFESSIONAL AND OTHER ORGANIZATIONS

In seeking to determine appropriate standards of care, courts have often looked to the statements published by professional organizations in health care. Statements regarding artificial feeding have been issued by the American Medical Association (AMA), the American Nurse's Association (ANA), the American Academy of Neurology, and the American Society for Parenteral and Enteral Nutrition. The AMA amended in March 1986 an earlier statement regarding patients who are imminently dying or permanently unconscious to include "life-prolonging medical treatment includes medication and artificially or technologically supplied respiration, nutrition, or hydration."[107]

The ANA's "Guidelines on Withdrawing or Withholding Food and Fluid" includes a strong presumption in favor of providing artificial feeding but also outlines specific instances when its withdrawal is permissible.[108]

The American Academy of Neurology has issued a position statement "On Certain Aspects of the Care and Management of the Persistent Vegetative State Patient." Included are guidelines for the diagnosis of PVS, a statement that PVS patients do not have the capacity to experience pain or suffering, and a statement that "the artificial provision of nutrition and hydration is a form of medical treatment and may be discontinued in accordance with the principles and practices governing the withholding and withdrawal of other forms of medical treatment."[109]

The American Society for Parenteral and Enteral Nutrition writes: "Specialized nutrition support should be terminated when the patient no longer benefits from the therapy. A patient no longer benefits from specialized nutrition support when its provision no longer has a meaningful effect on clinical outcome."[110]

Other statements permitting the withdrawal of artificial hydration and nutrition have been published by the Committee on Biomedical Ethics of the Los Angeles County Medical Association and the Los Angeles County Bar Association, the Medical Society of Milwaukee County, the New Jersey Chapter of the American College of Physicians, and the Massachusetts Medical Society.[111]

Statements against the withdrawal of artificial hydration and nutrition include the Association for Retarded Citizens Resolution on Cessation of Nutrition and/or Hydration, the Association for Persons with Severe Handicaps Resolution on Nutrition and Hydration, and the United Handicapped Federation Resolution.[112] A statement against the withdrawing of artificial feeding signed by more than a hundred prominent physicians, attorneys, and ethicists was also published in *Issues in Law and Medicine*.[113]

Courts have used statements by the AMA and other medical societies in their arguments that the state does not have an overriding interest in protecting the integrity of the medical profession since the withdrawal of care does not violate standards of medical ethics. Other courts, such as *Brophy* and *Cruzan*, have not seen such a clear consensus concerning the standards of medical ethics, and some have used the disagreement that is obvious in the above variety of statements to argue that professionals should not be forced to violate their individual moral conscience.[114]

ETHICS COMMITTEES

A few court cases have mentioned the use of ethics committees or ethicists in the resolution of these difficult cases. The *Jobes*[115] case in particular includes an interesting statement about the role of ethicists. The court writes:

> It is because of the unescapable moral ambiguity of these decisions [regarding "objective" or "best-interests" tests] that, before such approaches can be applied to right-to-die cases, appropriate decision-making processes must be developed. We should, I suggest, be able to turn to the persons regularly involved in life-and-death decisions. Such individuals are in the best position, borne of experience, training, and attitude, to evaluate fairly and impartially the numerous factors that are relevant to a decision based in whole or in part on patient best-interests. These persons should include those we turn to in a substituted-judgment approach case, namely, the doctors and health-care providers and responsible government and institutional representatives. Included should also be persons grounded in religious and ethical training.

The court goes on to say that nursing homes should give serious consideration to making available the services of ethicists or institutional ethics committees.

CONCERNS OF CAREGIVERS

A final area of interest in the court cases since *Conroy* is what happens when caregivers do not agree with the decision to withdraw artificial hydration and nutrition. Some caregivers believe artificial feeding is basic care that must always be provided. But beyond this level of disagreement, caregivers struggle to assess the benefits of artificial feeding and also struggle to live with the realities of death when artificial feeding is withdrawn. As one thoughtful author writes, "Gazing into the sunken, hollow eyes of a cachectic patient dying of cancer and into the hopeful eyes of his loved ones makes it very obvious that it appears to be easier to write these definitive statements [about withdrawing artificial feeding] than it is to apply them at the bedside."[116]

Courts have had a variety of responses to the concerns of health care professionals. Some courts insist that the caregivers must respect the patient's wishes regardless of their own moral beliefs, with no transfer of the patient allowed.

In the case of the *Application of the Plaza Health and Rehabilitation Center*[117] the court ruled that the health care facility was not obligated or responsible to attempt to perform such medical procedures (artificial feeding) nor would the court allow them to do so.

The *Jobes*[118] case upon appeal reversed the trial court's decision to let the nursing home refuse to participate. The court said the family had no reason to believe that they would surrender the right to choose any alternative when they initially entered the facility. But that did not mean that a policy, especially if it were known about, could never be enforced.

The *Requena*[119] case represents the most sensitive assessment of the competing claims of the patient and the health care providers. The court writes:

> I realize that by keeping Mrs. Requena in the Hospital I will be imposing a real burden on its nurses and technicians. I do not like to do that. But they are well and whole people. They have full and vibrant lives ahead of them. In the final analysis, it is fairer to ask them to give than it is to ask Beverly Requena to give.

The court ruled that the patient had no notice of the hospital policy and the sensibilities of the staff were subordinate to the psychological harm to the patient. They also said, however, that this was not a legal decision invalidating a hospital regulation against the withdrawal of artificial feeding, just a ruling that such a regulation did not apply to Mrs. Requena.

The majority of the cases permitted the transfer of patients if the health care providers did not agree with the decision to withdraw artificial feeding.[120] The presumption, however, seems to be in favor of honoring the patient's wishes, with transfer being permitted only if it is acceptable to the patient or the patient's guardian. As the court writes in the *McConnell*[121] case, to allow the institution to refuse compliance or to discharge patients when no transferring facility is found is to frustrate the patient's right of self-determination. Emphasis is also placed on trying to ensure that the patient still receives adequate care even when there is disagreement about the withdrawal of treatment.

A few cases seem to lean toward the rights of the caregivers in the balance struck between patient and provider rights. In a well-publicized case in California, *Gary v. California*,[122] the physician was first ordered to withdraw a feeding tube, but then the original order was amended and the physician was no longer compelled. The *Brophy*[123] case perhaps represents the strongest language in favor of caregiver rights, except that the institution was not allowed to interfere with the transfer of the patient. Citing substantial disagreement in the medical community over appropriate medical action in cases involving the withdrawal of artificial feeding, the court states that the patient's right to refuse medical treatment does not warrant unnecessary intrusion upon the hospital's ethical integrity. The court goes on to state that neither the Massachusetts patient's rights statute, nor informed consent, nor any other provision of the law requires the hospital to stop hydration and nutrition upon the request of the guardian.

SUMMARY

A consensus has emerged in court cases since *Conroy* in 1985 that artificial hydration and nutrition are medical procedures that can be forgone. Courts have supported decisions to refuse artificial feeding for patients who are competent or whose wishes are sufficiently clear. A few courts have supported decisions for incompetent persons based on a calculation of best interests. Several court cases have sufficiently challenged state living will statutes and nursing home regulations that prohibit the refusal of artificial feeding. Most courts have not ordered health care providers to comply with decisions to withdraw artificial feeding unless a transfer of the patient is not possible. Although the majority of health care organizations that have established guidelines permit the refusal of artificial feeding, the debate over artificial feeding continues. Much uncertainty continues regarding the application of a best interests standard and a standard for evidence of patient preference.

NOTES

1. *In re Conroy,* 98 N.J. 321, 486 A.2d 1209 (1985).
2. *Id.*
3. Three lower court cases make a distinction between artificial hydration and nutrition and other forms of life-sustaining medical treatment. In *Sullivan v. St. John's Mercy Medical Center* (Stoppe), No. 561631 (Mo. Cir. Ct. St. Louis County June 8, 1987) (Weinstock, J.) the court decided that a ventilator could be withdrawn from a 79-year-old woman who had suffered a massive cerebral accident. There was credible evidence that before she was incompetent she had expressed her desire not to be maintained in such a condition. But the court would not permit the withdrawal of hydration and nutrition or antibiotics, because such withdrawal was explicitly forbidden in the Missouri natural death statute. A recent Missouri Supreme Court decision would not permit artificial hydration and nutrition to be withdrawn from a PVS patient. The court ruled the trial court erred in declaring the state statute unconstitutional. The court also questioned whether nutrition and hydration are medical treatment. *Cruzan v. Harmon,* 70813 (Mo. Supp. Ct. Nov. 16, 1988). Two New York cases also do not allow the withdrawal of artificial hydration and nutrition, declining to follow a landmark New York decision to allow such withdrawal. *In re Vogel,* 134 Misc. 2d 395, 512 N.Y.S.2d 622 (Sup. Ct. Nassau County 1986), *declined to follow in Delio v. Westchester County Medical Center,* 129 A.D.2d 1, 516 N.Y.S.2d 677 (2d Dep't 1987). *Workmen's Circle Home and Infirmary for the Aged v. Fink,* 135 Misc. 2d 270, 514 N.Y.S.2d 893 (Sup. Ct. Bronx County 1987), *declined to follow in Delio v. Westchester County Medical Center,* 129 A.D.2d 1, 516 N.Y.S.2d 677 (2d Dep't 1987). In the Workmen's Circle Home decision the court said it was permissible to withhold a gastrostomy, but it was not permissible to withdraw antibiotics and intravenous nutrients.

4. The case of *Delio* relies only on common law principles, declining to address the question of a right to privacy grounded in the federal constitution until it is addressed by a court of appeals. See *Delio*, note 3 supra. *In re Gardner*, 534 A.2d 947 (Me. 1987) also does not mention state or federal constitutional rights of privacy, but grounds a personal right to refuse life-sustaining treatment firmly in the common law of informed consent. The recent Missouri Supreme Court ruling argues *against* a state or federal right of privacy. See *Cruzan*, note 3 supra. *Sanchez v. Fairview Developmental Center*, No. CV 88–0129 FFF (Tx) (C.D. Cal. March 30, 1988) (Fernandez, J.), *notice of motion for preliminary injunction filed*, No. 563–313 (Cal. Super. Ct. Orange County July 27, 1988) (McDonald, J.) also questions the existence of a federal right to privacy. A federal right to privacy is explicitly argued for in the recent *Gray v. Romeo*, Civ. 82–0573B-F. Supp.-(D.RI 1988).

5. Phyllis Schmitz and Merry O'Brien, "Observations on Nutrition and Hydration in Dying Cancer Patients" in this volume, pp. 29–38. *Brophy v. New England Sinai Hospital.*, 398 Mass. 417 at 426 n.20, 497 N.E.2d 626 at 631 n.20 (1986). *In re Guardianship of Grant*, 109 Wash. 2d 545, 747 P.2d 445, 453 (1987). Cox, "Is Dehydration Painful?" 9 *Ethics and Medics* 1–2 (1987).

6. American Academy of Neurology, "Position of the American Academy of Neurology on Certain Aspects of the Care and Management of the Persistent Vegetative State Patient," April 21, 1988.

7. *In re Requena*, 213 N.J. Super. 475, 517 A.2d 886 (Super. Ct. Ch. Div.), *aff'd*, 213 N.J. Super. 443, 517 A.2d 869 (Super. Ct. App. Div. 1986) (per curiam); *In re Application of Brooks* (Leguerrier) (N.Y. Sup. Ct. Albany County June 10, 1987) (Conway, J.); *In re Culham* No. 87–340537-AZ (Mich. Cir. Ct. Oakland County Dec. 15, 1987) (Breck J.); *In re Jane Doe*, 16 Phila. 229 (Pa. Ct. Com. Pl. 1987) (This patient did not request the termination of the feeding tube, but the court mentioned it in their ruling.); *In re Putzer*, No. P21–87E (N.J. Super. Ct. Ch. Div. Essex County July 9, 1987) (Margolis, J.); *In re Rodas*, No. 86PR139 (Colo. Dist. Ct. Mesa County Jan. 22, 1987, as modified, April 3, 1987) (Buss, J.); *Wilcox v. Hawaii*, Civ. No. 860116 (Hawaii Cir. Ct. 5th Cir. June 16, 1986) (Hirano, J.).

8. See *Putzer*, note 7 supra; *Bouvia v. Superior Court (Glenchur)*, 179 Cal. App. 3d 1127, 225 Cal. Rptr. 297 (Ct. App. 1986), *review denied* (Cal. June 5, 1986); see *Rodas*, note 7 supra. The *Rodas* court stretched the usual definition to call Mr. Rodas "terminally ill." Treatment could forestall his death for some years, but death would follow within a matter of days if treatment were withdrawn.

9. See *Brooks*, note 7 supra.

10. *In re Application of Plaza Health and Rehabilitation Center* (N.Y. Sup. Ct. Onondaga County Feb. 2, 1984) (Miller, J.).

11. See *Brophy*, note 5 supra; see *Delio*, note 3 supra; see *Gardner* and *Gray*, note 4 supra; *In re Strauss*, No. 8378/87 (N.Y. Sup. Ct. Bronx County July 1, 1987) (Tompkins, J.); *Hazelton [sic] v. Powhatan Nursing Home, Inc.*, No. CH 98287 (Va. Cir. Ct. Fairfax County Aug. 29, 1986), *order signed* (Sept. 2, 1986) (Fortkort, J.), *appeal denied*, Record No. 860814 (Va. Sept. 2, 1986), 6 Va. Cir. Ct. Op. 414 (Aspen 1987);

McConnell v. Beverly Enterprises, No. 0293888 (Conn. Super Ct. Danbury Jud. Dist. July 8, 1988) (Dranginis, J.), *on appeal*, Nos. SC 13477, 13478 & 13479 (Conn.); *In re Application of Licopoli* (Akullian), No. 1172–88 (N.Y. Sup. Ct. Albany County March 10, 1988) (Prior, J.); *In re Bayer*, No. 4131 (N.D. Burleigh County Ct. Feb. 5 and Dec. 11, 1987) (Riskedahl, J.); *In re Peter*, 108 N.J. 365, 529 A.2d 419 (1987).

12. The term "permanently unconscious" is used to include all conditions in which purposeful interaction with the environment, awareness of pain or pleasure, and any cognitive ability are permanently absent. It includes persistent vegetative state, anencephaly, and irreversible coma, but not brain death. President's Commission for the Study of Ethical Issues in Medicine and Biomedical and Behavioral Science, *Decisions to Forego Life-Sustaining Therapy*, U.S. Government Printing Office, Washington, D.C., 1983.

13. *Corbett v. D'Alessandro*, 487 So. 2d 368 at 369 (Fla. Dist. Ct. App.) *review denied*, 492 So. 2d 1331 (Fla. 1986).

14. American Medical Association Council of Ethical and Judicial Affairs, "Withholding and Withdrawing Life-Prolonging Medical Treatment," in *Current Opinions of the Council on Ethical and Judicial Affairs of the American Medical Association* 12–13 (1986).

15. See *McConnell*, note 11 supra.

16. See note 6 supra.

17. *In re Conservatorship of Drabick*, 200 Cal. App. 3d 185, 245 Cal. Rptr. 840 (Cal. Ct. App. 1988), *review denied* (Cal. July 28, 1988), *application for stay of remittitur filed* (Cal. Ct. App. July 28, 1988); see *Brophy*, note 5 supra; see *Corbett*, note 13 supra; see *Cruzan* and *Delio*, note 3 supra; *In re Jobes*, 108 N.J. 394, 529 A.2d 434 (1987); see *Gray* and *Gardner*, note 4 supra; *Gary v. California* (Hirth), No. 576 123 (Cal. Super. Ct. San Diego County March 5, 23), *modified in part* (April 15, 1987) (Milkes, J.); *In re Estate of Prange*, 166 Ill. App. 3d 1091, 520 N.E.2d 946 (Ill. Ct. App.), *vacated*, 121 Ill. 2d 570 (Ill. 1988); *In re Application of Alderson* (Kimbrough), No. 90193/86 (N.Y. Sup. Ct. N.Y. County Aug. 3, 1988) (Ciparick, J.); N.Y.L.J. Aug. 9, 1988 at 18, col. 2; *In re Jane Doe*, No. D. 56730 (Ga. Super. Ct. Fulton County July 13, 1988) (Williams, J.); *Barber v. Superior Court*, 147 Cal. App. 3d 1006, 195 Cal. Rptr. 484 (Ct. App. 1983); see *Licopoli*, *Peter*, and *Bayer*, note 11 supra; [LaSala] *In re Chetta* [Wickel], No. 1086/87 (N.Y. Sup. Ct. Nassau County May 1, 1987, Feb. 16, 1988) (Becker, J.); N.Y.L.J. March 9, 1988, at 15, *notice of appeal filed* (N.Y. App. Div. 2d Dep't March 17, 1988); *Rasmussen v. Fleming*, 154 Ariz. 207, 741 P.2d 674 (1987); *In re Zahn*, No. 85–3723 (Fla. Cir. Ct. Broward County Nov. 20, 1986) (Hare, J.); *Newman v. William Beaumont Army Medical Center*, No. EP-86-CA-276 (W.D. Tex. Oct. 30, 1986) (Hudspeth, J.).

18. "Cognitive and sapient life" comes from *Quinlan*, *In re Quinlan*, 70 N.J. 10, 355 A.2d 647 *cert. denied* 429 U.S. 922 (1976). Also see note 17 supra.

19. See *Cruzan* and *Delio*, note 3 supra.

20. There was disagreement between the trial court and the state supreme court in the *Cruzan* case, with the trial court finding the evidence of Nancy Cruzan's wishes sufficient, and the supreme court

challenging their reliability. Withdrawal was not permitted. See *Cruzan* and *Delio*, note 3 supra; see *Gardner* and *Gray*, note 4 supra; see *Brophy*, note 5 supra; see *McConnell, Licopoli, Peter*, and *Bayer*, note 11 supra; see *Corbett*, note 13 supra; and see *Jobes, Drabick, Jane Doe (GA), Barber, Rasmussen*, and *Zahn*, note 17 supra.

21. See Sanchez, note 4 supra; *Hoffmeister v. Satz*, No. 87–28451 CR. (Fla. Cir. Ct. 17th Dist. Broward County Feb. 22, 1988); see *Strauss*, note 11 supra; *In re Laws*, No. 226215 (Mass. Probate Ct. May 4, 1987) (Buczko, J.); *In re Application of Kerr* (O'Brien), 135 Misc. 2d 1076, 517 N.Y.S.2d 346 (N.Y. Sup. Ct. N.Y. County 1986); *in re Clark*, 210 N.J. Super. 548, 510 A.2d 136 (Super. Ct. Ch. Div. 1986); 212 N.J. Super. 408, 515 A.2d 276 (Super. Ct. Ch. Div, 1986), *aff'd*, 216 N.J. Super. 497, 524 A.2d 448 (Super. Ct. App. Div. 1987); *In re Visbeck*, 210 N.J. Super. 527, 510 A.2d 125 (Super. Ct. Ch. Div. 1986); *In re Hier*, 18 Mass. App. 200, 464 N.E.2d 959 (Ct. App.), *review denied*, 392 Mass. 1102, 465 N.E.2d 261 (1984); *In the Matter of Mary O'Connor, Westchester County Medical Center v. Helen Hall*, 312 (N.Y. Ct. App. Oct. 14, 1988).

22. See *Strauss*, note 11 supra; see *Hier* and *Laws*, note 21 supra. George J. Annas, "The Case of Mary Hier: When Substituted Judgment Becomes Sleight of Hand," *Hastings Center Report*, August 1984, pp. 23–25.

23. See *Kerr*, note 21 supra.

24. See *Clark*, note 21 supra.

25. See *Visbeck*, note 21 supra.

26. See *Hier*, note 21 supra.

27. See *Conroy*, note 1 supra; see *Grant*, note 5 supra; see *Drabick, Rasmussen*, and *Jobes*, note 17 supra.

28. See *Peter*, note 11 supra.

29. See *Jobes*, note 17 supra.

30. See *Conroy*, note 1 supra.

31. Hector M. Rodriguez, Acting Ombudsman, State of New Jersey Office of the Ombudsman for the Institutionalized Elderly, Trenton, New Jersey, August 30, 1988.

32. See *Kerr*, note 21 supra.

33. See *Visbeck*, note 21 supra.

34. See *Rasmussen*, note 17 supra.

35. See *Conroy*, note 1 supra.

36. See *Drabick*, note 17 supra.

37. *Id.* at 856.

38. *Id.*

39. *Id.*

40. See *Culham*, note 7 supra; see *Peter*, note 11 supra.

41. See *Prange*, note 17 supra.

42. See *McConnell, Licopoli, Bayer, Strauss*, and *Peter*, note 11 supra; see *Prange*, note 17 supra; see *Gardner* and *Gray*, note 4 supra; see *Delio*, note 3 supra; see *Laws*, note 21 supra; see *Brophy*, note 5 supra.

43. See *Conroy*, note 1 supra.

44. See *Brophy*, note 5 supra.

45. *Id.* at 632n22.

46. See *Delio*, note 3 supra.
47. See *Gardner*, note 4 supra.
48. See *Drabick*, note 17 supra.
49. See *Strauss*, note 11 supra.
50. See *Newman*, note 17 supra.
51. See *LaSala*, note 17 supra.
52. See *Delio*, note 3 supra.
53. See *LaSala*, note 17 supra.
54. See *Alderson*, note 17 supra.
55. See *O'Connor*, note 21 supra.
56. See *Hier*, note 21 supra. See especially, George J. Annas, "The Case of Mary Hier: When Substituted Judgment Becomes Sleight of Hand," *Hastings Center Report*, August, 1985, pp. 23–25. See *Conroy*, note 1 supra.
57. See *Laws*, note 21 supra.
58. See *Kerr*, note 21 supra.
59. See *Jobes*, note 17 supra.
60. *Id.* However, the court did allow artificial feeding to be withdrawn on the basis of the limited objective test. The court in the *Cruzan* case also relied upon this standard to claim Nancy Cruzan's comments were not reliable. See *Cruzan*, note 3 supra.
61. See *LaSala* and *Newman*, note 17 supra.
62. See *Jobes*, note 17 supra, at 444.
63. See *Grant*, note 5 supra.
64. *Id.* at 457; see *Conroy*, note 1 supra.
65. See *Visbeck*, note 21 supra.
66. See *Clark*, note 21 supra.
67. This specific list of four state interests is discussed in at least 14 of the cases and is cited to *Superintendent of Belchertown State School v. Saikewicz*, 373 Mass. 728, 370 N.E.2d 417 (1977).
68. See *Cruzan*, note 3 supra.
69. See *Culham*, note 7 supra.
70. See *Peter*, note 11 supra.
71. See *Delio*, note 3 supra.
72. See *Bayer*, note 11 supra.
73. See *Quinlan*, note 18 supra.
74. See *McConnell*, note 11 supra.
75. See *Grant*, note 5 supra.
76. See *Brophy*, note 5 supra.
77. See *Cruzan*, note 3 supra. At issue in the application of this ruling may be the fact that Nancy Cruzan is in a state facility.
78. See below, notes 107–112 on professional organizations.
79. See *Drabick, Rasmussen,* and *Jobes*, note 17 supra; See *Grant*, note 5 supra.
80. See *Grant*, note 5 supra.
81. See *Cruzan*, note 3 supra.
82. See *Drabick*, note 17 supra.
83. See *Culham*, note 7 supra.
84. See Rodriguez, note 31 supra.
85. See *Brophy*, note 5 supra.

86. John J. Delaney, "The Role of the Guardian ad Litem," in this volume.

87. The role of the guardian ad litem has been clarified by the New Jersey Supreme Court in the *Farrell, Peter,* and *Jobes* trilogy, published in late June, 1987 at 108 N.J. 335, 365 and 394 (1987).

88. See *Drabick,* note 17 supra.

89. See *Rasmussen,* note 17 supra.

90. Elena N. Cohen and Maynard M. Cohen, "Artificial Feeding and Patient's Rights: Recent Developments and Recommendations," *The Medical Staff Counselor* vol. 2, no. 3, Summer 1988, p. 24.

91. *Id.*

92. *Id.*

93. Oklahoma Statutes Ann. Section 3080.1-.5 (1987) "*Oklahoma Hydration and Nutrition for Incompetent Patients Act,*" Issues in Law and Medicine, vol. 3, no. 3, 1987, pp. 319–321.

94. See *Corbett,* note 13 supra.

95. See *Zahn,* note 17 supra.

96. See *Cruzan,* note 3 supra.

97. See *McConnell,* note 11 supra.

98. See *Gardner,* note 4 supra.

99. See *Rodas,* note 7 supra.

100. See *Jane Doe* (GA), note 17 supra.

101. See *Hazelton,* note 11 supra.

102. See *Drabick,* note 17 supra.

103. California Department of Health Services, "Guidelines Regarding Withdrawal or Withholding of Life-Sustaining Procedure(s) in Long-Term Care Facilities," August 7, 1987, states that withdrawal of artificial feeding should not be construed as a violation of California Administrative Code, title 22, section 72315, subdivision (h).

104. See *Hoffmeister,* note 21 supra.

105. Rules of State of Florida Department of Health and Rehabilitative Services *Chapter 10D-29, Florida Administrative Code Nursing Home and Related Facilities Licensure Amending Rule 10D-29.*

106. *Rekstad v. Florida Life Care, Inc.,* No. 87–4285-CA-01 (Fla. Cir. Ct. Sarasota County Sept. 18, 1987) (Walker, J.).

107. American Medical Association Council of Ethical and Judicial Affairs, Section 2.18 "Withholding or Withdrawing Life-Prolonging Medical Treatment," in *Current Opinions of the Council on Ethical and Judicial Affairs of the American Medical Association* 12–13 (1986).

108. American Nurses Association, "Committee on Ethics Guidelines on Withdrawing or Withholding Food and Fluid," Kansas City, Missouri, January 1988.

109. American Academy of Neurology, "Position of the American Academy of Neurology on Certain Aspects of the Care and Management of the Persistent Vegetative State Patient," April 21, 1988.

110. American Society for Parenteral and Enteral Nutrition, "Standards for Nutrition Support: Hospitalized Patients," January 1984.

111. National Reference Center for Bioethics Literature, *Scope Note: Withholding or Withdrawing Nutrition or Hydration,* Kennedy Institute of Ethics, Washington, D.C., p. 4, June 1988; *American College of Phy-*

sicians Observer, "Guidelines for Care of Hopelessly Ill Patients," p. 20, June 1984.

112. *Issues in Law & Medicine*, 3:315–317, 1987.

113. *Id.*

114. See *Brophy*, note 5 supra; see *Cruzan*, note 3 supra.

115. See *Jobes*, note 17 supra; see *Jane Doe* (PA), note 7 supra; see *Laws* and *Visbeck*, note 21 supra.

116. Susan C. Hushen, "Questioning TPN as the Answer," *American Journal of Nursing*, May 1982, pp. 852–854. TPN refers to Total Parenteral Nutrition.

117. See *Plaza Health and Rehabilitation Center*, note 10 supra.

118. See *Jobes*, note 17 supra. Justice O'Hern in a dissenting opinion argued against compelling health care providers to comply.

119. See *Requena*, note 7 supra.

120. George J. Annas, "Transferring the Ethical Hot Potato," *Hastings Center Report*, February 1987, p. 20–21. See *Gray*, note 4 supra; see *Gary*, note 17 supra; see *McConnell*, note 11 supra; see *Grant* and *Brophy*, note 5 supra; see *Gardner* and *Delio*, note 3 supra; see *Rekstad*, note 106 supra; *Cantor v. Weiss*, No. 626 163 (Cal. Super. Ct. Los Angeles County Dec. 30, 1986) (Newman, J.).

121. See *McConnell*, note 11 supra.

122. See *Gary*, note 17 supra. Allen Jay, "The Judge Ordered Me to Kill My Patient," *Medical Economics*, August 10, 1987, pp. 120–124.

123. See *Brophy*, note 5 supra.

SELECTED BIBLIOGRAPHY

George J. Annas, "Fashion and Freedom: When Artificial Feeding Should Be Withdrawn," *American Journal of Public Health*, 75:685–688, 1985.

George J. Annas, "Transferring the Ethical Hot Potato," *Hastings Center Report*, 20–21, February 1987.

Daniel Callahan, "Feeding the Dying Elderly," *Generations*, Winter 1985, pp. 15–17.

Elena N. Cohen and Maynard M. Cohen, "Artificial Feeding and Patients' Rights: Recent Developments and Recommendations," *The Medical Staff Counselor*, 2:23–25, 1988.

Congress of the United States, Office of Technology Assessment, *Institutional Protocols for Decisions About Life-Sustaining Treatments*, U.S. Government Printing Office, July 1988.

Rebecca Dresser, "When Patients Resist Feeding: Medical, Ethical and Legal Considerations," *Journal of the American Geriatric Society*, 33:790–794, 1985.

Sara T. Fry, "New ANA Guidelines on Withdrawing or Withholding Food and Fluid from Patients," *Nursing Outlook*, 36:122–150, 1988.

Hastings Center, *Guidelines on the Termination of Life-Sustaining Treatment and the Care of the Dying*, Bloomington: Indiana University Press, 1988.

Bernard Lo and Laurie Dornbrand, "Guiding the Hand that Feeds," *New England Journal of Medicine*, 311:402–404, 1985.

Barbara Mishkin, "Courts Entangled in Feeding Tube Controversies," *Nutrition in Clinical Practice*, 1:209–215, 1986.

Michael A. Nevins, "New Jersey's Right-to-Die Cases: Round Three," *Annals of Internal Medicine*, 107:927–929, 1987.

President's Commission for the Study of Ethical Issues in Medicine and Biomedical and Behavioral Research, *Making Health Care Decisions*, U.S. Government Printing Office, 1982.

President's Commission for the Study of Ethical Issues in Medicine and Biomedical and Behavioral Research, *Deciding to Forego Life-Sustaining Treatment*, U.S. Government Printing Office, 1983.

Richard Selzer, "Tube Feeding," in *Confessions of a Knife*. New York: Simon and Schuster, 1979, pp. 159–166.

Robert Steinbrook and Bernard Lo, "Artificial Feeding—Solid Ground, Not a Slippery Slope," *New England Journal of Medicine*, 318:286–290, 1988.

G. Janet Tulloch, "A Case in Which Suicide Is not Cowardly," *The Washington Post*, Sunday, January 29, 1984.

Sidney H. Wanzer, et al., "The Physician's Responsibility Toward Hopelessly Ill Patients," *New England Journal of Medicine*, 310:955–959, 1984.

INDEX

Milton Keynes UK
Ingram Content Group UK Ltd.
UKHW010252070224
437385UK00007B/382